D0873832

Training and
Conditioning of Athletes

Training and
Conditioning of Athletes

MAX M. NOVICH, M.D.

Diplomate, American Board of Orthopaedic Surgery;
Clinical Professor of Surgery,
Founder and Former Director of Sports Medicine,
UMDNJ/New Jersey Medical School;
Director of Sports Medicine, United Hospitals Orthopedic Center;
Member, Governor's Council on Physical Fitness

BUDDY TAYLOR, M.S., A.T.C.

Head Trainer, Winston-Salem State University,
Winston-Salem, North Carolina;
Trainer, 1968 and 1972 Olympic Games
and 1969 and 1973 Maccabiah Games;
Member, State of North Carolina Superintendent's
Sports Medicine Advisory Commission

2nd Edition

Lea & Febiger · Philadelphia · 1983

Lea & Febiger
600 S. Washington Square
Philadelphia, PA 19106
U.S.A

Lea & Febiger

Translations:
First Edition -
Hebrew Edition by Dr. Uriel Simri of the Wingate Institute in Israel, 1973
Spanish Edition by Nueva Editorial Interamericana, S.A. de C.V., Mexico, D.F., Mexico—1975

First Edition, 1970

Reprinted, April, 1972

Library of Congress Cataloging in Publication Data

Novich, Max M., 1914–
    Training and conditioning of athletes.
    Includes bibliographical references and index.
    1. Sports—Physiological aspects. 2. Sports medicine. 3. Physical fitness. 4. Physical education and training.
I. Taylor, Buddy. II. Title.
RC1235.N67   1982   613.7′1   82–17988
ISBN 0–8121–0833–7

Printed in the United States of America

Print number: 3 2 1

Dedicated to our wives, Jean Novich and Mildred Taylor, for their encouragement and patience during the preparation of this book.

Foreword

If I were to recommend anyone to write a book on the training and conditioning of athletes and the prevention and care of athletic injuries, I could not make a better choice than Dr. Max Novich and Buddy Taylor. Both men bring to this text their lifetime experience in the field in which they have established themselves as authorities. They both have Hall of Fame credentials. Max is in the World Boxing Hall of Fame and Buddy in the National Athletic Trainers Association Hall of Fame. The book has become a country-wide, easy-to-read reference not only on training and conditioning of athletes for various sports, but also on the prevention and management of athletic injuries attendent to these sports.

Dr. Max Novich, an eminent orthopedic surgeon who specializes in athletic injuries, has participated in sports as a top athlete, coach, and team physician. While attending the University of North Carolina, he played football, boxed, and was captain of the varsity boxing team; he has several boxing championships to his credit. He was selected as one of the top 60 athletes in the history of the University of North Carolina intercollegiate athletics. Besides having coached, refereed, and promoted boxing matches for high school, college, and military teams, he has also served as a team physician to these teams as well as to high school athletic teams. He has been a "bench doctor" for high school athletic teams since 1946. He also served as team physician for the Jersey Jays of the Atlantic Coast Professional Football League. He is presently team physician for Linden High School, which he has been for the past 10 years.

Max has persistently campaigned to return to athletics its vital and natural role in the physical and psychologic development of children and young people. To this end he has devoted much energy and countless hours seeking to bridge the communication and creditability gaps that have existed for too long between the medical, athletic, and educational professions in the United States. Even before the establishment of the A.M.A. Committee on the Medical Aspects of Sports in 1956, which no longer exists, he was writing articles on the necessity of developing safe and effective sports programs for young children and adults. A great deal has been accomplished, but a great deal more has to be done. Max was selected an alternate physician for the 1956 U.S. Olympic Team, and he presented several scientific papers before the International Congress of Sport Science in conjunction with the 1964 Olympic Games in Tokyo. He attended the 1968, 1972, and 1976 Olympic Games as a medical official and had a medical assignment for the 1980 Olympic Games in Moscow, which he declined in deference to the boycott by the U.S. Olympic Team. He was chief physician for the 1965, 1969, and 1973 U.S. Maccabiah Teams, which participated in the Maccabiah Games in Israel. An active member of his South Orange Community, his personally conducted boxing classes for young boys brought him national attention in a seven-page feature in Sports Illustrated.

Buddy Taylor ranks among the all-time greats in athletic training. He was the trainer for the semi-pro football team, the Richmond Rams, in 1948, and the assistant trainer of the professional team, the Richmond Rebels from 1949 through 1950. After serving as Post Athletic Trainer at Fort Campbell, Kentucky, in 1953, he attended the Chicago College of Swedish Massage and Morgan State University. At Indiana University, under the supervision of Dwayne "Spike" Dixon, Buddy received his master's degree in professional athletic training in 1958.

The success of a trainer is reflected in the success and quality of the athletes under his care. As athletic trainer at Tennessee State University from 1961 through 1968, Buddy Taylor handled more Olympic gold medal winners in track and field than any other trainer in the country. Such athletes as Ralph Boston, Wilma Rudolph, Edith McGuire, Madeline Manning, and Wyomia Tyus have all profited from Buddy's skills. He was appointed trainer to the 1968 and 1972 Olympic Games and to the 1969 and 1973 Maccabiah Games.

He established a great reputation as a trainer for professional basketball teams, first with the Los Angeles Stars (1970 Western Division Championship Team), then with the Utah Stars (1971 ABA Championship Team), and finally with the Carolina Cougars (1972–1973 Eastern Division Championship Team). All these teams were in the American Basketball Association. During his time with pros in basketball, he was selected as the trainer for the Eastern Division ABA All Stars Team and also became the trainer for the Western Division of the ABA All Stars Team.

Having already had successful experiences with Olympic teams in the past, he declined the offer to be manager for the United States Men's Track and Field Squad for the 1976 Olympic Games in Montreal.

In 1977, he received the 25-year award as Athletic Trainer and also served as athletic trainer for the U.S. Basketball Team touring Africa. In 1980 and 1981, he received the Cramer Award for Service to Athletic Training.

Buddy is now giving forth with his great expertise as head trainer and a member of the faculty of Winston-Salem State University. The care and training of an athlete requires considerable knowledge, skill, patience, and compassion. Buddy's competency as a trainer is well known and he is especially proud of his induction into the National Athletic Trainer's Hall of Fame. I personally know that Max Novich and Buddy Taylor have combined their talents to produce this book, which is a valuable contribution to sports.

Bill Stein
Director, Sports Advisory Board
Sales Executive Club, New York
Trustee, Lambert Trophy
Director, Volunteers of America

Preface

We are pleased by the favorable reception the first edition of this book was accorded. In recent years, there has been an explosion of interest and knowledge in the training and conditioning of athletes. We felt that the time was ripe for a new edition. In this second edition, we have made numerous changes and have added additional material without altering the level, philosophy, or tone of the book.

It is our purpose to give the reader an awareness in depth of the tremendous efforts put forth by the athlete and the athletic supervisory personnel and the many problems they encounter in the preparation of an athlete for his sport. We also wish to help the reader avoid some of the hazards associated with sports and to disseminate such information to physicians, coaches, and trainers that will ultimately lead to reducing the incidence of death, injury, and permanent disability that result from athletic participation.

Chapter 1, "The Value of Sports," cites the various physical, psychologic and social benefits to be derived by young people, both female and male, from participation in athletics. Reasons for including sports as an essential part of the educational process that contributes to the growth and development of young people are given, and the criticisms most frequently voiced in opposition to school athletic programs are refuted carefully and logically. The responsibilities of a school administration in the establishment and maintenance of viable athletic programs are meticulously outlined, as well as the responsibilities of the students themselves and their parents.

The inclusion of a physician as an integral member of the athletic program who can contribute to the intelligent management of a team by providing adequate medical supervision is discussed, as well as the need for physicians and medical groups to take a deeper interest in the medical aspects of sports. Areas of conflict between the medical and athletic professions are examined, and suggestions offered for their solution.

The responsibilities and qualifications of a trainer are discussed at length in Chapter 2, as well as the development of a staff of student trainers. Chapter 3, "The Training Room," discusses the planning and utilization of this most important facility, offering guidelines for equipping it adequately and economically. The necessary equipment and supplies are listed, along with those items that make up a well-stocked trainer's kit. The use of hydrotherapy and heat therapy in the training room is discussed in detail, and we have included a short section on massage.

"Equipment and the Equipment Room," Chapter 4, offers suggestions on selecting and ordering athletic equipment and its proper maintenance. The duties of the equipment manager and his student assistants are also discussed.

Chapter 5 discusses the responsibilities of a physician who supervises the medical aspects of an athletic program, and the background and orientation required to fulfill those functions.

Chapter 6 considers the conditioning of athletes, beginning with the preseason medical examination. Conditions leading to medical disqualification are considered, and a sample form is provided for the medical examination. Conditioning programs for various sports have been outlined, based on sound physiologic principles to develop strength, speed, endurance, flexibility, reaction, and agility training. Suggestions for proper conditioning in judo, ice hockey, and mountain climbing have been added.

Heat stress is an avoidable but frequent consequence of strenuous practice by unacclimatized players in hot, humid environments. A potentially fatal condition, it can be avoided by an understanding of fluid and electrolyte balance and proper methods of prevention. Should heat reactions occur, prompt recognition and management are essential. The information given here on this subject is invaluable. The keeping and interpretation of weight charts, also discussed, aids in establishing an index to the physical condition of the athletes.

The necessity of a well-balanced diet and the importance of proper nutrition are emphasized in Chapter 7, which also considers the role of food fads in athletics. Chapter 8 thoroughly investigates the use of drugs to enhance athletic performance, and gives suggestions on how to forestall this detrimental practice.

The diagnosis and treatment of injuries that commonly occur in athletics comprise Chapter 9. Since the trainer is frequently the first person to encounter the injured athlete, methods of obtaining a precise history of the injury and first aid techniques are outlined. Definitive treatment and follow-up care, exclusive of surgical intervention, are included.

Frequently, an athletic contest is stopped by an injury to an athlete on the field. Chapter 10, "Examinations and Decisions on the Field," will enable responsible personnel to come to a considered determination of whether an injured athlete can resume play, or what first aid and definitive care is indicated.

Chapter 11, "Training Room Tips," considers the management of minor complaints routinely encountered in the training room, such as "athlete's foot," corns and calluses, and minor abrasions. This chapter has been considerably enlarged to include information on the recognition of hernias, ganglion, varicose veins, swollen glands, and the treatment of such common conditions as cold sores, splinters, nausea, and vomiting.

The Glossary at the end of the book seeks to bridge the gap between training room jargon and medical terminology, and should prove invaluable to both physicians and athletic personnel.

We wish to acknowledge the help extended by the following people in the preparation of this text: Marvin C. Becker, Bernard Boodin, Phillip Brien, Rolando Cheng, Thomas Cuomo, Jack C. Kennedy, Paul J. Kiell, Joseph A. Lombardi, Robby Meijer, Carter R. Rowe, Mona Shangold, Myron J. Shapiro, Milton Singer, Nathan Smith, Vojin Smodlaka, Anthony J. Stefanelli, Irving Strauchler, Ernest Vandeweghe, and Martin Wortzel, physicians; Robert Schwartz, D.D.S.; Morton J. Holtzman, podiatrist; Aaron Rosner, optometrist; Gerald R. Appelbaum, Joseph J. Baraniecki, and Michael A. Maldony, pharmacists; Patricia Dunphy, Phil Dunphy, and Mark Wernecke, registered physical therapists; Sandy Biber and John D'Andrea, trainers; Gerald Sachsel, Dick Steadman, and Abner West, coaches; and Rhonda Dakelman, exercise physiologist.

Special acknowledgment is given to the late Gerald Balakian, M.D., Stephen H. Homer, M.D., and Jay Dakelman.

Perth Amboy, New Jersey   Max M. Novich
Winston-Salem, North Carolina   Buddy Taylor

Contents

1

The Value of Sports

In the sixteenth century the French author, Montaigne, in his essay Of the Education of Boys, recommends that games and exercises play a major role in the educational program for young men: "I would have a graceful exterior combined with a tactful manner; the body and the mind should be fashioned at the same time. It is not a soul; it is not a body that is being trained; it is a man; they must not be separated." That philosophy is just as valid today, applying equally to young women.

Athletics and the positive physical, psychologic, educational, moral, and social benefits derived from athletic competition provide the opportunity to fulfill some of the objectives recommended by Montaigne. This is supported by the experience of physical educators, physicians, coaches, and trainers. Most types of sports activities contribute substantially to the objectives of education, including good health and good health practices.

Since the first edition, there has been literally a fitness explosion at all age levels unprecedented in our society. Vast numbers of Americans have changed their social habits, which has led to health-oriented changes in eating, smoking, and exercise. With the passage of title IX, many programs have been instituted and implemented, bringing many females into health, fitness, and athletic programs.

Desirable traits of character are developed through sports, such as sportsmanship, discipline, observance of the rules of the game, self-control, and a spirit of fair play. Team playing encourages cooperation, leadership, fellowship, and a team spirit. It is not unusual for an athlete to subordinate his individual wishes for the good of the team. Participation in sports, individually or as a member of a team, is a preparation for life. The athlete prepares for a contest by training and conditioning just as we fit ourselves for a profession or trade. Both strive for excellence by vigorous training, self-discipline, and self-sacrifice. Athlete and nonathlete study and analyze opponents to prepare to meet the competitive problems of living.

The disappointments and frustration encountered in sports parallel those in life. In the highly emotionally charged climate of an athletic contest, decisions must be made with split-second timing to meet each new challenge as it appears. Sometimes, planned strategy is used; at other times, unplanned revisions must be made to meet unexpected challenges. It is in this setting that the athlete learns to give and take and to be able to accept success or failure and the joys or disappointments that go with them in a sportsmanlike manner.

The myth that girls involved in strenuous athletics are masculine in appearance is easily debunked by the many attractive, athletic females, such as Dr. Tenley Albright, gold-medal winner in figure skating in the 1956 Olympics, Tracy Austin, world-class professional tennis player, Mary Decker, world-record holder in middle-distance track, Donna DeVaronna, 1964 Olympic gold-medal winner in swimming, Dorothy Hamill, 1976 gold-medal Olympic figure skater, Nancy Lieberman of Olympic basketball fame, Chris Evert Lloyd, tennis star, Nancy Lopez, golfing champion, Ann Myers, member of the 1976 Olympic basketball team, Cathy Rigby, Olympic gymnast, and Wilma Rudolph, gold-medal winner in the 100-, 200-, and 400-meter relays in the 1956 and 1960 Olympics. We should not forget Judith Ann Ford, crowned Miss America of 1969, who gave a superb gymnastic performance as her talent offering. Women's athletic teams are composed of girls attractive of face and physique who perform techniques in a manner that is a pleasure to behold. The many hours devoted by the athletes to their sports lead to a harmonious synchronization of graceful and elegant movement. Sex stereotypes such as, "boys are athletic and strong," "girls are dainty and weak," and "it is unladylike to sweat," fly in the face of reality and are no longer valid.

Since the first edition of this book, a great deal of information concerning the effects of athletics on women has appeared in the medical literature. Menstrual dysfunction, galactorrhea, intermenstrual bleeding, and pregnancy are the gynecologic conditions that would cause a female athlete to stop training and seek medical help. According to Shangold, there is no evidence that exercise causes menstrual dysfunction. She points out that it is not at all clear whether the etiology involves the exercise itself, the physical stress of the training, the emotional stress of training or competing, weight loss, low weight, low body fat, or a combination of all these. She further points out that if a female athlete's menstrual interval (number of days from the beginning of one period to the beginning of the next period) is less than 20 days or more than 60 days, or if she has a breast discharge or bleeds between periods, she should consult her gynecologist. Attention is also warranted if menstrual irregularities developed in association with increased training. Continued training is not necessarily contraindicated.

A pregnant woman should consult her obstetrician before undertaking or continuing an exercise program. In a normal pregnancy, a woman can expect to continue safely any activity she practiced prior to pregnancy at the same level of exertion. Pain, bleeding, or ruptured membranes warrant prompt evaluation. Training should cease until the problem is assessed; it should not be resumed until the obstetrician agrees it is without danger.

A good athletic program should be available to all youth, starting with games and exercises. As a youngster grows and develops, he should be encouraged to engage in various sports just for the fun and the worthwhile experience that physical activity provides. Not only does this furnish immediate recreational pleasure, but athletic skills also are acquired, some of which may be carried over into adult recreational life. Sports enhance health and develop physical fitness of the participants, giving youngsters a healthful and socially acceptable physical and emotional outlet for aggressive and competitive needs.

Nothwithstanding the tangible benefits that stem from athletic competition, there are those misinformed and unsympathetic educators, teachers, sociologists, physicians, and laymen who oppose participation in organized athletics. Many of these critics have had no athletic experience themselves and invariably have the least understanding of the problems associated with sports. In their criticisms they greatly exaggerate the physical and emotional dangers that are associated with athletic participation. We will state their specific criticisms and refute each one.

1. **Overemphasis on Sports Lowers Academic Effort and Achievement.** This criticism is easily disposed of. An athlete on a high school or college team must maintain a satisfactory level of academic accomplishment if he is to remain on the team. If athletics is causing an unsatisfactory academic showing, there is no alternative but to remove him from the team until his studies improve. Many of the National-Collegiate-Athletic-Association universities that grant athletic scholarships have academic advisors assigned to athletic squads to assist athletes in their academic performances. The coach and school authorities must be firm about this, whether or not the athlete is on a scholarship.

Academic orientation should start in high school. An athletic scholarship should not be given to a superior athlete unless he has sufficient academic potential and motivation to acquire a higher education. The National Collegiate Athletic Association recognizes that an applicant for an athletic scholarship should project an ability to perform at a 1.6 on college level. If an athlete wishes to use college as a springboard to professional athletics, he should not be considered for scholarship help. There are other worthy athletes who should get financial aid because they have scholarly ambitions for an education.

2. Most Athletes Have an Inflated and Unrealistic Image of the Importance of a Sport. It's up to the coach to handle the obnoxious athletic participant. Team members also have various ways of reducing the "swelled head" to its proper size. Creating a positive image of the importance of a sport may be a bit more difficult and may require some professional help.

3. Too Much Emphasis is Put on the Concept of Competition. This criticism has no validity because athletics by its very nature demands that a participant properly balance his individual competitive and co-operative drives, both of which are facets of normal behavior.

4. Participants are Liable to Physical Injury. Critics feel that the preadolescent and adolescent child who engages in contact sports is especially susceptible to injury. In reality, most claims of bodily injury are greatly exaggerated. Youth is resilient and capable of rebounding quickly after sustaining injury or illness. This is particularly true in athletics, in which most injuries involve the musculoskeletal system, are usually minor, and rarely need extensive medical attention.

Injuries do occur, of course, and occasionally may be serious, even fatal. From 1959 to 1963, when 820,000 youths were exposed each year, the annual football fatality survey recorded 86 deaths as a direct result of playing football. From 1971 to 1975, when 1,275,000 players were exposed annually, 77 deaths occurred.

Many pediatricians and orthopedists claim that preadolescent and adolescent boys are susceptible to injury because the epiphyses of growing bones are insufficiently protected by incompletely developed periarticular muscles and ligaments. These physicians recommend that athletes refrain from organized sports until their epiphyses have closed; this theory is not supported by any scientific study. Children at early ages are now entering supervised training programs and preparing for competition. It is not unusual for young swimmers and gymnasts to be "burned out" during adolescence.

A physician I (M.N.) know has ruled out boxing for young boys, believing that epiphyses in the upper extremities will be injured with repetitive light or heavy bag punching. This is carrying the epiphyseal injury theory too far. My experience with boys engaged in boxing from 5 years of age through adolescence is in complete disagreement. An occasional epiphyseal injury of the wrist, knee, or ankle has occurred in the hundreds of high school athletes we have cared for, and the athletes made complete recoveries. However, epiphyseal injuries of the shoulder and elbow in Little League pitchers may lead to serious consequences if not managed properly.

"In Spain they kill bulls, in the United States they wreck knees." The knee is a remarkably engineered joint that nature never designed or intended for high velocity football. At least 5% of the 18,000 New York high school football players suffer knee injuries yearly and this compares similarly with injury figures from other states. Every year, high school, college, and professional football players undergo knee surgery as a result of football injuries. Direct viewing of football players being carried off the field with knee injuries and provocative newspaper and magazine accounts about them have overemphasized the problem.

The element of adventure in athletics appeals to all of us. This adventure involves a hazard—a calculated risk of injury. The risk cannot be completely removed from sports without removing the adventure. However, we can and must minimize the risk. The awkward, obese, or thin, slow moving, poorly trained, psychologically inadequate and unconditioned boy is the one who usually gets hurt.

Conditioning the athlete, using properly fitted protective equipment, and correcting faulty playing techniques—in that order—are the most important ways of minimizing the risk of injuries. Accidents inherent in all sports, and particularly contact sports, are the fourth most common cause of injuries. They are sometimes impossible to prevent. Bodily injury and an occasional death will always occur in athletics, notwithstanding all the preventive measures taken to eliminate them. But clinical disorders resulting from athletic participation in hot, humid weather, or in high altitudes need not occur if proper precautions are taken.

It is hoped that this book, by focusing on these hazards, will enable the reader to avoid some of the pitfalls associated with sports. This may be achieved by more frequent medical examinations, the use of scientific and sound physiologic methods of training and conditioning, better and safer coaching methods, and elimination of dangerous practices such as spear-tackling, goring, and variations of crack-back blocking.

Since the first edition, there have been a number of changes in safety-rules and equipment. Spearing, goring, and crack-back blocking techniques in football have been ruled illegal. The National Federation of State High School Associations has not banned blocking below the waist except in the free-blocking area close to the scrimmage line. Kickers will now be given additional protection by not allowing them to be hit unless they have advanced a minimum of 5 yards or unless the kick has touched ground, another player, an official, or anything beyond the scrimmage line. In baseball, helmets for batters and base runners as well as molded spikes for baseball shoes are recommended. By 1982, throat protectors will be required. Shin guards are now recommended. By 1984, metal cleats will be barred from high-school baseball. In wrestling, dangerous holds, such as the chicken wing, full Nelson, headlock with no arm, or any hold that extends a joint beyond its normal range of extension, have been outlawed.

Research in protective equipment for athletes is an ongoing operation under the guidance of the National Operating Committee on Standards for Athletic Equipment (N.O.C.S.A.E.). Improvements of protective equipment in coordination with rule changes are continuously being implemented to reduce the incidence of risks and hazards in athletics. If an injury does occur, the ability to arrive at an early diagnosis and to start definitive care will help the athlete achieve full recovery. Dissemination of such information to the physician and key athletic leaders will ultimately lead to reducing the incidence of deaths, injuries, and permanent disabilities that result from athletic injuries.

PREVENTION OF ATHLETIC INJURIES

Supervisory athletic personnel on every level have always been aware of the hazards and risks inherent in sports. Yet, they have been hampered in their efforts to reduce the incidence of athletic deaths, injuries, and permanent disability because of the apathy of the medical profession, insincere and superficial cooperation from educators, the scarcity of trained coaches with degrees in physical education, and the small number of qualified trainers.

All of these factors certainly existed prior to World War II, when the medical profession was not as involved or concerned with sports as it is today. Although new concepts of exercise physiology first developed in Europe were vigorously pursued by many European scientists, only a few United States investigators showed interest in them. Coaches now have an awareness and better understanding of the benefits that can be derived in the coaching of athletes by the application of the principles of exercise physiology and biomechanics. The medical aspects of training and conditioning of athletes were hardly ever mentioned in American medical annals, and literature about the various branches of sports medicine in the United States was scant. Thorndike's Athletic Injuries, published in 1938, was the first work of any moment by an American medical author on the prevention, diagnosis, and treatment of athletic injuries. It was an oasis of practical information in a desert of indifference exhibited towards sports medicine by many members of the medical profession. There was also a noticeable lack of dissemination of available athletic medical information to team physicians and to doctors called upon to treat athletic injuries. Moreover, protective equipment in use had not really been developed to the point of meriting the label "protective."

However, the most significant deterrent toward the rendering of the best medical care to the athlete was the friction and lack of cooperation between the coaching and medical professions, compounded by the feigned interest of school administrators. The duties and responsibilities of these three groups toward the athlete had never been firmly established, especially at the high school level, which encompasses about one million young people. This discord militated against effective methods of prevention and treatment of athletic injuries. Even in this enlightened era, such attitudes still prevail.

In pre-World War II days the preseason or pregame examination of the high school athlete was almost unheard of. Physicians did not concern themselves with the manner in which coaches conditioned their athletes, including their nutrition. Doctors almost never appeared on a practice field, either before the season or during the regular season of play. Had they done so, physicians might have learned a great deal about the coach and his influence on the athletes in his charge. (The coaches' zeal, or lack of it, is responsible for many clinical conditions exhibited by the players.) If a player became sick or injured, there was no guarantee that the coach would see to it that the athlete consulted a physician. If he did get the athlete to a doctor, communication was apt to be tenuous between the doctor and coach about the athlete's follow-up care and fitness to return to play.

Although we believe in hard-nose conditioning and coaching, we are also aware that many coaches drive their teams too hard. The modern coach is better informed about the scientific basis of training and conditioning of his athletes. In most cases, they have a better understanding, appreciation, and attitude toward their trainers and physicians. With this information and medical backup, coaches are less apt to drive their charges and/or make excessive demands. They know that this can be counterproductive and lead to less-than-maximal performance of the athlete as well as to states of anxiety, resentment, and even fatigue that will result in higher incidence of injuries. Most modern coaches know that they need to condition their athletes mentally, emotionally, and physically to get maximum performance.

Doctors have complained that too many coaches are concerned more with the success of their teams than with the health and safety of their athletes. Some coaches will ignore the advice of a doctor not to play an injured athlete, especially one with a sprained ankle or knee, apparently in the mistaken belief that activity is the best treatment for an injured joint, regardless of the pathologic condition. Fortunately, this is happening less and less because of the better rapport between the medical and coaching professions and the threat of a malpractice action against the coach.

Training-room jargon was foreign and confusing to most doctors, so they found it difficult to communicate with coaches, trainers, and even the athletes themselves. This state of affairs, however, worked well for the coach and trainer, by reinforcing the bond that already existed between them. Trainers, in many instances, practiced a sort of "twilight zone" medicine, including manipulation, injections, dispensing of drugs, physical therapy, and homespun psychotherapy. Because of the indifference and apathy of so many physicians towards athletics in general as well as the abdication to the trainer of many responsibilities properly the concern of the physician, coaches gave more credence to the opinions of trainers than to those of doctors.

Much information concerning the medical needs of athletes has been made available to the trainer. Companies that sell athletic equipment and supplies also publish magazines, newsletters, posters, and other materials. These contain scientific information about adhesive strapping and bandaging, first-aid measures, and emergency procedures for the injured athlete, including methods of transportation off the field and the use of physical and chemical agents. Protective equipment, fashioning and fit of protective pads, uniforms, and the mechanism of athletic injuries are also covered. Most coaches abreast of their profession provide strength coaches (specialists) for their sport. Certification of coaches much like physicians and trainers is a future consideration.

Articles written by physicians about human anatomy, physiology, and kinesiology, accompanied by appropriate illustrations, charts, drawings, and pictures are also distributed, complemented by articles about the prevention, diagnosis, and treatment of illnesses and injuries attendant to athletics. Such publications as the First Aider, by the Cramer Company, Journal of the National Athletic Trainers Association, Scholastic Coach, Athletic Journal, and Athletic Purchasing and Facilities represent positive influences that have continued upgrading the knowledge and skills of the coaching and training professions.

Dr. S.E. Bilik, a physician and physical educator who specialized in training, conditioning, rehabilitation, and treatment of athletic injuries, wrote his first Trainers' Bible in 1916. This book was directed to the training profession in an effort to institute scientific training techniques and methods to upgrade the trainers' services to the athlete. These many publications, which were directed to trainers, would have been equally beneficial to the medical profession had doctors been aware of their existence.

Just as the medical profession developed from sparse beginnings into the science it is today, the training profession is developing to produce men soundly educated in the physical and paramedical care of the athlete. Many trainers now have academic degrees, and some hold faculty rank at institutions with which they are affiliated. A large number are registered physical therapists. The National Athletic Trainers Association exacts high standards for membership.

Because the medical profession had not yet taken a position on defining the separate duties and responsibilities of the school administration, coach, and physician and what was expected of each concerning the prevention of athletic injuries among high school athletes, one of us (M.N.) wrote an article on the subject for the Journal of the Medical Society of New Jersey in 1953. In this article the following areas of responsibilities were clearly set forth:

1. The academic administration should be supervised by the principal and faculty, with the cooperation of the Board of Education.

2. The athletic administration should be supervised by the athletic director and the coaches.

3. The medical department should be supervised by a physician with experience in handling athletic injuries.

Role of the Academic Administration. Leadership of the academic administration is essential to the establishment of a complete athletic program for students, and is no less important to the academic program. In our complex society we attach too much awe to the intellectual and the creative that overbalancing occurs in this direction. It is lamentable if overemphasis on sports mocks the concept of the school as a center of learning; however, it is no less regrettable if preoccupation with intellectual matters results in a man being ill-prepared to cope with the hard facts of existence.

School administrative authorities who are not exactly sold on the educational values of athletics might be impressed by the statement of James B. Conant, a well-known and respected educator. In a 1951 report to the Board of Overseers of Harvard University about expenses for athletics, he said: "This sum is not to be regarded as an athletic deficit but is as much a proper charge against the resources of the Faculty as the maintenance of the library or laboratory."

The ideal of a "sound mind in a sound body" is just as valid today as it was when promulgated by the Greeks. Therefore, school authorities are obligated to provide the best of the following for their athletes:

1. A competent coach and staff who know not only the fundamentals and intricacies of the sport, but how to get athletes into proper condition for participating in it. The coach must know how to avoid fatigue states and be sufficiently knowledgeable to recognize them when they appear. He must be able to react to and handle the personality of each athlete. He must also know all phases of uniforming, equipment, and proper fitting, how to fashion and fit protective pads when the need arises, and when to give first aid. He must teach athletes how to avoid or minimize injury.

It has been established that the incidence of athletic injury is definitely related to the years of training and experience of the head coach. The coaching staff should give to their athletes as much mental, emotional, and physical effort as it expects from them. It is the coach's duty to advise a boy to change his sport, if the athlete's expectations exceed his abilities. The attitude of a coach toward academic achievement has already been stated.

The coach must also regard the doctor's decision as final, since it is made in the best interest of the athlete. Victory is not worth the candle if it is won at the expense of any athlete's health. Competent coaching can prevent athletic injuries provided the coach is concerned with even the smallest details, from graduated muscular exercises to the proper fit of a mouthpiece. A good coach and his staff will maintain a proper balance between the objectives of winning and the health and safety of his athletes.

2. A suitable playing field for each sport, with proper supervision and policing of these facilities, such as removal of stones and other hazards from outdoor fields, proper chlorination of swimming pools and proper amount of floor padding for boxing rings.

3. The best protective equipment and fitted uniforms should be provided for each member of the team in each sport. Improper equipment stands second in a list of four causes of football injuries.

4. Adequate health and accident insurance for each athletic student, whether he competes interscholastically or intrascholastically.

5. A competent physician who is genuinely interested, sympathetic, oriented toward sports, and available when needed. Although there are some advantages to selecting a physician trained in traumatic and orthopedic surgery, such a background is not mandatory. However, the physician must have facilities available for x-ray studies, physical therapy, and consultation (or know where to get them) if they are needed. His duties and responsibilities must be agreed upon in advance.

6. A competent trainer who can not only do his job for the athlete but can also act as an able assistant to both the coach and the team physician without compromising his important position with the athlete.

7. Adequate, well-equipped lockers and training room facilities.

8. A dietician to regulate and instruct coaches, players, and parents concerning proper diet, during the season as well as off-season.

These responsibilities of the academic administration are as valid today as when first written in 1953. However, in high school and college sports, the parents and athletes themselves also have duties and responsibilities.

Role of the Parent. Parents can play a vital role in the development of a school's athletic program without interfering with its administration. Once a parent is satisfied that the program is conducted in the best interest of his child, he should and usually does give his wholehearted support to the coach and school authorities.

1. A parent should encourage his child's participation in a sport if such is the child's desire, and not the parent's acting out of his own

unconscious needs. The parent must not push his child into an athletic activity to vicariously realize his own unresolved fantasies or ambitions. He must honestly examine his own motives.

2. A parent must be concerned with the following:
   a. The coach—his qualifications, his experience, his knowledge of the human body, whether or not he is a physical educator (because of their knowledge and training in anatomy, physiology, and kinesiology, physical educators usually make the best coaches for school teams, particularly in high schools), the coach's reputation with his athletes, and his attitudes and practices.

   Since most parents do not have the background to judge a coach's fitness to teach a sport, they have a right to expect the school to make inquiries into such considerations before engaging a man. The school must select a person qualified to be a coach. However, if the parent has a suspicion that a coach may be exploiting his youngster or is coaching in a manner that is not in the child's best interest, he has the obligation to reveal these suspicions to the proper school authorities. It is the parents' responsibility to see that sports are conducted for the good of the athlete, with the health of the athlete at all times a primary consideration. However, in coming to a conclusion as to whether or not a coach is fit for his position, only objective yardsticks must be used, not hearsay or emotionalism.
   b. Equipment—the school must provide the best protective equipment, especially for contact sports. The wearing of worn out, outmoded, or improperly fitted gear should not be tolerated.
   c. Facilities—suitable playing fields, adequate, well-equipped locker and training rooms.
   d. Medical care—
      (1) Preseason history and physical examination.
      (2) Attendance of a physician at every game, particularly in contact sports.
      (3) Competent medical care for sick or injured players; a careful examination by the doctor and the issuance of a permit from him should be demanded before any athlete is allowed to practice or compete following an injury or illness.
      (4) Accident and health insurance.

3. Parents must be concerned with the effect of sports participation on the child's education and must keep the two objectives in balance.

4. Parents must assist the child in adhering to the rules of training and conditioning, which include:

    a. Eating a palatable, balanced, and nutritious diet.
    b. Sleeping a minimum of 8 hours a night, and possibly more.
    c. No smoking.
    d. No alcoholic beverages.
    e. Use of drugs as prescribed by the physician.
    f. Restricted use of automobile.

Role of the Athlete. The athlete must recognize that he has certain obligations to fulfill toward his teammates, his coach, and his school, which are no less important than the bill of rights he expects as an athlete. He is required to follow certain regulations and training rules that, of course, vary depending upon whether he is a candidate for a high school, collegiate, or professional team.

1. He must act like a gentleman at all times on and off the field so as to bring credit to himself, his parents, his school, and his team.

2. He must abide by the rules of training and conditioning established by the coaching staff:
    a. Train precisely as advised by the coaches.
    b. No smoking.
    c. No drinking of alcoholic beverages.
    d. Use of drugs as prescribed by the physician.
    e. Home and in bed by 10:30 P.M.; at least 8 hours' sleep a night, and possibly more.

3. He must keep up with his education. This is best accomplished with an organized study program.

4. He must maintain his equipment and uniform in good working order and return all items in good condition at the end of the season.

5. He must report illnesses and injuries to his coach and trainer regardless of the nature and extent. These men will decide if they warrant the attention of a physician. Many athletes are reluctant to complain to coaches because they fear being criticized as a "gutless wonder," as some coaches tend to do. Others fear they may be benched. Such fears should not be allowed to predominate.

6. He must strive for excellence in his sport through determination, dedication, and hard work.

7. He must be aware that cooperation and discipline benefit not only the team but himself.

8. He must show respect for his coaches and teachers.

9. He must cooperate for group effort.

Developing Cooperation Among the Professions. In 1956 one of us (M.N.) wrote an article in the Journal of the American Medical Association in which he expanded and elaborated on the differences of opinion between coaches and school administrators on the one hand, and between coaches and team physicians on the other, and suggested how these differences could be reconciled. One of the main points of contention was that physicians who lacked a sincere interest in athletics were too quick to disqualify athletes. Because there was some validity to this complaint, the article listed disqualifying medical conditions of the various body systems as well as the functions of the team physician, concepts of conditioning players, protective equipment, and the treatment of athletic injuries. Also listed were duties and responsibilities of the physician at the ringside and on the football field.

Great strides were made in the medical care of the professional boxer by the various state athletic commissions that existed a generation before the enormous prestige of the American Medical Association was brought to bear on the medical supervision of athletics. Not until 1956 did the A.M.A., through its Committee on the Medical Aspects of Sports, step in to exert necessary leadership in ensuring the health and safety of athletes. Although there has been a remarkable upgrading of medical supervision for athletes, this has not kept pace in professional boxing. The professional boxer still receives periodic physical and neurologic examinations, including encephalograms and brain scans when indicated, maintenance of his complete medical records and pre-bout examinations, but the quality of this care varies from city to city.

When a boxer is examined, it is important that his win-loss record and prior medical records be renewed by the examining physician. It is also important that a ringside physician maintain constant communication during a bout by means of manual and vocal signals in an effort to protect the fighter from needless injury. The recent rash of deaths in 1980 confirms my (M.N.) prior statement that administratively much remains to be done and much reform is still necessary.

Before the recent fitness boom, the amount of medical literature available on sports medicine was small considering the tremendous opportunity for scientific research into human activity under a variety of stress conditions. The situation happily has changed and there is now a steady flow of information from team physicians, physical educators, physiologists, trainers, physical therapists, recreation specialists, dentists, and others. Sources of information are easily available to all interested health professionals for them to keep abreast of current thinking and practices in sports medicine. The two major journals are the American Journal of Sports Medicine and The Journal of the Physician and Sportsmedicine. In addition, there are a variety of other journals and newsletters such as the Journal of Sports Medicine and Physical Fitness, Medicine and Science in Sports and Exercise, Journal of Orthopaedics and Physical Therapy, InfoAAU, Sportsmedicine Digest, Sports Medicine Bulletin, Sports Medicine Update, United States Sports Academy News, Physical Fitness/Sports Medicine, published by the President's Council on Physical Fitness and Sports, and the yearly book on sports medicine published by the Year Book Publishers of Chicago. The A.M.A. News and the Medical Tribune periodically publish material on sports medicine. These are recommended reading for health professionals interested in sports medicine.

The physician is faced with many problems concerning the complete health care of an athlete since so much depends on the dedication, knowledge, and skills of nonmedical athletic supervisory personnel. These medical problems could be more effectively met if an amiable, understanding, and cooperative relationship existed between the practicing doctor and the physical educators, including coaches and trainers. On professional and big-time college levels, this rapport has been achieved because of the availability of highly qualified physicians, coaches, and trainers who are oriented to the use of physiologic principles of training and conditioning, the best protective equipment, preseason medical examinations, and sound medical therapy and follow-up care of the sick or injured athlete. Such a situation, however, does not generally exist on the small college and high school levels.

The A.M.A., through its Committee on the Medical Aspects of Sports, put forth tremendous efforts to make the practicing physician aware of the various branches of sports medicine and how he can best apply his medical skills for the care of the athlete. This was done through conferences, publications, and statements of position on important issues in sports medicine. The A.M.A. sponsored and conducted studies on subjects pertinent to athletics. Although this committee was discontinued in 1974, it still has one staff member Jack A. Bell, M.P.H. who keeps contact with the members of the last committee, which enables them to run a yearly national conference on sports medicine. Because of the A.M.A.'s mutually beneficial liaisons and cooperative activities with local medical societies and national medical and athletic governing bodies, its influence caused a number of county and state medical committees on sports medicine to be established. Nationally, the Sports Medicine Committee of the American Academy of Orthopaedic Surgeons, the American Orthopaedic Society of Sports Medicine, and the American College of Sports Medicine are the major sports-medicine societies in our nation. They are making more clinical and scientific research contributions in sports medicine than any other scientific organizations in the free world. These bodies develop and disseminate a wealth of information on athletic medicine.

Notwithstanding the prodigious efforts put forth by these groups, the community physician's relationship with physical educators, coaches, and trainers—although improved—still has some way to go. Although physicians may display some familiarity with achievements of nationally famous athletes, the community and the medical profession would be benefitted if more physicians "got the message" from their state and county medical societies' committees on the medical aspects of sports and became more involved with the local school athletic programs. There is too little contact between these professional groups at the county and state levels, where it is most needed. More conferences, meetings, consultations and workshops are needed to bring these people together on a grass-roots supervision of athletics.

Local physicians, physical educators, athletic directors, coaches, and trainers should get together and discuss matters related to health supervision in sports. The officials upon whom the proper conduct of an athletic contest depends are usually physical educators. Such conferences will enable these concerned individuals to become better acquainted with one another's viewpoints and problems. The more informal the meeting, the greater the flow of discussions and ideas. Many physicians would be surprised to discover the difficult decisions and problems that confront coaches in their daily routine. Conversely, coaches and other athletic supervisory personnel would better appreciate the physician's problems, which are both medical and legal. Once cooperation is established between the physician and the allied sports personnel, an integrated and coordinated attack can follow on administrative and medical problems that adversely affect the health and safety of the athlete. This would reduce the incidence of serious injuries and deaths resulting from athletics.

Many pertinent topics, questions, and problems concerning the health supervision of athletes need further discussion, inquiry, and resolution. Some of the more immediate and pressing ones are:

1. Agreement on disqualifying medical conditions for each sport.
2. Prevention and management of head and neck injuries.
3. Prevention and management of knee injuries.
4. Prevention of clinical disorders commonly associated with athletic participation in environmental conditions of high temperature, high humidity, and high altitude.
5. Weight control, particularly in boxing and wrestling.
6. The role of diet and nutrition.
7. The use and misuse of drugs.
8. The value of weight-training and the use of mechanical body building aids and gadgets.
9. Examination on the field and first-aid decisions.
10. Research into and development of more effective protective equipment.
11. Rule changes to eliminate situations and conditions that lead to injuries.
12. Upgrading the qualifications and competency of officials so that they can properly interpret and enforce the rules.
13. Use of administrative safety controls as promulgated by the

American Football Coaches Association and National Federation of State High School Associations.

14. Value of various physical therapy modalities in the management and treatment of athletic injuries.

15. Emphasis on individual combative sports such as boxing, wrestling, and judo, for students in the public school systems.

Everyone concerned with the fielding of an athlete or a team must integrate and coordinate his individual duties and responsibilities into a joint effort aimed at making athletics pleasurable and safe. Full cooperation must exist among physicians, coaches, trainers, and administrators to ensure that sports are conducted in the best interest of the participants. If channels of communication between all concerned parties are kept open at all times, conditions will improve and many perplexing problems will be resolved.

REFERENCES

Blyth, C.S., and Schindler, R.D.: The forty-eighth annual survey of football fatalities: 1931–1979. Prepared for American Football Coaches Association, The National Collegiate Athletic Association, and The National Federation of the State High School Associations, 1980.

Clarke, K.S.: Football head and neck injuries. *In* Athletic Injuries to the Head, Neck, and Face. Edited by J.S. Torg. Philadelphia, Lea & Febiger, 1982.

Jensen, C.R., and Fisher, A.G.: Scientific Basis of Athletic Conditioning. 2nd Ed., Philadelphia, Lea & Febiger, 1979.

Koynovsky, N.: The Joy of Feeling Fit. New York, E.P. Dutton, 1971.

McArdle, W.D., Katch, F.I., and Katch, V.L.: Exercise Physiology: Energy, Nutrition, and the Physiology of Human Performance. Philadelphia, Lea & Febiger, 1981.

Novich, M.M.: Our Olympic success is in your hands. Medical Times, *105*:1d–3d, 1977.

Shangold, M.N.: Sports and menstrual function. The Physician and Sportsmedicine, *8*:66–72, 1980.

Torg, J.S., et al.: The National Football Head and Neck Injury Registry. JAMA, *241*:1447–1479, 1979.

Football Rule Book 1980. Kansas City, The National Federation of State High School Associations, 1980.

2

Responsibilities of Training Personnel

THE ATHLETIC TRAINER

It is the joint responsibility of the athlete, coach, trainer, and team physician to get and maintain an athlete in top-notch condition. The degree of physical fitness achieved is directly related to the time and the manner of the conditioning; maintaining physical fitness for a sport depends on the prevention and prompt treatment of athletic injuries. The trainer cooperates not only in developing the body of the athlete, but in building and maintaining the emotional stability and spirit necessary to handle the tensions and anxieties encountered in athletic competition.

Qualifications*

The best educational background for a trainer is one that would provide him† with the necessary credentials to teach physical education or to function as an athletic coach. Studies in methods of physical therapy are desirable. He should have gained experience under the supervision of physicians versed in athletic medicine and of experienced trainers, from whom he obtained the practical knowledge necessary to follow his profession. By attending clinics and conventions, sponsoring clinics for student trainers and coaches, and reading the latest publications on the training profession, he improves himself as a trainer and stays abreast of new trends within the profession. The trainer can contribute to his profession by writing articles. Membership in the National Athletic Trainers Association affords a wealth of information and benefits.

The trainer assists the coach in getting the athletes in top condition; this is his primary function. He also assists the team physician in ren-

*For information on how to become a NATA certified athletic trainer, consult the 1982 Procedures for Certification, which is prepared by the National Athletic Trainers' Association, Board of Certification, P.O. Drawer 1865, Greenville, N.C. 27834.
†The masculine pronoun is used throughout the text for simplicity of style.

dering first aid, and in carrying out therapeutic procedures prescribed by the doctor for the athlete. He should have a working knowledge of the human body and its functions, a complete understanding of the common athletic injuries, methods of taping and massage, and physical therapy equipment and techniques. He must know when these techniques are indicated and when they are contraindicated.

The trainer must hold a certificate in Red Cross first aid, cardiopulmonary resuscitation (CPR) and be a certified athletic trainer. He is familiar with the amount of time required for an athlete to recuperate from a specific injury and the manner of recuperation. Despite his knowledge of anatomy and physiology and his skills in physical therapy, he immediately refers to the team physician all significant and disabling injuries. Rendering care other than first-aid may hurt a player more than help him. The trainer's activities are always conducted in the best interest of the athlete. In his unique position, the trainer can do much to keep the lines of communication open between the coach and the physician, to the benefit of the athlete.

The responsibilities of the job and the necessity of working with many people require high personal standards of the trainer. He must be in good health and possess manual strength and dexterity—"a good pair of hands." The ability to improvise and to work effectively on a limited budget and under all conditions is necessary. He must be able to work and to make competent decisions under pressure, both during practice and actual games. The hours are long and the work hard, and he cannot limit the rendering of his services to a rigid schedule.

One of the trainer's greatest assets is a congenial personality: he is cheerful, friendly, patient, and emotionally mature and demonstrates self-control, an even temper, prudence, and a sense of humor. He works cooperatively with, and under the supervision of, the team physician and the coach.

As an executive of the athletic department, the trainer's activities and public contacts should reflect creditably on himself, his profession, and the school or organization that he represents. As a leader, he has wholesome personal habits that will inspire and encourage the athletes in his care. He treats each athlete fairly. Because of his close association with the athletes, the trainer frequently knows everything that is going on. He hears the gossip, finds out about academic troubles, and learns the names of sweethearts and the degree of their involvement. The trainer often becomes a father image and hence, a trusted friend and counselor. In such a role he must listen, be empathetic, encourage, motivate, and inspire. The coach frequently relies on information given to him by the trainer, which must be considered a privileged communication.

The training of women is a new and unique experience to most trainers. In many instances, the trainer of female athletes is much closer to the athletes than the coach, and the coach relies on the trainer for more intimate and necessary information far more than he would if he were working with males. A woman in competitive athletics, especially on a college campus, must endure the criticism and frequently, the isolation imposed by traditional thinking. She must have the desire to endure the rigors of conditioning to an extent surpassing that of the male athlete.

A trainer of women athletes deals with states of tension that differ in degree, but not in kind, from those experienced with males. Pains brought on by menstruation may cause alterations and modifications in training schedules and plans. The key factors in being a successful trainer for women are understanding and especially tolerance. Women are more responsive to the types of assistance that trainers can render; they frequently are more appreciative and seek counsel more often. There seems to be no real difference in the time needed to get them into top physical condition as compared to males. The assumption that women athletes heal more slowly is incorrect.

The suggested responsibilities of the athletic trainer are as follows:

1. Remains available throughout the day and on call at other times when he is not attending practice sessions or games.
2. Assists in the application of protective equipment, including strapping and bandaging.
3. Renders first aid and refers injured athletes to the physician for diagnosis and treatment.
4. Uses therapeutic equipment and techniques as prescribed by the physician for the treatment of athletic injuries.
5. Assists the physician in conducting medical examinations.
6. Serves as a liaison between sick or injured players and the team physician, seeing to it that the players carry out the prescribed treatment.
7. Maintains records of the medical examinations of athletes, together with precise notations of injuries, treatment, and results obtained.
8. Refrains from diagnosing or stating his opinion about injuries to anyone except the team physician or the coach.
9. Cooperates fully with the coaches to field the strongest possible team.
10. Helps build team morale through the activities of the training room.
11. Purchases, stores, and keeps a record of all training-room supplies.
12. Maintains all training-room equipment in good operating condition at all times.
13. Reports (in writing) any defects in machinery or equipment immediately.
14. Supervises student trainers.
15. Refers athletes to team dentist.

Undergraduate Athletic Training Curriculum*

I. Educational requirements

    A. A college degree with a teaching license.

    B. Completion of the following required courses:
1. Anatomy
2. Physiology
3. Physiology of Exercise
4. Applied Anatomy and Kinesiology
5. Psychology (2 courses)
6. First Aid and CPR
7. Nutrition
8. Remedial Exercise
9. Personal, Community, and School Health
10. Techniques of Athletic Training
11. Advanced Techniques of Athletic Training
12. Clinical Experience (600 clock hours) over a 2-year period

    C. Recommended, but not required, courses:
1. Physics
2. Pharmacology
3. Histology
4. Pathology
5. Organization and Administration of Health and Physical Education
6. Psychology of Coaching
7. Coaching Techniques
8. Chemistry
9. Tests and Measurements

Graduate Athletic Training Curriculum*

I. Educational requirements

    A. Proof of a Bachelor's degree being awarded by an accredited college or university.

    B. Completion of the specific undergraduate course and clinical requirements either before or during graduate level studies.

    C. Completion of the specific course work and clinical experience requirements at the graduate level:
1. Advanced Athletic Training (2 courses)
2. Clinical experience—minimum of 300 clock hours at the graduate level.
3. At least one course in one of the following areas:
    a. Advanced Anatomy
    b. Advanced Physiology
    c. Advanced Physiology of Exercise
    d. Advanced Kinesiology or Applied Anatomy

*There are more than 70 colleges and universities with NATA approved curricula; a list of these schools may be obtained by writing to the National Athletic Trainers Association, P.O. Drawer 1865 Greenville, North Carolina 27834.

A CODE OF ETHICS*

A code of ethics specifies the acceptable standards of conduct for members of a profession and protects those members, as well as the individuals they serve. It establishes standards that ensure a high level of professional service and it permits the profession to exercise some control over the conduct of its members.

The National Athletic Trainers Association has developed a "Trainer's Code of Ethics," which indicates the acceptable patterns of conduct. The main qualities stressed in the code are *honesty, integrity,* and *loyalty.*

The following suggestions, based upon the code, will help the trainer to build desirable patterns of conduct:

1. Be honest with yourself and with others. Avoid attempting to bluff your way through situations that demand answers you do not possess. Admit your lack of knowledge. Doing so will make you seem more human and increase the athlete's respect for you.
2. Under no circumstances should you attempt to carry out a procedure that is a prerogative of the physician, unless you have been given instructions to do so. Do not proceed beyond the limits of your responsibility.
3. Cooperation is a constant watchword. It is your responsibility to create a congenial relationship between yourself and the coaches, parents, administrators, and medical personnel.
4. Be thorough. Administer your respective duties with attention to detail and with professional exactness.
5. Observe the rules of good sportsmanship and fair play in respect to all your associates—colleagues, athletes, and opponents. Avoid making criticism or speaking disparagingly about coaches or other staff members. Avoid discriminatory practices.
6. Refrain from giving testimonials or endorsements of commercial items. It is unprofessional and unethical and against the law in some areas.
7. Be courteous and considerate to visiting competitors. Do all you can to render assistance. Remember, they are your guests. Treat them accordingly.
8. Do your best to instill the qualities of good sportsmanship in the athletes by precept and example.
9. Encourage and promote scholastic achievement among the athletes.
10. Use common sense in all public relations. Refrain from making statements that are critical or misleading or that may be misconstrued and so reflect unfavorably upon the school, your colleagues, or the athletic program.
11. Conduct yourself as a responsible, mature member of the community and as one who reflects professional competence and integrity. By your actions, earn the respect and confidence of those about you.
12. The unauthorized and/or nontherapeutic use of drugs for any purpose is not to be condoned.

*Adapted from Klafs, C. E., and Arnheim, D. D.: Modern Principles of Athletic Training. 5th Ed. St. Louis, C. V. Mosby, 1981.

THE STUDENT TRAINER*

The formation of a good school athletic department, as stated in Chapter 1, depends primarily on the school administration, who must make available to the student a competent coaching staff, proper equipment, and game areas for each sport. The administration is also responsible for providing an effective program to prevent athletic injuries. To this end, they must provide medical supervision of athletes and engage a coach knowledgable in ways to prevent athletic injuries. College and professional teams usually employ an experienced trainer to assist the coach and the team physician in preventing and treating injuries, but many high schools rely on the coach and his assistants to assume the functions of a trainer. Frequently, students are recruited to assist the coach in some of these activities.

A few suggested duties and responsibilities of the student trainers' staff are:

1. Assist the team physician and coach at all times.
2. Keep daily treatment records of athletes.
3. Keep the training room in a hygienic condition at all times.
4. Give daily treatment under proper supervision.
5. Be concerned with overall safety of the team at all times.
6. Welcome visiting student trainers and inform them of the availability of your facilities.
7. Check first aid kit to see that it is well stocked and in an orderly fashion for practice, game, and/or trips.
8. Prepare training equipment for road games.
9. Keep a want list of needed supplies.

Note that this list does not mention that the student trainer accepts responsibility for determining the extent of injuries or for their treatment, except under the direct supervision of the team physician or coach. While the student may be taught certain first-aid procedures, such as giving artificial respiration or controlling hemorrhage, he immediately notifies the coach or the team physician of any suspected injuries and follows their directions. First-aid techniques, though sometimes life-saving, may cause additional harm if improperly used. Only the physician possesses the background sufficient for diagnosing injuries and for prescribing treatment.

To set up a student trainers' staff, the head coach selects students to work with him in developing a program of injury prevention. Ideally, the group of student trainers would consist of four students: freshman, sophomore, junior, and senior. After the initial program has been established, the coach would have at his disposal three well-trained students

*Adapted in part from Taylor, B.: The high school student trainers' staff. The First Aider, *36*:122, 1967.

and one apprentice—the freshman. Since the freshman's first year is a period of adjustment to a new academic environment, his duties and responsibilities should be limited. He should be taught the use of the therapeutic equipment found in the training room and should not be allowed to work on any athlete alone. He may be permitted to assist the upperclassmen on the staff in their routine work. If possible, have the student work out with the athletic trainer of a nearby college or university.

During his first year, the student may be enrolled in the Cramer's Student Trainer Course in Athletic Training given by Cramer Products, Inc. of Gardner, Kansas. This course is mailed to the student at his home address. The course will give him insight into simple treatment techniques of all kinds of athletic injuries. After an adequate instruction period, these student trainers will form a nucleus for a strong injury-prevention team.

A young man selected for the student trainer's staff should be one who is interested in sports, but who may not have the ability, desire, size, or other qualifications to participate in competitive sports. He should possess a congenial personality, a good sense of humor, good judgment, a good attitude, a willingness to learn and to work hard to improve himself, the team, and his school. Above all, he must be able to work cooperatively with his fellow student trainers under the supervision of the team physician and head coach.

The student trainers of today will be the certified trainers of tomorrow. With the extensive growth of athletics nationally, more administrators will become aware of the need for competent and qualified trainers. The following are suggestions for conduct of student trainers[*]:

1. Be the first man on the job and the last one to leave.
2. Keep the training room clean and neat but do not spend time housekeeping when there are players in need of attention.
3. Let the coach make and enforce rules. They are his responsibility.
4. Put supplies away before going home at night. Get them out in the morning after putting the room in order.
5. Find things to do in slack moments.
6. Prepare a "want list" of needed supplies; make this a daily practice. Bring the list to the attention of the coach, who will be responsible for ordering them if he feels they are necessary.
7. Always keep the first-aid kit properly packed for use.
8. Your hands are your most important tool; keep them clean. Keep your nails trimmed and clean at all times.
9. A special uniform is not necessary but neat dress is. Prove you are worthy of the respect of the squad, and you will get it.
10. Do not tell off-color stories or anecdotes that slander a man's race,

[*]Adapted from Athletic Training in the Seventies. Gardner, KA, Cramer Products, Inc., 1970.

religion, or culture. It is not only unprofessional but can lead to trouble.

11. When in doubt, ask the coach.
12. Always be loyal to the coach. When things get tough (as they often do), prove that you are a part of the team.
13. Plan trips with the coach and let him advise you on extra supplies that may be needed.
14. Do not get involved in local "quarterback club" discussions. Let the coach handle the news on player conditions and prospects.
15. Your job is to lessen the physical and mental load of the coach, and he will be surprised how well you can do it if you work at it properly.
16. Do not experiment with new methods until you have learned the merits and disadvantages of the old ones.
17. The only time you or anyone else can decide whether or not an injury is "minor" is after it has healed.
18. You may not have as good a training room as your neighbor, but do the best you can with what you have. Do not acquire the habit of being a complainer or grumbler.
19. Do not play favorites. Every star and scrub should rank equally in the training room unless the coach instructs you differently. (Today's scrub may be next year's star!)
20. Do not play practical jokes in the training room.
21. Close to 60% of your time will be spent preventing injury. Thoroughness will save time and pay large dividends.
22. During practice sessions or a game, pay particular attention to those athletes known to have some sort of injury and check every player at half-time or as occasion permits.
23. Do not be guilty of letting "a little knowledge become dangerous." The coach and team physician must be responsible for the athlete's welfare.
24. Use your ears and eyes to improve the efficiency of your hands. In other words, read and observe what other trainers and coaches are doing.

3

The Training Room

One of the most significant developments in the medical supervision of athletes has been the expansion of facilities in the training room. Once it was a room furnished sparely with a long treatment table, adhesive-tape wall rack and antiseptic solutions, distinguished by a pervasive odor of oil of wintergreen. Now it is replete with modern equipment and supplies, and in some instances rivals hospital emergency-room set-ups. Formerly, trainers massaged the athlete, did some taping, and rendered some crude (often questionable) first aid. Presently, the most scientific methods of conditioning, training, and emergency care are given by highly qualified trainers under the direct supervision of the team physician. The training room is usually the first medical facility to receive the injured or ill athlete. The physician, coach, trainer, and athlete should have an intense interest in this facility, which should be provided with the best equipment.

PLANNING A TRAINING ROOM

Location. Modern architectural designs for sports stadiums and buildings, high school and college gymnasiums make adequate provision for training and first-aid room facilities. This is exemplified by the Delmar Stadium, Houston, Independent School District, Texas (Fig. 3-1). The training-room area is an important component of the total architectural sports design, which also includes the playing area, squad locker room, shower and toilet facilities, and coaches' quarters. Unfortunately, most athletic areas currently in use were not designed to include training-room facilities, so the trainer must find appropriate space. Because he must start somewhere, the trainer modifies and rearranges the available space to suit his needs.

The following basic prerequisites may serve as a guide in locating a training room:

1. Convenient location, accessible to both outdoor and indoor playing areas (ground level).

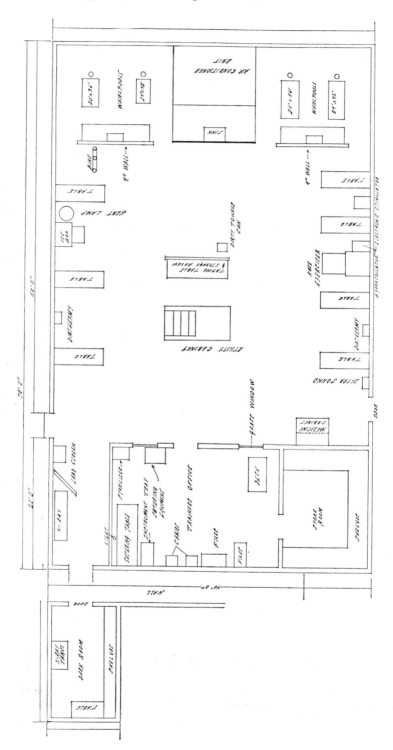

Fig. 3-1. Training room layout, Delmar Stadium.

2. Adjacent to but separate from the team dressing room.

3. Has facilities for central heating, hot and cold water, adequate lighting, electrical outlets,* and ventilation.

4. Allows the maintenance of scrupulous cleanliness.

5. Provides adequate storage space.

Determination of Size. The ideal training room allows 3 feet of working space around each piece of equipment. A minimal room size of 15 × 20 feet is recommended for high schools, although smaller rooms have proven adequate (*e.g.,* the training room at Columbus Senior High School, Columbus, Indiana, measures approximately 14 × 15 feet). Rooms measuring 20 × 22 feet or larger are recommended for colleges and universities. The following guidelines may be used in determining the size of the training room:

1. The number of athletes to be accommodated (one long treatment table is sufficient for 20 athletes).

2. The type and quantity of equipment and supplies that can be purchased or improvised within the existing budget.

Efficient Utilization of Space. Proper utilization of space for the equipment and supplies aids the trainer in rendering maximal service.

1. Place the training tables at the front of the training room; this discourages excessive traffic.

2. Locate the work tables and therapy equipment near electrical outlets.† Establish good overhead lighting (fluorescent).

3. Keep sensitive electrical instruments against the wall and away from the flow of traffic.

4. Equipment should not be located in drafty areas.

5. Locate the training room cabinets near the taping and treatment tables.

6. If the room is small, space can be conserved by hanging cabinets and shelves on the wall. Also, taping tables may be shorter than treatment tables.

7. Place the wash-up and whirlpool areas toward the back of the room, out of the way of normal traffic.

8. Keep whirlpool baths near wall outlets and drains.

EQUIPPING THE TRAINING ROOM

A training-room budget depends upon many factors, including the following:

1. Whether the team is amateur, semiprofessional, or professional.

2. Whether it is a high school, college, or university team.

    a. Geographic location.

---

*All electrical outlets in the training room must have ground-fault interrupters as required by code.

†Electrical equipment, especially hydrotherapy equipment, and wiring must be installed and checked by a competent electrician to prevent fatal accidents.

    b. Role of the Department of Athletics in the total educational
      program.
  3. The space, equipment, and supplies that are available.
  4. The quality of the coaching staff and the awareness of its members of the importance of the training room.

Obviously, the training room of a professional team with the most modern and sophisticated medical and physical therapy equipment and supplies will bear little resemblance to a training room set-up in a college or even a large university, because their budgets are thousands of dollars apart. Some high schools and colleges have to build and improvise part of their equipment. Other small schools might depend on donated equipment from neighboring and patronizing colleges and universities. Many high school teams have no training-room facilities.

Inasmuch as training-room set-ups vary with the size of the budget, only general guidelines can be stated. The most important allocation must be for a qualified trainer with an excellent pair of hands who is also knowledgeable in the techniques of physical therapy. Depending on the budget, the trainer must select the equipment and supplies that will enable him to render the best care to the athlete (Tables 3–1 to 3–4). The initial outlay required to establish a training room may be large, but much of the equipment purchased will have a long life expectancy. Later, most of the expense is incurred for expendable items, such as medications and supplies.

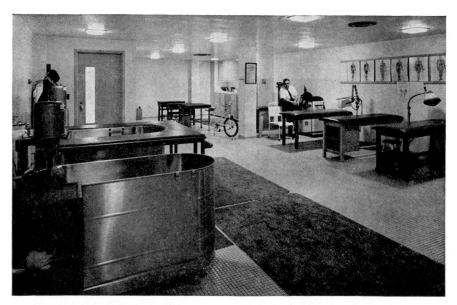

Fig. 3-2. A well planned and equipped training room. (Courtesy of the late Joe Abraham, Hobart College, Geneva, New York.)

Table 3-1.   Suggested Training Room Equipment

Autoclave, small
Basins, hand, stainless steel
Baths
    Paraffin unit
    Whirlpool, large, stationary
    Whirlpool, small, portable
Bench, waiting
Bulletin board
Cabinets
    File
    Metal, with sink
    Wood, for overhead placement
Chairs
Cutters, for adhesive tape
Desk
Exercise equipment
    Bike (isotonic)
    Quadriceps boot w/50 lbs of weights (isotonic)
    Progressive resistive and assistive exercise unit (isokinetic)
Hot pack unit, portable (e.g., Hydrocollator)
Ice machine
Lamps
    Gooseneck
    Infrared heat lamp, caster base
    Spotlight, battery-operated
Oxygen tank and face mask, portable
Refrigerator with a freezer compartment, 10 cu ft
Rotary wrist machine
Scale, beam type
Scissors, bandage
Shoulder wheel, adjustable height
Sink
Spine board
Stretcher, folding
Tables
    Dressing, stainless steel with casters
    Taping, short
    Treatment, long
Wall rack, for adhesive tape
Wall shelves
Waste can, covered, enamel

Each training room must have a treatment table, physical-therapy equipment for heat applications, and a first-aid dressing cart on casters that contains sufficient instruments, medications, and dressing supplies to provide a sterile dressing for an injured part. A refrigerator with a freezer compartment for biologic supplies and ice cubes and a file cabinet are necessary.

The treatment table is the most important piece of training room equipment because it can be used for a variety of purposes. This table may be used for examining, treating, taping, and massaging athletes.

Table 3-2.   Suggested Instruments for Training Room

Clippers, electric
Forceps, for splinters
Hemostat
Medicine droppers
Needles, disposable syringe, 20, 22, 25 gauge, short and medium
Oral screw
Probe, metal
Scalpel, handle and blades
Scissors, bandage
Syringes
    Asepto, bulb, disposable, 2 oz
    Hypodermic, disposable, 2½, 5, 10 ml
    Ear
Thermometers, oral and rectal
Tweezers

The athlete may use this table himself to exercise joints and muscles, as well as for resting from the day's activities. Because of its multipurpose functions and its reasonable price, the treatment table should be the first piece of equipment installed in the training room. One long table per 20 athletes is sufficient. The dimensions recommended for a table are 78 inches long, 24 inches wide, and 30 inches high; however, individual trainers may prefer other sizes. It is wise to get a table with which the trainer is familiar and with which he functions best. When the budget is increased, additional, shorter-sized tables may be installed primarily for taping.

The ability of heat to improve circulation and aid resorption of swelling, induration and relief of pain in traumatized soft tissues of the musculoskeletal system by increasing tissue metabolism is well-documented. This modality is enhanced when local swelling is first minimized by compression dressings, ice packs, and elevation of the injured part when feasible. Therapeutic heat for training room purposes may be produced by various types of apparatuses (see pp. 34–38). In each instance, the attending physician prescribes the type and amount of heat therapy to be used.

Infrared and microwave units are not recommended for training room use. There is no proof that these apparatuses produce any better results than other forms of heat therapy. The proper application of these devices demands the experience and knowledge of a trainer skilled in their use and the ease with which they may be self-administered makes them, in our opinion, undesirable in a training room. Ultrasound units should not be placed in a training room unless the trainer is thoroughly qualified and experienced in the use of such machines. Ultrasound therapy must never be self-administered by an athlete.

A whirlpool bath is an excellent therapeutic device that also affords psychologic benefits in the treatment of an injured athlete. If funds are available, a large whirlpool bath should be purchased, to enable treatment of several athletes at one time. If there is no monetary provision for a whirlpool bath, substitutes can be improvised (see p. 37).

From the athletes' point of view, the ultimate in training-rom facilities is the sauna bath. This is quite popular but is found mainly at the collegiate and professional levels. The trainer also has available other therapeutic modalities outside the training room but within the school environs that can be used effectively to rehabilitate the injured athlete. For instance, a swimming pool is excellent for providing exercises by eliminating the effects of gravity. Gymnastic equipment, such as stall bars, are useful for stretching. The presence of a nearby weight room with free barbells, isotonic and isokinetic equipment can be used to increase the strength, power, and endurance of an injured part as well as noninjured parts of the body. This equipment is equally useful in reaching and maintaining condition.

When a budget is particularly limited, donations of training-room equipment and supplies should be actively solicited. Potential contributors of such items include doctors, hospitals, pharmaceutical houses, and manufacturers of physical-therapy equipment. As soon as the budget is expanded, we recommend purchasing new equipment to replace second-hand items. Some items, particularly storage units, work tables, benches, and stools, may be built in school or home workshops, allowing considerable savings. Also, government surplus materials may be bought at discount. Access to complicated and expensive equipment often results in the fitting of the athlete to the equipment, rather than vice versa.

More modern and sophisticated equipment and supplies should be purchased as the demand arises and the budget allows. However, high-school training rooms have no need for expensive paraffin bath units,

Table 3-3.   Suggested Training Room Supplies

Adhesive tape
  Elastic, 3″, 4″ × 5 yds
  Elastic tape, 1″, 2″, 3″, 4″ × 5 yds
  For sensitive skin
  Standard, 1″, 2″, 3″ × 5 yds; 1½″ × 15 yds
Adhesive tape remover
Alcohol
  Rubbing, 70%
  Swabs, packaged
Antiseptic solutions and sprays
Applicators, cotton-tipped, sterile
Aromatic ammonia, breakable ampules
Aspirin, 5 gr tablets

Table 3-3.   Suggested Training Room Supplies (Continued)

Bandages
 Elastic, 2½″, 3″, 4″, 6″
 Gauze, self-adhering (Kling), 2″, 3″, 4″
 Plaster of Paris, 3″, 4″, 5″, 6″
 Roll, ready-cut
Band-Aids
 Assorted, patch, spot, and strips ¾″ × 3″, 1″ × 3″
 Butterfly closures, medium and large
Cold packs, chemical or ice cubes
Collodion
Combination roll, cotton and gauze
Cotton
 Absorbent, sterile and nonsterile
 Balls, sterile
Counterirritant salves
Cups
 Medicine
 Paper
Deodorant spray
Detergent
Disinfectant
Envelopes, for pills
Ethyl chloride spray
Fungicidal liquids and powders
Gauze pads
 Sterile, 2″ × 2″, 3″ × 3″, 4″ ×3″
 Sterile, nonadherent (Telfa)
Hot water bottle
Hydrogen peroxide
Ice bag
Jars, medicine
Massage lotion
Mouthpieces
Petrolatum
Petrolatum gauze dressing
Safety pins
Sheets
 Felt, 6″ × 12″ × ¼″
 Foam rubber, 6″ × 12″ × ¼″
Skin adherent spray
Skin lubricant
Slings, triangular
Soap, antiseptic liquid (tincture green soap, pHisoHex, etc.)
Sodium bicarbonate tablets, 5 gr
Sodium chloride tablets, 10, 15½ gr
Splints
 Air
 Wooden
Stockinette, orthopedic (may also be used beneath adhesive tape
  for sensitive skin)
Strawberry ointment
Talcum powder
Tincture benzoin compound
Tongue blades
Vitamin C tablets

Table 3-4. Suggested Contents of Trainer's Kit*

Item	Amount
Adhesive tape, 2″ × 5 yds; 1½″ × 15 yds	6 rolls
Elastic tape 2″ × 5 yds	6 rolls
Adrenalin chloride, 1:1,000 (for topical application)	1 fl oz
Applicators, cotton-tipped	1 doz
Aromatic ammonia, breakable ampules	10
Aspirin tablets, 5 gr	100
Bandages	
Elastic, 6″ × 5 yds	1
Elastic, 3″ × 5 yds	3
Gauze, 1″, 3″ × 10 yds	6
Gauze, self-adhering, 2″, 3″ × 10 yds	6
Triangular, with safety pins	1
Band-Aids	
Assorted strip, patch and spot	1 box
Butterfly closures, medium and large	1 doz
Cold packs, chemical, instantaneous	3
Collodion	1 oz
Cutters	
Nail	1
Tape	1
Envelopes, for pills	
Ethyl chloride spray	1 can
Gauze pads, sterile, packaged, 2″ × 2″, 3″ × 3″, 4″ × 3″	1 doz
Liniment, heating (oil of wintergreen, etc.)	4 oz
Medicine droppers	2
Merthiolate spray, aerosol	6 oz
Nasal spray	1 bottle
Oral screw	1
Rosin, powdered, in can	6 oz
Scissors, bandage	1
Sheets, foam rubber, 6″ × 12″ × ¼″	6
Smelling salts	1 oz
Sodium bicarbonate tablets, 5 gr	100
Sodium chloride tablets, 10, 15½ gr	100
Strawberry ointment	2 oz
Thermometer, oral in protective case	1
Tincture benzoin compound	4 oz
Tongue depressors	1 doz
Tweezers	1

*When possible, use plastic containers instead of glass.

electrical muscle stimulators, or progressive resistive exercise units. Moreover, the experience, training, and qualifications of the trainer bear a direct relationship to the type and amount of equipment ordered and used in the training room. A trainer must beg, borrow, build, and improvise to make his work area the most complete, efficient, and inviting place for the conditioning and training of athletes. The success or failure of a training room is mainly the trainer's responsibility.

Each trainer must carry a trainer's kit at all practice sessions and scheduled contests. This kit should contain sufficient training-room equipment, medication, and supplies to enable him to cope with emergency situations that may occur with athletes in competition. It must be inclusive, practical, yet not bulky (Table 3-4). Each coach and trainer may have favorite supplies, especially for such sports as gymnastics, wrestling, boxing, and swimming.

RATIONALE AND USE OF THERMOTHERAPY EQUIPMENT IN THE TRAINING ROOM

Thermotherapy equipment being considered for purchase for use in a training room should satisfy many of the following prerequisites:
1. Relieves pain.
2. Stimulates circulation.
3. Relaxes muscle spasm.
4. Helps soften adhesions.
5. Aids absorption of waste products.
6. Offers some psychologic benefit in its application.
7. Its projected use warrants the expenditure.

Hydrotherapy. Hydrotherapy has become the most popular and effective modality in the treatment of clinical conditions encountered in athletes. Hydrotherapy techniques may range from the simple application of a warm, moist towel for a contusion to a sauna bath for

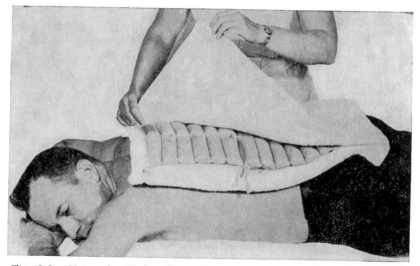

Fig. 3-3. Using the Hydrocollator Steam Pack for moist-heat therapy. The pack is wrapped in a heavy Turkish towel to avoid injuring the skin. (Courtesy of Chattanooga Corporation, Chattanooga, Tennessee.)

generalized muscle soreness. Other forms of hydrotherapy include immersion baths, with water temperatures ranging from lukewarm to hot, sitz baths, contrast baths, salt glows, steam cabinets, whirlpool baths, and hot packs.

Hot Packs. Every training room should have moist heat-pack equipment (Hydrocollator), because it is the simplest and most economical way to apply moist heat for the relief of pain and muscle spasm. The packs are contoured to fit different parts of the body and are especially good for necks, shoulders, backs, and the musculature of the arms and legs. Wrapping the hot pack in a heavy Turkish towel before applying it diminishes the risk of injuring the skin. The heat penetrates 3 cm, compared to the 0.1 cm penetration of infrared heat. A 20- to 30-minute treatment is sufficient; the steam packs maintain effective heat for at least 30 minutes. A master unit with an 8- or 12-pack capacity is a real time-saver because it allows a trainer to handle several athletes at one time. After 10 minutes, the trainer must check the skin to avoid burns.

Whirlpool Bath. The whirlpool bath is a popular piece of equipment for giving hydrotherapy, and is probably the apparatus most familiar to athletes. Training room scenes in books and newspapers invariably include the whirlpool bath. Most athletes consider a whirlpool bath a necessary part of a well-equipped training room. A whirlpool bath should definitely be purchased if funds are available; otherwise, the trainer can use substitute methods to accomplish similar results (see p. 38). After the initial investment, the cost of the operation is low.

Benefits of Whirlpool. The whirling water has the effect of gentle massage, which helps reduce swelling, relieves pain, and relaxes muscles. Tissues become soft and pliable and joints move with less difficulty. The whirlpool action provides certain psychologic benefits: it is a type of therapy that may be seen, heard, and felt by the athlete, and it has a sedative, comforting, soothing effect.

As with any form of physical therapy, the treatment of specific conditions with the whirlpool must be prescribed by the physician. The use of warm water in the whirlpool stimulates circulation through the dilatation of superficial blood vessels (range of heat between 99° to 112° F). The average water temperature is best held between 101° to 105° F for 30 minutes. A warm whirlpool stimulates phagocytosis and helps to reduce inflammation. It usually reduces pain, relaxes certain muscle spasm due to trauma, and aids absorption of waste products. It is also an excellent debriding agent for open wounds. Mobility of a limb is increased as a result of decreased swelling and pain. Cold water constricts superficial blood vessels. It may be used in the whirlpool to reduce swelling in acute sprains, but other methods exist (Table 3-5).

Table 3-5.   Whirlpool Bath Treatment

	New Injury		Old Injury	
	Time	*Temp.*	*Time*	*Temp.*
Hands, Feet, Elbows	*Without Swelling*		*Without Swelling*	
	Up to 30 min	Less than 100° F	Up to 45 min	Up to 110° F
Legs, Arms	*Without Swelling*		*Without Swelling*	
	12 min	100° F	30 min	110° F
Hips, Pelvis	*Without Swelling*		*Without Swelling*	
	15–18 min	95°–100° F	30 min	Up to 105° F
Full Submersion	*Without Swelling*		*Without Swelling*	
	20 min	Up to 103° F	20–30 min	Up to 103° F

NOTE: In old injuries, to utilize the whirlpool bath to its best advantage, start with a mild temperature and build the heat level upward to the athlete's tolerance.

The following conditions may be treated by the whirlpool method in the training room when prescribed by the attending physician:

1. Adhesions.
2. Ankle swelling.
3. Arthritis.
4. Before applying electrical treatments.
5. Bone bruises.
6. Bromidrosis (odorous feet).
7. Burns (healed or healing).
8. Bursitis.
9. Circulatory disturbances (peripheral)—water temperature usually should not be higher than 99° to 100° F (around body temperature).
10. Cleansing wounds, lacerations, etc.
11. Contusions.
12. Hyperhidrosis (excessive sweating).
13. Myalgia.
14. Periostitis.
15. Postfracture care.
16. Postoperative care.
17. Scars.
18. Sprains.
19. Strains.
20. Tenosynovitis.

The whirlpool is an efficient form of therapy. It saves treatment time and prepares muscles and joints for massage and manipulation. Moreover, it is easily applied and handled by someone trained in its use, and the temperature and duration of treatment may be regulated at will. Depending on the model, it may be a mobile unit and have a self-emptying tank.

Prevention of Adverse Effects. A few adverse effects may occur with the use of a whirlpool bath. A dirty tank becomes a carrier of disease; several cases of dermatitis and spread of infection have been reported. Occasionally, a person may faint if the water is too warm. If a person with an acute condition is unwisely treated too long in hot water, with too much agitation, and a high temperature, his ailment may become worse. Transient swelling may occur.

To keep the tank clean, add Betadine, according to manufacturer's direction, to each tank of water. When the tank is drained, spray the inside of the tank, rim, and seat with an aerosol germicide. Do not depend on the heat of the water to kill bacteria. Athletes should be instructed to use the whirlpool only after they have thoroughly showered with soap. Persons known to have a skin infection should not be allowed to use the whirpool unless they use it alone and the water is drained and the tank disinfected afterwards. Frequent use of the whirlpool dictates frequent draining and disinfecting; used water should not be allowed to stand overnight.

If the water is hard, a detergent may be added, but one should check with the athletes for possible allergies to such chemicals.

Tips From the Trainer's Table

1. Keep the hydrotherapeutic equipment grounded by running a ground wire from the chassis to a nearby faucet. Use an alligator nose on the wire, which is easy to remove and hook up.

2. Use hydrotherapy to prepare for massage, and range-of-motion exercises. The whirlpool bath can be quite soothing to the athlete.

Substitute Methods for Whirlpool Bath

1. Epsom Salt Soak: Use an empty bucket of 2 to 5 gallon capacity. Dissolve 2 tumblerfuls or 4 cups of Epsom salts to a gallon of hot water from the faucet and soak the following injured parts: ankle, foot, toe, calf of leg, hand, finger, wrist, forearm, elbow.

2. Shower: A hose attached to a shower connection can direct warm water on an injured part, wrapped in a towel, to accomplish the same purpose as a whirlpool. Adjust the noozle so that there is a forceful direct spray on the following injured parts: shoulder, neck, back, knee, thigh, hip, arm, ribs, groin muscles.

There are many forms of hydrotherapy. The type to use depends mainly on the attending physician's prescription and the training, experience, and ingenuity of the trainer.

MASSAGE

Massage is an ancient and well-documented therapeutic modality useful for the treatment of athletic injuries and as part of a preliminary warm-up for an athlete prior to competition. In his book, How Ancient Healing Governs Modern Therapeutics (New York, G. P. Putnam's Sons, 1937), Kleanthos A. Ligeros, a physician from Athens, Greece, states the following: "Naturally, such practices as laying one's hands over the patient's head and manipulating his forehead for relief of headaches or other pain or massaging the spine or the entire body and thus relieving the sufferer of his affliction have been known to man from remote times. All ancient records point straight to the fact that these methods were instinctively practiced in the stone age and have been transmitted and transplanted by man everywhere." Dr. Allan Ryan, Editor-in-Chief of the Journal of the Physician and Sportsmedicine, bemoans the fact that massage, one of the oldest and time-proven methods of treatment, is being neglected by the modern trainer-therapist. He further emphasizes the fact that massage is an excellent warm-up exercise modality prior to athletic competition that is not practiced by most athletes. He further states that, in American athletics, the masseur has been given a back seat, unlike the masseur in European athletics. He recommends that the practitioner of the art of massage be given a specialty rating within the framework of the training profession.

Massage can be beneficial for many of the soft-tissue and joint injuries suffered in athletics. This includes sprains, strains, contusions, as well as other injuries. Massage is used to assist in removing edema and facilitates recovery after the initial inflammatory reaction due to the athletic trauma has subsided. In clinical conditions in which there is muscle spasm or painful muscular contractions due to prolonged tension, strenuous exercises, or immobilization, deep-stroking or kneading massage are useful in relaxing muscle spasm and in relieving discomfort by increasing the athlete's pain threshold. In regard to adhesions and scars, friction massage is often used in combination with stretching to help free the tissues and gain mobility. In giving massage for adhesions, it should be remembered that only the thumbs massage over the adhesions or scar tissue, gently giving friction massage in the hopes of lessening the scar without any lubricant.

Massage should be used along with other forms of treatment as soon as bruising and swelling have ceased; this may take 24 to 72 hours postinjury depending on the severity of the trauma. Massage is only one part of the total treatment and does not replace other modalities, such as immobilization, cryotherapy, heat, and exercise. Massage and therapeutic exercises are also used following cast or dressing removal for dislocations, fractures, and operations. Following the massage, the injured limb should be elevated for 10 to 15 minutes to encourage further drainage of the injured part using the force of gravity. Isometrics of the muscles of the elevated limb further encourage drainage, which results in reduction of the swelling as well as improved muscle strength. Range-of-motion exercises of the surrounding joints lessen the potential for adhesions and assist the total rehabilitation of the injured athlete. Massage is indicated when the following are sought:

1. Relief of pain.
2. Improvement of circulation.
3. Improvement of circulation of the skin and underlying soft tissues.
4. Accelerated removal of waste end products.
5. Dissolution of adhesions.
6. Reduction of swelling and induration of tissues.
7. Loosening and stretching of contracted tendons,
8. Soothing of the central nervous system and peripheral nerves.

J. Cyriax, in his classical textbook, Massage, Manipulation and Local Anaesthesia (London, England, 1941) lists the following principles governing massage of striated muscles:

1. Massage the area causing pain.
2. The fingers of the masseur and the skin of the athlete must move as a single unit.
3. The hand must move longitudinally to the long axis of the affected structure.
4. Massage must be forceful enough to reach the deepest fibers of the muscle.
5. Prewarming the area with moist heat softens tissues and assures deep penetration with less force.
6. Use of a skin lubricant prior to massaging is helpful except when friction massage is used.
7. All stroking in massage must be rhythmic and relaxing to the athlete; the masseur should move his hands towards the heart to encourage the return flow of the venous circulation without causing pain to the athlete.

Contraindications to massage are the following:

1. Inflammations due to bacterial action (obviously the infection may become disseminated).

2. Skin eruptions, infections, abrasions, and varicose veins.
3. Calcifications of soft structures such as the quadriceps muscle, medial collateral ligament of the knee, and others.
4. Rheumatoid or gouty arthritis.
5. Traumatic arthritis of the elbow.
6. Acute bursitis.
7. Pressure on nerve as in a carpal tunnel syndrome.
8. Phlebitis and cellulitis.

Effleurage

Effleurage, or stroking, is accomplished by passing the hands slowly, gently, and rhythmically over a portion of the athlete's skin. This is a superficial type of massage usually affecting the subcutaneous level. It is the type of massage most frequently used for athletes. It is usually performed with the palm of the hand. To obtain maximal benefits from superficial effleurage, the movement of the hands must be deeper centripetally. The movement is slow, rhythmic, continuous, and in the same tempo, with the hands always remaining in contact with the athlete. Approximately 15 strokes per minute is the usual rate. The movement must be gentle because this is essential in obtaining the desired effect.

Petrissage

This is a kneading and/or compression type of technique. The tissues are picked or lifted off the bones by the thumb and fingers and kneaded, compressed, or wrung. This type of massage assists arterial and venous circulation and accelerates lymphatic flow and hastens the removal of waste products from the muscle. This technique also stretches retracted muscles and tendons and assists in breaking adhesions. One or both hands may be employed. In addition to improving circulation it is frequently used to relieve muscle spasm.

Friction

Friction massage is a deep, circular, rolling movement employed around bony prominences or joints. It is used in loosening adhesions and promoting absorption of exudate. Friction massage may also be useful in lessening scar tissue. The fingers of the trainer-therapist remain on one point of the skin, and the skin is rolled over the underlying tissue. This movement tends to loosen superficial scars and adhesions. Most of the motion is carried out with the thumbs over the treated area. Friction movements are usually followed by effleurage.

Tapotement

This type of massage is not recommended for athletes. It consists of sudden, blow-like contacts by the ulnar side of the hands to the patient, such as in clapping, hacking, and cupping. It is used to encourage drainage from lungs with patients afflicted with bronchitis, emphysema, and chronic pulmonary disorders. There are potential, harmful effects with its use.

Vibration

This type of massage is also not recommended for athletes. It is an inward, trembling pressure exerted by the hands and fingers to any part of the body to stimulate nerve activity.

THERAPEUTIC COLD

The use of ice (cryotherapy) has been used as an immediate therapeutic agent for many years, principally for arresting and reducing swelling. It can also be used to interrupt the pain-spasm cycle, which is present in a wide variety of injuries to the neck, shoulders, or lower back. The changes observed in the muscle during ice therapy are the firm hardness at the onset and jelly-like consistency at the end of the treatment. The local application of cold decreases neural activity locally and studies have shown that cold raises the threshold stimulus of the muscle spindles, thereby greatly enhancing the relaxation of muscle spasms. Along with the visible relaxation, ice produces a mild anesthetic effect on the area being treated. This effect provides the athlete with the opportunity to perform exercises with a minimal amount of pain and if the exercises are too strenuous or cause more damage to the injury, enough pain will be exhibited by the athlete that the limits will be known.

Physiologic Effects:
1. Superficial anesthetic effect.
2. There is a depressing effect on the stretch reflex allowing the muscle-spindle threshold to rise. This decreases the spasticity that usually accompanies injury, and that then causes some loss of range of motion in the area.
3. Initial vasoconstriction, then secondary vasodilation, which may last from 30 minutes to an hour (with heat application, there is a return to normal in 10 to 15 minutes; cold penetrates deeper than heat).

For muscle injuries, cold facilitates increased blood flow via two mechanisms: by cold vasodilation and by allowing use of the injured muscle by light exercise (which may increase body metabolism by 300%). These two processes have a greater effect on increasing muscle blood flow than heat has, and they allow the athlete to perform exercises with less pain.

ULTRASOUND

Ultrasound is the deepest form of heat currently available for therapeutic use. Ultrasound waves are of the same nature as sound waves but have such a high frequency (in excess of 20,000 cycles per second) that they are inaudible. After experimental work, it was found that waves 700,000 to 1 million cycles per second were desirable for therapeutic application. The electrical energy produced by the generator is converted into mechanical vibrations by means of a quartz crystal. The mechanical vibrations produced by the ultrasound must be propagated through a coupling agent between the transducer head and the patient's skin in the form of an oil, cream, or water. The mechanical vibrations produce a liberation of heat in the body tissues, which is greatest at interfaces between heterogeneous tissues, such as bone and muscle or muscle and tendon. There also seems to be selective heating of bones, joints, tendons, and nerves.

Though the thermal effects of ultrasound account for the majority of its use, there are mechanical, chemical, and biologic effects that add to the versatility of the apparatus.

Clinically, ultrasound produces a mechanical effect of dispersion and agitation of the deep cellular tissues, which may be referred to as the micro-massaging effect. In addition, electron microscopy studies have shown ultrasonics capable of separating collagen fibers from each other.

Certain effects of ultrasonic energy can be considered chemical, such as acceleration of enzyme activity and the increase in cell-membrane permeability.

Studies on tendon extensibility have been conducted revealing that ultrasonic energy can produce changes in frog tendon that make for greater extensibility; thermal denaturation of proteins of the tendon is offered as a possible explanation. Ample evidence exists to demonstrate that ultrasound affects the nervous system, including the autonomic portion, which produces a vasomotor response.

Indications

Generally speaking, ultrasound seems to have proven successful in the treatment of neuromuscular and musculoskeletal diseases including:
1. Periarthritis, myositis.
2. Adhesive capsulitis and other joint constrictions.
3. Arthritic conditions.
4. Inflamed joints to reduce swelling.
5. Bursitis.
6. Neuromas.
7. In cases of joint limitation due to scar formation.

8. Sprains, strains, contusions, plantar warts, and various other conditions.

Ultrasound is contraindicated in the following areas:

1. Epiphysis of growing bones.
2. Reproductive organs.
3. Pregnant uterus.
4. Heart.
5. Anesthetic areas.
6. Eye.
7. Directly over spinal cord.

BIBLIOGRAPHY

Balakian, G., et al.: So your patient wants a sports doctor. Patient Care, 10–20: 90–107, 1976.

4

Equipment and the Equipment Room*

The equipment to be purchased for an athletic department and the elaborateness of the equipment room depend in great measure on the available funds and vary from school to school. Most schools finance athletic expenditures from gate receipts, funds appropriated from the general budget, and donations. The percentage of funds from each source depends upon the individual school's fiscal set-up. It is obviously important, especially when the school is small, that each dollar be expended wisely.

SOME SUGGESTIONS ON BUDGETING

The athletic budget, as a rule, is broken down into individual sports and is estimated by each coach for the sport he sponsors. The estimate should be accurate and carefully itemized and should cover operations for an entire year. The coach who continually requests additional funds because he has budgeted improperly will soon lose the faith of the school administration.

Inventory guides are useful in estimating the new equipment necessary. The coach and athletic director should thoroughly familiarize themselves with new equipment and its costs and may find it advisable to enlist the aid of the school purchasing manager. The budget may be drafted by the athletic director or, in small schools, the head coach. Before it is submitted to the chief school administrator, it should be thoroughly discussed with the full coaching staff, the school principal, and the school business manager.

An accurate account should be kept of all financial transactions involving athletics, such as scouting, publicity, transportation, new equipment, laundry and dry cleaning, medical expenses, insurance, guarantees, awards, and repairs. The record, if kept properly, serves as a basis for estimating the needs of the following year. Some provisions

*Adapted in part from Athletic Goods Manufacturers Association: How to Budget, Select and Order Athletic Equipment. Chicago, Ill.

should be made in the budget for unforeseen contingencies, but it must never be "padded." There may be reasons for cutting the budget, but a charge of padding should not be one of them. Purchases of athletic equipment should be made as soon as possible after the budget has been approved and funds made available.

An accurate record should also be kept of all athletic receipts, including gate receipts, donations, and advertising revenue. This information helps to determine what portion of the budget for the coming year must be financed from the school's general fund (if one is available).

SELECTION OF EQUIPMENT

The selection of equipment is a problem that plagues almost every beginning coach and many a seasoned coach, as well. However, it usually becomes easier with experience. Every person devises his own formula for selecting equipment, but in general, there are six basic categories for a buyer to keep in mind when he goes shopping: (1) design and material; (2) utility and cost of maintenance; (3) safety factors in protective equipment; (4) quality and workmanship; (5) source of supply; (6) price. An effective selection of equipment rests upon the individual buyer's talent to analyze correctly these six "measuring sticks for sound purchasing." Most coaches admit readily that they are not experts in all categories and that they must rely heavily upon the advice of salesmen or manufacturers to guide them. The following "selection tips" may prove helpful.

Design and Material. The design of equipment and the material used in the product go hand-in-hand. Design must be practical and the material must be thoroughly serviceable. One should be skeptical of a dressed-up item in which basic design and utility may be sacrificed for eye appeal. Extras and frills often serve no functional purpose. Most experienced coaches agree that, without technical assistance and considerable experience, the material standard is the most difficult aspect to analyze. The coach who wants additional counsel on materials, other than that of the manufacturer, should consult the dealer or salesman for assistance. Naturally the experiences of other coaches can be helpful as well.

Many of the basic materials used in the manufacture of athletic equipment are readily judged, but, it is the buyer's knowledge, based upon experience and in-use field testing, that assures an intelligent evaluation of the product. The coach should never be reluctant to test new products. Many coaches prefer to buy or try new items in a limited way, possibly during spring practice or during the training period. If it does not meet his needs, the coach can give his reasons to the dealer.

Utility and Cost of Maintenance. Utility is an important consideration in purchasing equipment. Not only should it meet game and safety standards, but be of such quality and construction that it is easily and economically maintained. In other words, equipment should be practical and playable.

When considering the utility and cost of maintaining a new piece of equipment, be sure to check the following: (1) Are there frills on the equipment that will make it difficult to maintain? (2) Will the equipment clean easily and well? (3) Must the equipment be repaired and reconditioned after normal use? (4) Is the cost of maintaining the equipment too great for effective use?

Safety Factors in Protective Equipment. In buying protective equipment, a coach's first consideration must be the safety of the wearer, which should be maximal. Through careful selection of equipment with the assistance of the salesman, the coach can be assured that he is buying the safest possible gear.

Quality and Workmanship. In athletic equipment, quality has no substitute. The buyer should look for consistent quality in a manufacturer's line of products, no matter what the material.

Workmanship is an equally important feature. Superb design and good material do not constitute quality if the item is not expertly manufactured. By purchasing a single item first, before ordering large quantities, a coach can compare that item with his present equipment. Results thus obtained supplement the research efforts and opinions of manufacturer's representatives and other coaches.

Source of Supply. A coach can come to recognize reputable dealers through experience and seeking the advice of others. Reputable dealers show samples upon request and offer a large variety of items from which to choose. They also service the account, thus ensuring complete satisfaction with the product.

Price. High price does not necessarily indicate high quality, but, in general, the athletic equipment of finest quality is the most expensive. Side-by-side comparison usually reveals the difference between a low-priced item and a higher priced one. A careful analysis of the construction, design, quality, and utility of a product provides a basis for evaluating its cost.

Never sacrifice quality for price. Although not expected to be a manufacturing expert, the coach is expected to spend athletic funds wisely and equip his team with safe, well-constructed equipment. Good equipment costs a little more, but it pays dividends in the long run. Never take a chance with untested, low-cost equipment.

HOW TO ORDER ATHLETIC EQUIPMENT

The ordering and purchasing of athletic equipment should be a systematic procedure. The use of purchase forms saves time and avoids problems, and copies give an exact record of the quantity, description, and date of items ordered. No matter who actually purchases equipment, the same general buying procedure should be followed:

1. Someone is appointed to determine what is to be purchased. Usually, this is the coach of the individual sport concerned. He makes recommendations based upon a report of an inventory of equipment on hand.

2. After deciding what is to be purchased, he passes the order on to the one who is to place it.

3. The purchase order should always have proper approval of the chief school administrator.

4. The order is then placed with the dealer, and a duplicate copy is given to the coach. If a duplicate copy is *not* given to the coach, he should request some type of memorandum to keep in his files. This assures him that the equipment has actually been ordered and indicates when.

5. The invoice is received either prior to, with, or after the shipment of goods. It should be examined, approved, and sent to the paying official.

6. The goods, when received, should be examined and approved as to the quantity and the quality ordered. After the coach or buyer is satisfied that the goods are in order, they should be placed in the current inventory.

Athletic equipment must be ordered as early as possible. Frequently, coaches do not allot time for this important function far enough in advance, and then they unjustly blame the manufacturers for late deliveries, when actually they have placed the order too late.

CARE AND MAINTENANCE OF ATHLETIC EQUIPMENT

There are ten basic principles for good maintenance of athletic equipment:

1. The head coach is directly responsible for proper maintenance.

2. The equipment manager must have a clear understanding of his duties and responsibilities to the coach.

3. Draw-up a definite policy for the care of all equipment.

4. Instruct players in the rules of care.

5. Keep an accurate record of all equipment, including its condition, size, and age.

6. Mark all equipment with size, identification number, and date of issuance for service.

7. Draw up a definite policy for the issuance, use, and return of all equipment.

8. Correctly clean equipment and launder, if possible, after every

game. Practice equipment should be cleaned every 2 or 3 days. Air-dry equipment after use.

9. Store, repair, and maintain equipment according to manufacturer's directions.

10. Determine and utilize proper methods of off-season storage.

Properly interpreted, "the care of athletic equipment" encompasses the time from when an item is first unpacked to the time it is destroyed. This involves all personnel who handle the equipment, including coach, manager, trainer, athlete, and cleaning and repair personnel.

FITTING THE HELMET

The helmet should fit tightly and there should be no motion of the helmet on the head with the hair either dry or wet. The front edge of the helmet should be one finger breadth above the orbital ridge, and its posterior edge should rest on the occiput. The lateral hole of the helmet should be directly opposite the external auditory canal. The chin strap should be centered, and the athlete admonished about the practice of playing without his chin strap in place.

If one is using a suspension helmet, the crown cord should be tight —that is, the helmet should not be able to be depressed when the chin strap is in place.

Those teams using the so-called "water helmet" should follow this inflation sequence:

1. Crown.
2. Front.
3. Back.
4. Neck.
5. Sides.

Any helmet of the air-inflatable type (for example, Bike) should be checked daily for correct amount of air by the athlete and advisory personnel.

It is advisable that a neck roll be used to limit neck extension and that a double roll be placed on the lateral aspect to limit lateral flexion. The use of a full face mask should be encouraged by all parties to limit forward flexion.

If these criteria are followed closely and if a mouth guard (which is mandatory) is used, the incidence of head injury will be significantly reduced.

THE EQUIPMENT ROOM

A good equipment room is essential to the proper care of athletic equipment. A sloppy, carelessly-kept room can be harder on athletic equipment than many hours of service on the field.

The size of the room depends largely upon the number of sports and athletes to be serviced. It should be large enough to store adequately all the equipment, with room for handling and repair. Above all, the room should be dry, free from sweaty walls and pipes, and well ventilated. An ideal location would be away from the shower room but close to the locker and training rooms. Both natural and fluorescent lighting are desirable, and the temperature should range around 70 to 72° F. Safeguards against moths, roaches, and rodents are essential.

Nothing should be stored on the floor. Racks must be available for hanging equipment up to dry. There should be large shelves for cartons and bulky articles, and narrow shelves for shoes and smaller articles.

THE EQUIPMENT MANAGER

An important position on the athletic staff is that of the equipment manager in charge of equipment. It is recommended that this individual be an adult faculty member with student assistants. The equipment manager should possess the knowledge and experience necessary to perform responsibilities properly.

He has the responsibility of outfitting all athletes, and in some schools he is in charge of all equipment used in the health and physical education classes. It is important that accurate records of all equipment be kept, and generally speaking, an adult is more qualified in this respect. The equipment manager should inform the athletic director and the head coach of each sport of the condition of the equipment at various intervals.

Suggested Duties and Responsibilities of the Equipment Manager.

1. Have equipment ready to issue 2 days before the first day of practice.

2. Assist the head coach in supervising student managers.

3. Prepare equipment cards at time of issuance and assign lockers.

4. Collect laundry and issue clean equipment weekly, or more often, if necessary.

5. Fit and issue game uniforms.

6. Wash and dry equipment, as soon as possible after it has been soiled.

7. Make changes in faulty or improperly fitting equipment.

8. Send out dry cleaning when necessary. Check and sort the dry cleaning when it is returned.

9. Check and collect all equipment at the end of each sports season. Prepare equipment for shipment to a reconditioning company or to storage.

10. Report stolen or misplaced equipment to the head coach.

11. Stress that the reissuing of equipment will be based upon the return of previously issued equipment.

12. Assist the coach in determining equipment needs for next season.

13. Check in all equipment that is ordered and report immediately all discrepancies.

14. Assume responsibility for security of the equipment and locker rooms.

15. Make certain that the equipment room is in a hygienic condition at all times.

16. Issue game equipment according to the coaches' information.

17. Have all necessary game equipment, supplies, and traveling bags ready for issuance 12 hours prior to the departure of the team.

18. Have the visiting team room ready for use a day before the visitors arrive and provide the normal or usually agreed upon services to the visiting team.

19. Provide housing security for visiting teams when necessary.

20. Make a yearly inventory of all movable equipment.

THE STUDENT MANAGER

The student manager staff should consist of one freshman, one sophomore, one junior, and one senior. The senior manager is the manager in charge of the equipment.

Following are a few suggestions of duties and responsibility of student managers, which may change for different seasonal sports.

Practice Sessions.
1. Assist the equipment manager at all times.
2. Keep up with all equipment on the field.
3. Have equipment on field half-hour before start of practice.
4. Keep daily attendance record of players.
5. Have ice, water, and towels available for players at all times.
6. Keep tools and supplies handy for minor repairs.
7. Establish rapport with all players.
8. Be physically and mentally alert at all times.
9. Be concerned with overall safety features of all practice sessions.

Home Games.
1. Be on hand when visiting teams arrive, and explain procedure to visitors for handling valuables.
2. Provide the necessary materials and services for both teams prior to and during game.
3. Check all equipment that you are responsible for on the field (down box, chains, flags, and game balls).
4. Make materials and supplies available for pregame warm-up.
5. Keep extra equipment available for replacements and repairs.

Road Games.

1. See that each member of traveling squad receives an itinerary.

2. See that all players' traveling and game-uniform bags are loaded.

3. Load equipment on bus.

4. Check seating arrangement of team to see that each member of traveling squad is seated.

5. Make a room roster available to all traveling personnel.

6. See that a meeting room is in order before the start of a meeting.

7. Notify players of all meals, practice sessions, and meetings.

8. Assist coach or trainer in making bed check.

9. Upon departing for home, double check to see that nothing has been left behind.

10. Upon arrival home, unload, check, and store equipment.

5

Responsibilities of the Team Physician*

Scientific proof shows that until recently the physical fitness of American youth has progressively declined. At present there are positive signs that this decline is slowing down. Efforts have been expended on many levels to expose more and more young people to physical education programs and sports activities as a means of achieving physical fitness. A national program has been developed that tests the ability of children to perform certain exercises.

European physicians are no longer ahead of us in the concepts of sports medicine and aiding in the promotion of the physical fitness of their youth. In the United States, the physician in the past concerned himself mainly with the prevention and treatment of disease, and there is no doubt that he has done an excellent job. For years, physicians maintained a "hands off" attitude toward physical education and sports, leaving these vital considerations completely in the hands of nonmedical personnel, such as physical educators, coaches, and trainers. Physicians have looked with a mixture of disdain and resentment on professionals who have been working to ensure healthy growth and development, including health practices and sports skills. This is no longer true.

In the past two decades, the medical profession has shown a new awareness of the importance of physical education and sports to the growth, development, and physical fitness of our youth, resulting in the concept of the "team physician." School and team administrators, along with the coaching and training staffs, call upon physicians to assist in the training and conditioning of athletes as well as to prevent and treat athletic injuries and nontraumatic medical conditions peculiar to athletes.

QUALIFICATIONS

The proper medical care of an athlete demands the services of a physician. However, obtaining the services of an interested and quali-

*Marvin C. Becker, M.D., provided special assistance in preparing this chapter.

fied physician is easier said than done. Physicians in general are in short supply, and many are not suited by training or temperament for a position as a team physician. Small schools and organizations especially may experience difficulty in obtaining a team physician, whereas large universities and professional, Olympic, Pan American, and Maccabiah teams have no problems in engaging physicians with training and experience in the medical and surgical care of the athlete. General and orthopedic surgeons with experience in trauma usually predominate on such teams, and many are former athletes themselves. Many physicians who are called on to be team physicians for small colleges and high schools have no experience in trauma or in treating athletes. They have not been athletes themselves, and they assume these duties as a civic responsibility. Little League baseball and midget football teams suffer most, often having little or no medical surveillance.

A team physician should be interested, understanding, sympathetic, and cooperative towards athletes and athletics. He must be aware of the psychologic and physical drives of boys and girls to participate in sports. He can acquire the necessary medical knowledge by exposure to sporting events, reading, and by taking postgraduate courses.

The team physician should be in complete charge of the medical care of the athlete. Basically, he must prevent illness and injury whenever it is possible and restore the sick and injured athlete to optimal function.

Sound medical care for the athlete centers about the preseason and in some instances, the precontest examination. This examination includes a detailed history and physical examination and indicated modern laboratory and diagnostic adjuncts, such as modern advances in radiology, cardiology, neurology, and vascular diagnostic techniques. Included among these, in addition to the conventional ECG's, are cardiac stress testing with treadmill or bicycle ergometers and radionuclear imaging techniques, such as thallium and technetium scans and echocardiography.

Nuclear imaging of the heart with thallium 201 can determine myocardial perfusion and cell viability. Thallium 201 imaging along with stress testing can show poor perfusion and insufficiency. Echocardiography is most useful in the diagnosis of mitral disease such as "floppy" mitral valves, aortic valvular disease, pericardial effusion, idiopathic hypertrophic subaortic stenosis and atrial myxoma.

From a neurologic standpoint, the team physician must be familiar with the conventional EEG. However, the brain scans and CAT scans are now more frequently used.

For peripheral vascular disease, the Doppler ultrasound technique is commonly used. A history of transient ischemic attacks should immediately alert the physician to the latest in vascular diagnostic techniques, such as the ophthalmoplethysmography and digital vascular imaging for carotid-artery abnormalities. Gargantuan-appearing basketball players with large and arachnodactyly fingers should be checked out for Marfan's syndrome because of its association with dissecting aortic aneurysms as well as other vascular abnormalities. The findings must be recorded in full and filed in the office of the director of athletics. Such an examination ensures the physical fitness of the athlete and eliminates those who are unfit for a sport.

Since the preponderance of athletic injuries involves the musculoskeletal system, the team physician should have a more intimate knowledge of the muscles, circulation, and nerve supply of the extremities, trunk, and neck than some physicians might consider necessary. He should be thoroughly aware of muscle origins, insertions, and actions as well as joint anatomy, kinesiology, and biomechanics. He notes joint restrictions and muscle weakness and corrects them with remedial exercises when applicable. He knows that an athlete who functions with unbalanced muscles is prone to injuries. He must have some familiarity with the loose and tight-joint syndrome described by Nicholas. He should be familiar with the Ehlers-Danlos syndrome, in which dislocations are frequent. Although he is familiar with the use of x-rays he should also know that a bone scan may pick up a fracture more quickly than a conventional x-ray in selected cases.

A sports physician is aware that the knee joint is the most vulnerable to injuries because of its location and anatomic bareness (this subject is more fully discussed in Chapter 9). The best protection for this joint, as well as for others, is a balanced development of the surrounding muscles. A program of resistance exercises for the quadriceps and hamstring muscles using isotonic and isokinetic equipment when available is absolutely necessary in preseason conditioning of the athlete. The same can be said of the ankle and its muscles. If the muscles about these joints are developed and protective strapping is wrapped about the ankles, the incidence of ankle injuries will decrease. (Hockey players develop unusually strong ankle muscles and are not plagued by these injuries as often as football players). Physicians must be familiar with stress testing of the knee and ankle joints clinically and radiographically when ligamentous damage is suspected. He must also be familiar with the use of arthrograms of the shoulder, knee, and ankles when ligamentous and capsular damage are suspected. Arthroscopy for knee injuries is now commonly used for suspected internal derangements. Arthroscopic surgery is being used currently.

The team doctor must have a thorough understanding of and familiarity with trauma and its by-products. He must have the patience to exact from his patient the precise mechanism of the injury so that he can visualize how the anatomy has been distorted by the traumatic forces. He can then plan appropriate treatment. The bulk of athletic injuries require immediate application of ice-packs and compression for 24 to 48 hours. This regimen reduces local swelling and hemorrhage, allowing speedy maximal recovery after definitive therapy has been instituted.

The team physician must be familiar with athletic equipment and be able to improvise protective padding. Although a physician should not be expected to be as familiar with protective equipment as the coach, he should understand the physiologic basis of such equipment and the hazards attending its use (as with the new face guard of the football helmet). Coaches and trainers seem to do a better job of taping ankles, knees, and other portions of the body than doctors. However, the physician is in a far better position to check on the safety of such strappings than a coach or a trainer. Inefficient knee tapings not only fail to protect the knee from injury, but give the wearer a false sense of security.

The team physician must be conversant with the training techniques that coaches employ to bring their charges to peak physical condition. In addition to developing sports skills, the athlete must develop wind and endurance. These can only be accomplished through hard work and systematic exercises; adequate rest and nutrition are also parts of the conditioning program. The physician should become familiar with the concepts of circuit training, interval training, and weight-training programs.

Last but not least, a team physician must be familiar with emergency medicine, especially when taking care of adult and older athletes and spectators who, in a rare instance, suffer a cardiac arrest or ventricular fibrillation and require cardiopulmonary resuscitation while waiting for an ambulance to arrive for possible cardioversion and/or transportation to the hospital.

The sports-minded physician will be sympathetic and cooperative with all personnel who administer physical education, intramural, and interscholastic sports programs, but will be primarily concerned with the athlete. The team physician should seek to understand the difficulties and responsibilities of the coaching staff and the athletic department. By attending conferences with the coach and the trainer, he encourages cooperation between the professions, to the benefit of the athlete. Working together, they can formulate recommendations to the administration concerning the athletic program.

SUGGESTED RESPONSIBILITIES OF THE TEAM PHYSICIAN

1. Makes sure that all candidates for an athletic team have passed a meticulous preseason or precontest medical examination consisting of a detailed history, physical examination, indicated laboratory proce-

dures and diagnostic adjuncts. These examinations may be performed by physicians other than the team doctor, depending on local custom. For example, physicians on the medical staffs of boards-of-education, university and college medical dispensaries, and medical schools may perform them. In some areas, family doctors can certify to the medical fitness of their patients. Regardless of who examines the athlete, the team physician must have on file a written record from the doctor who performs this vital and important prerequisite for sports participation.

2. Cooperates with the coaching and training staff in order to field the physically best-conditioned team, giving his advice on matters of conditioning, diet, protective padding, water and electrolyte balance. His ideas and recommendations on equipment as it relates to prevention of injuries and other clinical conditions are welcomed by the coaching staff.

3. Examines all reported cases of injuries or illnesses as soon as possible. He treats only those medical and surgical conditions he is capable of handling, and refers to consultants beyond his scope of training or experience.

4. Notifies the coach, trainer, and athletic director in writing his impression of the athlete's fitness. If the athlete is injured, he reports the progress of therapy and the prognosis. He may have to do the same for the parents of a high school player who is ill or has been injured.

5. Directs the trainer by prescription as to the type of physical therapy to be instituted and the type of protective strapping and padding that may be necessary.

6. Notifies the coach by telephone or written note when an athlete may return to play. He gives the athlete written permission to do so. Meticulous records are kept of these decisions.

7. Is always in attendance at home football and hockey games and boxing matches. When his team plays out of town, arrangements must be made to have another physician in attendance. Although injuries also occur in track, soccer, lacrosse, swimming, tennis, basketball, and other sports, a doctor is not required on the bench for these events; it is sufficient to have a trainer in attendance. However, the team doctor should be near enough to respond quickly if necessary.

8. Is exceptionally competent in making examinations and decisions on the field. Although it is better for the doctor to err on the side of safety, to take an athlete needlessly out of a game because of the physician's faulty judgment does much to sap the strength and morale of a player and his team.

9. Periodically takes an inventory of the medical bag in company with his trainer, so as to have the proper type and amount of medical supplies and equipment always on hand.

10. Is in immediate communication with first-aid men in charge of the ambulance that should always be in proximity during contact-sports contests.

11. Checks the work of his trainer, who acts as his right-hand man, to see that his orders regarding physical therapy, protective strappings, and paddings are being carried out.

12. Remains the final authority when matters of health are concerned, determining who may or may not participate at any given time.

A team physician understands that natural competitiveness and aggression in many children are fulfilled through sports outlets. He is also aware that playing a sport provides educational features that can be obtained nowhere else except in the battle of life, which at best is no bed of roses. Possessing unique skills and a sympathetic attitude, the team physician, with the cooperation of administration, coaching, and training professions, can reduce the incidence of athletic injuries, permanent residuals, and other medical risks attendant to athletic participation.

REFERENCES

American College of Sports Medicine (ed.): Guidelines for Graded Exercise Testing and Exercise Prescription. 2nd Ed. Philadelphia, Lea & Febiger, 1980.

Apple, D.F., and Cantwell, J.D.: Medicine for Sport. Chicago, Year Book Medical Publisher, 1979.

Balakian, G., Eliert, R.E., Krause, H., and Novich, M.M.: So your patient wants a sport doctor. Patient Care, 10–20: 90–107, 1976.

Frankel, V.H., and Nordin, M.: Basic Biomechanics of the Skeletal System. Philadelphia, Lea & Febiger, 1980.

Krakover, L. J.: Yearbook of Sports Medicine 1981. Chicago, Year Book Medical Publisher, 1981.

McArdle, W.D., Katch, F.I., and Katch, V.L.: Exercise Physiology: Energy, Nutrition, and the Physiology of Human Performance. Philadelphia, Lea & Febiger, 1980.

6

Conditioning of Athletes

Competitive sports make a tremendous demand on the physical condition, vitality, endurance, and mental powers of the participant. Only athletes in the finest condition can withstand the wear and tear of a competitive season; only the fittest can play to the best of their ability. Athletes not in condition are prone to injury or "going stale," and might never make the team. Thus, proper conditioning not only is necessary in preparing for sports participation, but is of great importance in preventing injuries. The athlete who is properly trained and conditioned will sustain a lower incidence and severity of injuries and a higher level of performance. Individuals who are obese, awkward, considerably underweight, or ill-trained suffer the greatest number of injuries. The athlete who is well muscled and properly conditioned rarely requires medical treatment for injuries. Proper conditioning requires the joint effort of the physician, coach, trainer, and athlete.

PRESEASON PHYSICAL EXAMINATION

The conditioning of an athlete is based upon well established physiologic principles, but results can only be expected if the athlete is of sound mind and body. This is determined by a detailed preseason history and physical examination; sometimes, a precontest examination is indicated. Preferably, the examination is performed by a physician who understands sports medicine and is sympathetic to athletics. Although personal experience in sports on the part of the examining physician is advantageous, it is not a prerequisite. A family physician* familiar with a candidate's prior medical history may contribute information that has a bearing on the athlete's fitness for a sport, but he may also be less thorough and objective in his examination. Nevertheless, in the best interest of the athlete, the team physician and family

*It has become clear that the best physicians to do such examinations are the family physicians who perform the examinations in the privacy of their offices and follow established preparticipation physical examination guidelines. This information is sent to the school or team doctor.

physician should be in communication about the athlete's past and present state of health.

Purpose of the Examination. The basis for sound medical care of the athlete is the preseason and in some instances, the precontest medical examination. School administrator, athletic director, coach, trainer, or team doctor should not presume an athlete to be physically fit merely because he "came out for the team." A complete medical examination is mandatory prior to all participation to prevent potential tragedies. The preseason examination has several purposes:

1. To determine the physical fitness of the athlete and eliminate candidates who are unfit for a sport.
2. To screen out silent diseases, congenital abnormalities, and residuals from injuries, of which the athlete and even the parents may be completely unaware. This is an important part of an athletic-injury prevention program.
3. To establish a baseline profile of the athlete's state of health, which is especially useful to a physician in the treatment and follow-up care of injury or illness. This information should be available to the athlete, the doctor, and the athletic supervisory personnel throughout his athletic career.
4. To demonstrate the school's concern for the candidate's health and welfare.

The physical examination of athletes prior to participation is a medical, legal, and moral obligation of the administrators, athletic directors, coaches, and physicians. It is not subject to the whims, interference, or control of the coach or others.

Extent of the Examination. Before any conditioning program begins for an athlete, a medical examination is performed, which includes a history of past illnesses and injuries as well as emotional and psychiatric difficulties. In addition, all indicated laboratory and electrodiagnostic adjuncts are performed. If a history or medical examination reveals evidence of potentially disqualifying medical conditions, the athlete must be referred to an appropriate consultant for an opinion on his fitness to participate in a particular sport. Dental, visual, and auditory surveys are also an integral part of the examination.

The following conditions might be causes for disqualification depending on the sport:

1. *Medical*
   a. Uncontrolled diabetes mellitus.
   b. Hypertension.
   c. History of/or active heart disease.
   d. History of/or active nephritis and other renal disease.

e. Tuberculosis, if active or arrested for less than 5 years.
f. Asthma, emphysema, bronchiectasis.
g. Syphilis, active or untreated.
h. Other active venereal diseases.
i. Narcotics addiction.
j. Blood dyscrasias, hemophilia, sickle cell disease or trait.
k. Athletes with one organ, such as an eye, kidney, or testicle, or severe deafness in one ear (disqualified in contact sports).
l. Prior cardiac surgery for acquired or congenital heart disease.
m. Enlarged liver or spleen.
n. Acute infections, respiratory, genitourinary, infectious mononucleosis, and rheumatic fever.

Some recent judicial decisions have permitted an athlete with one eye to participate in basketball and an athlete with an undescended testicle to play football. In such cases, appropriate protective equipment must be used. A boxer possessing sight in only one eye, an epileptic, and a deaf-mute are disqualified from international amateur boxing under International Amateur Boxing Association auspices.

Primary aortic disease or a combination of aortic and mitral disease, unusual rhythm changes, conduction disturbances, and coronary artery diseases are sufficient reasons for disqualification. "Functional" heart murmurs must be thoroughly investigated to determine whether or not they are disabling. This can be done by using noninvasive techniques, such as an exercise tolerance test (stress test) using a bicycle ergometer, treadmill, or radionucleotide stress testing with thallium 201, or technetium. The use of echocardiography is extremely valuable for evaluating murmurs. Of course, the conventional electrocardiogram and determination of heart size clinically and by x-ray should be done first when heart disease is suspected. This can be followed by the more expensive, sophisticated, and time-consuming noninvasive techniques noted earlier.

Diabetic teenagers and adults are encouraged to participate in athletics and exercise programs such as calisthenics, baseball, basketball, golf, and tennis. Diabetics have been known to play varsity college football. The diabetic must be instructed in regulating his food and insulin intake in the proper amounts because strenuous exercises result in an increase of endogenous insulin. The athlete must learn to neutralize anticipated episodes of hypoglycemia with extra carbohydrate intake during athletic activity.

2. *Neurologic*
    a. Convulsive disorders not completely controlled by medication.
    b. Tremors, tics, fasciculations, and other abnormal involuntary movements.

   c. Ataxic, spastic, or cerebellar gaits.

   d. Cerebral hemorrhage, concussion, or history of serious head injury.

   e. Labyrinthine disturbances.

   f. Chorea.

Candidates with a history of convulsive disorders require individual evaluation, but should be barred from participation in those sports where chronic recurrent head trauma may occur.* History or clinical findings of injury following a fractured skull or brain concussion indicate electroencephalography to rule out the presence of intracranial damage. An athlete who sustains a head injury in a contact sport other than a minor concussion should be disqualified for the rest of the season. In the case of a boxer, who has been knocked out with a loss of consciousness, two months' rest is mandatory, and if he has suffered three or more such injuries within a year, he should be disqualified for life from the sport. Athletes who sustain head injuries require follow-up by frequent clinical examinations, brain scans, CAT scans, and electroencephalograms.

Athletes with lantern ("glass") jaws are easy prey to knock-out blows in football and in boxing, and should be discouraged from participating in sports in which the chin is especially vulnerable.

3. *Ophthalmologic*

   a. Severe myopia (minus 6 diopters or more in boxing).

   b. The presence of only one eye or useful vision in only one eye.

It is extremely important that both normal peripheral vision and central visual acuity be present. The need for corrective lenses is not in itself disqualifying, but is determined by the extent of visual deficiency and the type of sport. In recent years, the soft lenses (hydrophilic) are commonly used in athletic pursuits. They are even worn in contact sports in which glasses are not commonly seen.

4. *Orthopedic†*

   a. Klippel-Feil syndrome.

   b. Myelomeningocele.

   c. Instability of the atlantooccipital joint.

   d. Anomalies of the odontoid process.

   e. Incapacitating clinical conditions of the axial or appendiceal skeleton.

---

*See *Joint Statement on Convulsive Disorders and Participation in Sports and Physical Education* for further considerations. JAMA, 206:1291, 1968.

†National Federation of State High Schools Association rule on amputees with artificial limbs: "Artificial limbs, which, in the judgment of the rules-administering officials, are no more dangerous to players than the corresponding human limb and do not place an opponent at a disadvantage may be permitted."

A physical examination is directed to the musculoskeletal system to check out the muscles, joints, and bones of the athlete. Balance, gait, and coordination ability during the performance of certain exercises in the examination are noted. Muscle strength and weaknesses are tested. Girth measurements of extremities are taken if atrophy or hypertrophy is suspected. Joints are examined for range of motion, restrictions, and laxity. Leg lengths should be measured when shortening is suspected. Extremities showing residual weakness or imbalance, joint restrictions or laxity from prior injuries, disease, disuse, or overuse may be prone to recurrent injury.

Athletes with long necks should not be encouraged to play football or box unless they can build up strong neck and shoulder muscles. An athlete may be unaware of congenital anomalies of the vertebral column until he has been injured. Such backs heal less satisfactorily than spinal columns with normal bony architecture. Unless the restoration proceeds normally and fully, the athlete should be directed to a less-demanding sport.

A consultation must be requested whenever the examination causes the examining physician to suspect a clinical condition beyond the scope of his training and experience. This also applies to mental and emotional difficulties.

Physicians must not be restricted by inflexible rules in determining the fitness or unfitness of an athletic candidate. Individuals vary considerably in their capacity for adjustment and achievement. Sports lore is replete with stories of severely handicapped men and women who have competed with nonhandicapped players, often winning prominence in highly competitive sports. A great deal of psychologic damage can be done to an athlete who has been unnecessarily restricted. When the physician forbids a candidate to participate in sports, the reasons must be made clear to the candidate and to all those concerned with the program. Much misunderstanding and resentment will be avoided if the team doctor maintains a policy of frankness and clarity in his dealings with the coaches and players.

When a candidate is a minor, the parents must be advised of the reason for the disqualification. If the candidate is in need of medical care, the instructions must be imparted to those concerned. On occasion, parents may insist that their child is capable of playing a sport in spite of medical disqualifications. At no time may the coach take it upon himself to set aside the doctor's decision. In such a situation, the coach should direct the athlete and his obstinate parents to the athletic or school administrators, who should refer the matter to their legal representative. It may be necessary to adjudicate legally. However, a candidate with physical conditions that disqualify him from one sport is not automatically disqualified from all sports. For instance, a youth with mild mitral insufficiency may be permitted to participate in a sports program that does not require constant strenuous effort or body contact. Rigorous sports, such as swimming, track, tennis, football, boxing, wrestling, soccer, and hockey should of course be forbidden; but golf, baseball, and volley ball, in which effort alternates with relaxation, may be permitted.

Setting Up a Physical Examination

Step One. Obtain the services of a licensed physician who is interested in and sympathetic towards athletics and athletes. Spell out in precise terms the exact medical coverage you expect from the doctor. The doctor must know whether he is to be the examining physician for the preseason or precontest examination, the game physician, or the team physician (the medical responsibilities for each category differ significantly). A financial arrangement for the doctor's services must be arranged in advance.

The physician in charge of attending the medical needs of the team must have free rein in the choice of consultants. However, if a parent insists upon a different consultant or examining physician for the child, this request must be honored, but a note of it should be made on the athlete's medical file.

Step Two. Provide a satisfactory examination area. Doctors prefer conducting examinations for a large number of athletes in a large area, such as a gym, rather than in a private office. A satisfactory area may be arranged by providing a few examining tables, screens, weighing scale, and eye chart.

Step Three. Provide the doctor with assistants, such as a nurse and perhaps a trainer who can take height, weight, temperature, pulse, and respiration readings. Blood pressures may be taken by nurses. Student managers and stenographers can record the observations and facilitate the working of the project. Scheduling the examinations over several periods of time instead of crowding them all into one afternoon would alleviate pressure on the doctor and perhaps allow a more thorough, unhurried examination of each athlete.

Record-keeping. All medical records should be typed in triplicate. The physician, coach, and athletic director each keep one copy.

It is absolutely essential that a candidate for an athletic team sign an athletic participation form, wherein he states he is familiar with the eligibility rules and believes he is eligible to represent the team. He also agrees to abide by rules and regulations of the school authorities as well as the training rules established by the coach and his staff. (Members of professional teams sign contracts covering such matters, frequently under the direction of legal representatives.) Parental con-

(*Text continued on page 66.*)

Highland Park High School Athletic Department
Highland Park, New Jersey

Athletic Permission

Dear Parent:

Your son/daughter has requested the privilege of taking part in our athletic program of which we are very proud. However, before he/she may take part it is necessary for you to be aware of certain facts and for us to have your consent for him/her to participate.

The Board of Education is not responsible for any injury incurred while participating in school activities. For many years students who were injured paid their own bills. In order to protect the students the Board of Education has set up an insurance plan so that the greater portion of the expense is taken care of.

We have been able to pay most of the bills in full through this policy. However, due to past injustices, we have been forced to adopt a policy whereby the injured student will be sent to a doctor with our consent.

We have selected excellent doctors with the help of our school physician and I am sure that they will be most competent. However, the student may be cared for by the family doctor with one stipulation, that all expenses incurred over the insurance limit will be accepted by the parent. We have always taken excellent care of our athletes and intend to do so in the future. We will go to the limit to insure the health and safety of the students taking part in our programs. We trust you will understand our position and will appreciate your cooperation.

To further enhance athletic-insurance coverage for student athletics the state of N.J. has passed a first payment clause of insurance, where the insurance is fully funded by the local Board of Education. This means in the event of hospitalization or surgery, if you have an insurance plan that plan would make the first payment, and whatever this did not pay, the Board Policy would pay for. In the event you carry no hospitalization, the Board Policy would pay the bills as stipulated in the policy limits. If an injury requires no hospitalization or surgery, the Board Insurance would pay all bills as stipulated in the limits of the policy.

To further protect your son/daughter during his/her participation, the Board of Education has also adopted a policy whereby all participants in contact sports must receive tetanus inoculations prior to participating in the interscholastic athletic program.

The inoculations will be provided by the Board of Education and will be administered by the school physician at no expense to you. If you prefer to take your child to your own physician, you must bear the expense and we must receive a statement from your doctor that the inoculation has been given.

Please read the above notice very carefully, then I would appreciate your reading the other side of this notice very carefully. After you have done this, please fill out the spaces provided for you under the section labeled "Parent's Consent." Have your youngster return this slip to us so that we may have it on file in our office. No one will be permitted to participate in the program without a signed permission slip on file with his/her coach.

I will be most happy to answer any questions or comments that you may have concerning this matter of participation and consent. You may call me at the Highland Park High School Athletic Department Office (572-2402) or write me in care of the school. (Please turn to other side to sign statement to parent consent.)

Sincerely yours,
Jay H. Dakelman—Athletic Director

Student Athletic Participation Request

I, _____, hereby apply for the privilege of trying out for the _____ team at the Highland Park High School. I realize that playing athletics at Highland Park is a privilege provided by the Board of Education. I recognize my responsibilities if I try out for the sport, and even greater responsibilities if I am selected to play. I will make it my duty to govern myself so that my connection with the Athletic Department will bring honor to it and to the school and I will be expected to be penalized for my failure to comply with the regulations.

If extended the privilege to play, I will further:

1. Train consistently as directed by the coaching staff of my sport.
2. Follow closely and not violate any of the training rules set down by the coaches.
3. Make a serious endeavor to keep up in my academic program.
4. Do all in my power to keep the athletic program a desirable one.
5. Make it a point to abide by the regulations of the school administration and the student council.
6. Conduct myself at all times, at other schools and on trips, on the playing field and off, so as to bring credit to my school, my town, and myself.
7. Agree to take proper care of all equipment loaned to me and to return all such items in good condition at the close of the season. I agree to pay for loss or damage of said items.
8. I agree to uphold the tradition of the Athletic Program of Highland Park High School, for this program is not to be entrusted to the timid or the meek.

I promise, on my word of honor, to do the above.

Signed _____
                                    Athlete

Date of birth _____ Place of birth _____
DOCTOR'S APPROVAL This student was examined by Dr. _____
on _____ and was passed as qualified to participate.
The above candidate received a tetanus inoculation on _____.

Parent's Consent

Parents, please fill out and sign the below, so that your son/daughter may participate. We, the undersigned, do hereby grant permission for my son/daughter ___
_____ (name) to play _____ at Highland Park High School according to the stipulations on the other side of this note and to the above statements signed by my son/daughter.

HOME ADDRESS _____
HOME PHONE _____
BUSINESS PHONE _____
FAMILY DOCTOR _____   Signed: _____
                                                 (parent or guardian)

                                         Date: _____

Fig. 6-1.   An athletic permission form. (Courtesy of Highland Park High School, Highland Park, N.J.)

(To be completed by athlete, assisted by parents and/or family physician. Return to team physician, athletic trainer, or coach)

Name _____   Date of birth _____

Home Address _____   Telephone _____

Parents' Name _____

Circle One

1. Have you ever been told not to participate in any sport?   No   Yes
2. Have you ever been unconscious or lost memory from a blow on your head?   No   Yes
3. Have you ever had a fracture or dislocation?   No   Yes
4. Have you had a knee or ankle sprain?   No   Yes
5. Have you had other injuries?   No   Yes
6. Are you under a physician's care now?   No   Yes
7. Do you take any kind of medicine every day?   No   Yes
8. Have you had an illness lasting longer than one week?   No   Yes
9. Do you have allergies (Hay fever, hives, asthma, or to medicines)?   No   Yes
10. Have you been in a hospital for an operation or any other reason?   No   Yes
11. Do you have any worries about your health or other questions you would like to discuss with a physician?   No   Yes

Explain any of the above questions you have answered with "Yes" _____

Have you had poliomyelitis ("polio") immunization? _____

Date of last tetanus toxoid booster _____

Approximate date of last examination by a physician _____

_____
Parent or physician

Fig. 6-2, A.   Sports candidate's questionnaire. (Reprinted with permission from *Pediatric Annals*. Copyright © Insight Publishing Co., New York, N.Y. October 1978.)

sent is necessary for minors, and a parental consent section may be incorporated with the physician's examination certificate on a single form, such as that used by Highland Park High School Athletic Department.

At this time, no standard physical examination form for athletes is available. In general, the form should include all past and present medical history that might have a bearing on the physical fitness of the candidate. Any injuries or illnesses, old or new, and the degree of res-

Athletic Medical Examination

Athlete's Name: _____ Date of Examination: _____ Age: __

SECTION I:

HISTORY: Previous illnesses, injuries, operations, accidents: _____

_____

_____

IMMUNIZATION RECORD:

Diphtheria _____	Polio _____	Smallpox _____
Pertussis _____	Measles _____	Other _____
Tetanus _____	Mumps _____	_____

SECTION II:

Height: _____ft._____in.   Pulse: At rest_____2 min. postexercise _____

Weight: _____lbs._____oz.   Blood Pressure: _____

Temperature:_____

1. HEAD: Any bruises, scars, discolorations, swellings or tenderness? _____

_____

_____

_____

Eyes: Distance vision: Right_____   Left_____
With glasses: Right_____   Left_____
Do pupils react to light and accommodation? _____

Ears: Hearing at 20 feet: Right_____   Left_____

Nose: _____

Mouth: Does tongue protrude in midline? _____
Is gag reflex active? _____
Does uvula elevate normally? _____

Teeth: Dental work needed? _____
Are prostheses present or needed? _____
Periodontitis? _____

2. NECK: Is it freely movable and without pain? _____
Is muscle spasm present? _____
Is normal cervical lordosis present? _____
Evaluation of lymph glands and thyroid _____

3. CHEST: Any deformities? _____
Does compression of rib cage cause pain? _____
Is configuration of breast-budding developing symmetrically? __
Lungs: What is quality of breath sounds? _____
Are rales present? _____
Heart: Is normal sinus rhythm present? _____
Are any murmurs present? _____
What is the size of heart? _____

4. ABDOMEN: Any masses, scars, tenderness, rigidity, enlarged liver or spleen?

_____

_____

_____

_____

5. UPPER EXTREMITIES: Scars, swellings, discolorations, tenderness, muscular atrophy, hypertrophy, deformities, restrictions or laxity of any joints, injury of bones, or peripheral nerve injuries? Is there axillary hair?

_____

_____

_____

_____

6. LOWER EXTREMITIES: Check as for upper extremities. Are there any lumps, varicosities, or ulcerations?

_____

_____

_____

Can athlete squat down and arise easily without complaints? ___

_____

7. BACK: Is there muscle spasm, loss of normal spinal curves, deformities, or restriction of spinal mobility? _____

_____

_____

_____

Straight-leg-raising test: _____
Patrick test: _____

8. NERVOUS SYSTEM: Any tremors of the eyelids, tongue or outstretched finger?

_____

_____

Romberg test: _____
Are deep tendon and significant skin reflexes present and active? Any sensory changes? _____

9. GENITALIA: Pubic hair distribution, absent or undescended testicle, hydrocele, varicocele, inguinal or femoral hernia _____

_____

10. RECTUM: Hemorrhoid, pilonidal cyst, pruritus ani _____

_____

11. Gait and neuromuscular coordination _____

_____

SECTION III:

Complete blood count: RBC:_____ WBC:_____ Platelet:_____
Urinalysis _____
Blood serology _____
Sickle cell prep _____

RECOMMENDATIONS: _____

Signature of Examining Physician _____

Fig. 6-2, B. Physical examination form used and recommended by M.N.

toration are significant data to a physician in assessing an athlete's fitness to play. The athlete must be thoroughly and completely examined from head to toe, front and back. Normal and abnormal findings must be recorded.

The short but comprehensive physical examination form included here is especially useful in assessing the physical fitness of an athlete. It not only includes all body systems, but also covers those parts of the body that have special significance in athletics. General practitioners and specialists will find this form easy to handle and informative in evaluating an athlete's physical fitness. In drawing up an examination form, it may be advisable for the physician to consult a lawyer familiar with state and school regulations.

CONDITIONING

Introduction

Getting into condition or "shape" for a sport is the athlete's goal. The athlete reaches this goal when he can make specific musculoskeletal movements repeatedly and efficiently without becoming unduly fatigued, and when fatigue does set in, a quick recovery is anticipated. Such bioefficiency results from the interrelated development of the musculoskeletal, respiratory, and circulatory systems coordinated by the central and autonomic nervous systems. All body functions contribute to the quality of the athlete's performance. Only the athlete in the finest condition can stand the wear and tear of a competitive season.

The main features of a conditioning program are:
1. Stretching/flexibility training.
2. Strength training.
3. Speed training.
4. Endurance/stamina training.
5. Equilibrium (balance).
6. Agility training.
7. Reaction training.
8. Percent body fat.

Since the first edition, flexibility/stretching training is a prime effort in the training and conditioning program. This type of training not only prepares the athlete for maximum performance, but also prevents many types of musculoskeletal injuries. Examples of this will be stated later. Too flexible a knee joint (loose joint) in sports such as football, soccer, and hockey should be strengthened if possible.

Strength, speed, stamina, and endurance are developed by the physiologic overload principle, which utilizes graduated muscular exercises, and interval and circuit training. All of these should be achieved in off-season programming and maximized during preseason and seasonal activities. Physicians, coaches, trainers, and athletes have become increasingly aware that only through strenuous exercises and play can an athlete reach his best playing form: that when the arms and legs begin to hurt, you know they are being strengthened. The heart muscle also benefits from overloading by beating more slowly and more efficiently, delivering a greater volume with each stroke. The capacity of the lung increases by utilizing many dormant alveolar sacs as well as developing accessory muscles of respiration, thus supplying larger amounts of oxygen to the blood and removing waste metabolites more efficiently. Getting the cardiovascular and respiratory systems in shape should be the first order of business; the best way to do this is by running.

Each sport has its own patterns, muscle loads, tempo, and duration. The skills and the conditioning necessary to participate in one sport are not interchangeable with another sport. For example, a well conditioned football player might run out of steam quickly in a boxing match, and a high-scoring bowler might be a duffer at golf. Participation in the particular sport is the best way to become proficient and conditioned for that athletic activity. However, despite the differences among sports, some generalizations can be made about getting into condition and maintaining it.

Although we now recognize that keeping in condition is a year-round objective, it may be divided into preseasonal, seasonal, and off-seasonal activities. During off-seasons, bicycling, running, and rope jumping are excellent exercises for maintaining tone of the muscular and cardiorespiratory systems. Supervised weight training based on weight-pushing, pulling, lifting, and pressing is an excellent activity for maintaining condition. Weights of varying sizes may be attached to various parts of the anatomy to develop general muscle tone, or to a specific group of muscles used in a particular sport. During the season, these off-seasonal activities are generally relegated to a lesser role in the training program. Progressive overloading is carried out through one or a combination of interval, circuit, or weight-training techniques.

Interval Training. Interval training originated in Europe as a scientific method of developing speed and endurance in trackmen. It is a method of overloading the athlete by the use of aerobic and anaerobic exercises, thus developing a high oxygen debt. A quick recovery of the cardiovascular and respiratory systems is sought for and expected. In this method, an athlete runs a prescribed course in a specified time for a prescribed number of times. Fast runs are interspersed with short recovery periods of jogging. The athlete becomes fatigued many times in a single training session, depending on his fitness and his ability to handle many states of high oxygen debt. In this manner, he is able to progressively increase his endurance by increasingly stressing the cardiorespiratory system. Besides developing endurance and strength, interval training has the added advantage of allowing large numbers of athletes to train at the same time.

Circuit Training. This method was devised by G. T. Adamson and R. E. Morgan of Leeds University, England. A scientific arrangement of proven exercises are performed systematically and repeatedly as a circuit, then repeated twice more as a circuit. Circuit training is designed to elicit maximal overall balanced development. A circuit may consist of the following exercises:

1. Steps on and off chair.
2. Trunk curls.
3. Hops 25 yards on alternate legs.
4. Dips between chair backs.
5. Squat jumps.
6. Press-ups.
7. Situps and twists.
8. Squat thrusts.
9. Shuttle run.
10. Dorsal lifts, supported by a partner.

Because of the strenuous nature of the exercises, circuit training is usually done at the end of a training session. The entire session should not last more than 20 minutes. Sebastian Coe, gold-medal winner for the 1500 meter in the 1980 Moscow Olympics, is a devotee of circuit training.

Weight Training. Today the people of our country are more concerned with physical fitness than ever before. Each year, manufacturers of fitness equipment introduce to the coaching and training professions and to the public new apparatus that can be used to build strength and improve cardiovascular endurance. Weight training is used by many athletes to get into top condition for a particular sport; it is an integral part of every athlete's training program. It is physiologically and psychologically sound.

A general program of weight training for conditioning must include exercises that will develop muscular power (strength) and muscular endurance. Muscular strength is the ability to work against a specified resistance without injuring the muscle; it is best developed by using high resistance with a low number of repetitions. Muscular endurance is the ability of a muscle to respond repeatedly for a long period of time; this is best developed by using low resistance with a high number of repetitions. The athlete tries progressively to exceed his limits in lifting, and also stresses movements that must be done repeatedly with enough weights to make the muscle work. All lifting motions require timing, snap, and explosive power, which are desirable in athletic training.

Weight training for athletes is not the same as lifting weights for body building. In body building, isolated muscles or muscle groups are exercised to produce large muscle mass (a muscle-bound look) and strength—reaching total conditioning is not the goal. Generally, conditioning is not enhanced when body building is the main concern, although some body builders achieve total conditioning through the intelligent application of weight lifting exercises.

Isotonic and isometric muscle exercise programs with and without apparatuses are popular because of their time-saving features. When finances are a problem, the same routines can be used without apparatus, although the desired results may take a little longer to attain. In isotonic exercises, the muscle is contracted under constant tension. Performed with full range of motion of the adjoining joint and using the power rack, isotonic exercises provide an efficient means of *achieving* general bodily development.

In isometric exercises, one muscle or one part of the body is pitted against another or against an immovable object. The pushing, pulling, pressing, and flexing activities are strong but motionless. Isometric exercises are valuable only if the athlete expends 100% effort to develop strength in specific muscles or to *maintain* general muscular strength. The isometric rack may be used, and the exercises may be done daily at the beginning of football practice.

The most popular muscle-strengthening program is performed by using isotonic apparatuses. We refer to the Nautilus and others. The Cybex and Orthotron machines are isokinetic devices used therapeutically to strengthen and rehabilitate injured limbs. Isometric exercises have lost favor with the strength programs for athletes. However, they still play a significant therapeutic role in the rehabilitation of the injured athlete. If budgetary deficits preclude those apparatuses, isometrics are still useful.

Only through hard work can an athlete develop his strength potential from a weight-training program. The athlete should start off with a general body-building program during the off-season. During the preseason, he must focus on those muscle groups that are most involved in his sport. However, the athlete should not overdevelop one set of muscles to cause an imbalance with the antagonistic muscle groups, since this could cause an uncoordinated joint movement. Experience has shown that there is a need to place more emphasis on strengthening the shoulder and upper extremities, although this should not be done at the expense of strengthening the legs. The amount of weight to be used is somewhat a matter of trial and error, and each athlete must experiment to find the baseline from which his weight training program is launched.

The best results in a weight training program can only be realized when the program is fitted to the individual's need and he is conscientiously involved in it. If an athlete is presently working on a weight training program and getting good results, there is no need to experiment with a new method until its advantages and disadvantages have been evaluated. Records should be kept of the individual's progress, and adjustments in the program made in accordance with the athlete's newly acquired strength. An individual progress chart—much like a diary—should be kept by each athlete.

Weight training is no replacement for running in the conditioning program. During the season, weight training should be used sparingly; however, it has a place as a supplement to regular workout activities (e.g., 2 days a week) to maintain strength and endurance that might be lost during a season. If a coach insists on weight-training exercises during the season, they are best done after stretching/flexibility exercises.

Weight-training exercises are also useful as therapy following injuries to athletes. This completely differs from conditioning routines and is prescribed by the team physician as rehabilitative therapy.

Flexibility Training. One only has to watch a football game to see the unusual positions in which a joint may be placed in the course of a game. Flexibility allows uninhibited joint motion and perfection of movement, giving an added margin of safety to the joint and its surrounding connective tissue structures when it is needed most, without tearing, which could lead to sprains, subluxations and dislocations, or fractures. Flexibility training is designed to increase the range of motion of joints; this requires stretching of the tissues, especially connective tissues, beyond their normal limits. Connective tissue periodically shortens with aging, and unless it is actively stretched, it will remain shortened, thus cutting down on the range of motion of the joint. This is especially noticeable in the shoulders and low back, as well as other joints.

Flexibility is best achieved with slow, controlled movements, as is seen in ballet, rather than with ballistic or bouncing-type movements. Since pain is a factor in inhibiting movement, controlled movements are not likely to exceed the extensibility of muscle tissue and cause injury. A simple way to maintaining a full range of motion, and even slightly more, is for the athlete to go through those motions associated with his sport daily and even during the off season. Each sport has its own particular activities that help in obtaining suppleness of the joints. For example, the golfer and the batter should practice swinging; the boxer shadow boxing; the hurdler and the punter, leg and groin stretching. The following sketches (Fig. 6-3) are examples of stretching/flexibility exercises that can be used by the athlete in his sport.

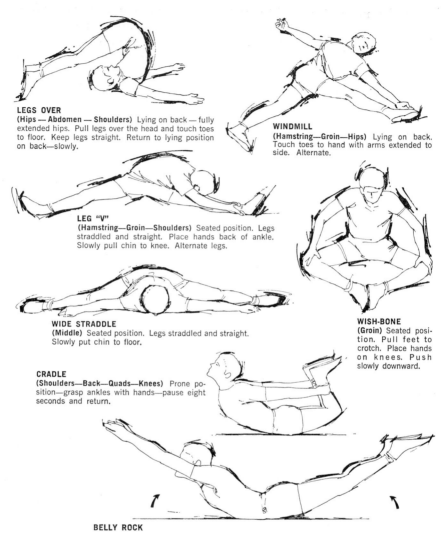

LEGS OVER
(Hips — Abdomen — Shoulders) Lying on back — fully extended hips. Pull legs over the head and touch toes to floor. Keep legs straight. Return to lying position on back—slowly.

WINDMILL
(Hamstring—Groin—Hips) Lying on back. Touch toes to hand with arms extended to side. Alternate.

LEG "V"
(Hamstring—Groin—Shoulders) Seated position. Legs straddled and straight. Place hands back of ankle. Slowly pull chin to knee. Alternate legs.

WIDE STRADDLE
(Middle) Seated position. Legs straddled and straight. Slowly put chin to floor.

WISH-BONE
(Groin) Seated position. Pull feet to crotch. Place hands on knees. Push slowly downward.

CRADLE
(Shoulders—Back—Quads—Knees) Prone position—grasp ankles with hands—pause eight seconds and return.

BELLY ROCK
(Shoulders—Back—Quads). Prone lying position. Raise both arms and legs. Rock on abdomen by lowering chest as legs are raised, then lowering legs as chest is raised, then repeat several times.

Fig. 6-3.   Stretching/flexibility exercises. (From Flexibility Exercises. *In* A Coach's Guide to Safe Football. Edited by Bill Murray and Dick Herbert. Durham, The American Football Coaches Association, p. 15.)

Reaction Training. Reaction training is designed to shorten the delay between the perception of a stimulus and the athlete's response to it. The objective is to make the musculoskeletal system move almost automatically, in a reflex manner, thus bypassing the decision-making functions of the brain. In effect, each muscle has its own "mind." Automatic response in anticipating the stimulus reduces reaction time. Continuous training of this type will improve performance. Reaction training and agility training are combined to increase mobility in the quickest possible time.

Fluid Balance and Weight Charts

Coaching and conditioning athletes demands complex skills that go far beyond the teaching of offensive and defensive plays. The coach must correlate and utilize large amounts of personal and environmental

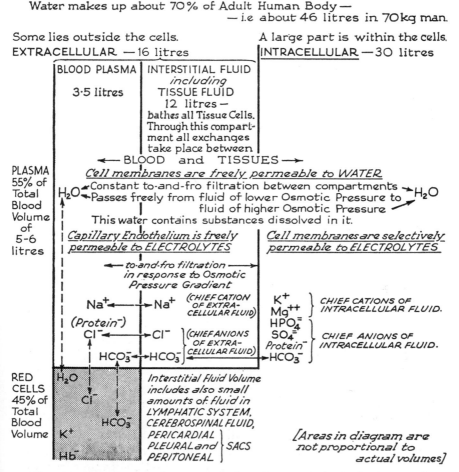

Fig. 6-4. Distribution of water and electrolytes in body fluids. (McNaught, A., and Callander, R.: Illustrated Physiology. Edinburgh, E. & S. Livingstone, Ltd.)

data to get his charges into condition. He depends on information from his assistants, trainer, and the physician as well as his own daily observations to determine the level of conditioning that an athlete has reached.

The weight of the athlete is an important indicator of his physical state. The training room should have a scale, and daily weight records should be kept for each athlete. Weight loss or gain is related to environmental conditions as well as bodily conditions. Therefore, weather facts such as temperature and humidity, as well as the type and severity of the workout, should be noted along with the daily weight record: the coach uses all this information to form an educated opinion of the athlete's state of conditioning.

Fluid and Electrolyte Balance. Maintenance of adequate body fluids and proper balance between extracellular and intracellular fluid volume is a complex concept, often neglected, yet indispensable for an effective conditioning program because it affects weight loss, and the musculoskeletal, cardiorespiratory and neurologic systems. An understanding of these relationships by the coaching and training staffs will reduce the casualties that occur from water, electrolyte, and acid-base disturbances.

Water comprises about 70% of the adult body, i.e. 46 L in a man weighing approximately 154 pounds (70 kg). Obese people have relatively less water than thin people, and their water content may be as low as 45%. Some of this water (extracellular) lies outside the cells, as in blood plasma, and also between the cells (interstitial), and some lies within the cells (intracellular). Dissolved in this water are electrolytes, which are ions that carry an electric charge and are involved in the chemical reactions that occur within the body. In order to function properly, the body must maintain a proper balance in the amount and distribution of water and electrolytes. Homeostatic mechanisms regulate this balance.

About 86 to 90% of weight loss from muscular activity is due to water loss and only about 10 to 15% is from heat and caloric dissipation. The increased heat produced escapes from the body. It is dissipated mainly through the skin and the lungs and a small amount through the kidneys. As the superficial blood vessels dilate, heat is lost from the skin by way of radiation, convection, and conduction, except when the external temperature is high. In addition, the sweat glands excrete a fluid composed mainly of water and salt (perspiration) although it also contains other minerals, including potassium, which is important. Evaporation of perspiration allows cooling of the skin surface. Rapid breathing also allows evaporation of water from the lungs, thus reducing heat. Evaporation cannot take place effectively in a humid atmosphere. Therefore, the water and electrolyte balance is affected by heat, such as that generated by muscular activity, and by the external temperature, humidity, and environment. Reducing the amount of clothing, which tends to insulate body heat, and lessening the physical activity also help to stabilize the body temperature (Figs. 6–5, 6–6).

Losses of water and electrolytes, as occurs in dissipating increased heat, must be compensated by fluid and electrolyte intake. Since heavy perspiration causes a loss of water and salt, both must be replaced. An average adult requires 1500 to 2000 ml of water a day; he needs an additional 500 to 1000 ml to compensate for slight to moderate sweat-

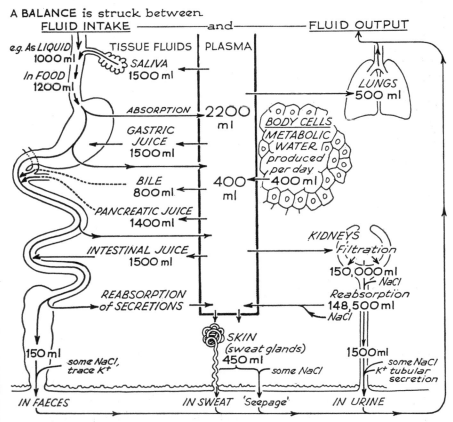

In health the *total amount of body water (and salt)* is kept *reasonably constant* in spite of wide fluctuations in daily intake.

A BALANCE is struck between
FLUID INTAKE ————————and———————— FLUID OUTPUT

e.g. As LIQUID 1000 ml
In FOOD 1200 ml

TISSUE FLUIDS PLASMA
SALIVA 1500 ml

ABSORPTION 2200 ml
GASTRIC JUICE 1500 ml
BILE 800 ml
PANCREATIC JUICE 1400 ml
INTESTINAL JUICE 1500 ml
REABSORPTION of SECRETIONS

LUNGS 500 ml

BODY CELLS (METABOLIC WATER produced per day) 400 ml

400 ml

KIDNEYS Filtration 150,000 ml — NaCl
Reabsorption 148,500 ml — NaCl

150 ml some NaCl, trace K+

SKIN (sweat glands) 450 ml some NaCl

1500 ml some NaCl
K+ tubular secretion

IN FAECES   IN SWEAT 'Seepage'   IN URINE

Except in Growth, Convalescence or Pregnancy, when new tissue is being formed, an INCREASE or DECREASE in INTAKE leads to an appropriate INCREASE or DECREASE in OUTPUT to maintain the BALANCE.

Fig. 6-5. Water balance. (McNaught, A., and Callander, R.: Illustrated Physiology. Edinburgh, E. & S. Livingstone, Ltd.)

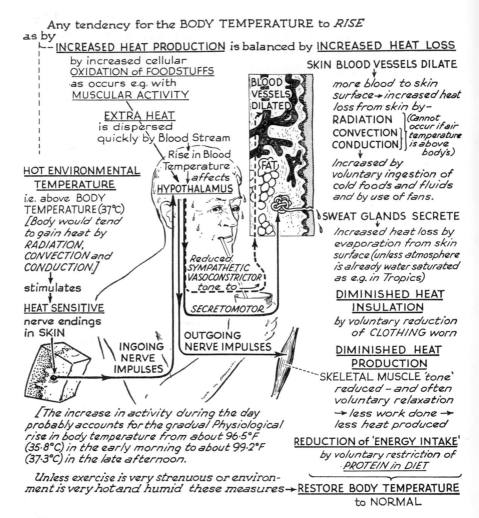

Any tendency for the BODY TEMPERATURE to *RISE*
as by
└ INCREASED HEAT PRODUCTION is balanced by INCREASED HEAT LOSS

by increased cellular
OXIDATION of FOODSTUFFS
as occurs e.g. with
MUSCULAR ACTIVITY

EXTRA HEAT
is dispersed
quickly by Blood Stream

Rise in Blood
Temperature
affects
HYPOTHALAMUS

HOT ENVIRONMENTAL
TEMPERATURE
i.e. above BODY
TEMPERATURE (37°C)
[Body would tend
to gain heat by
RADIATION,
CONVECTION and
CONDUCTION.]

stimulates

HEAT SENSITIVE
nerve endings
in SKIN

Reduced
SYMPATHETIC
VASOCONSTRICTOR
tone to

SECRETOMOTOR

INGOING
NERVE
IMPULSES

OUTGOING
NERVE IMPULSES

BLOOD
VESSELS
DILATED

FAT

SKIN BLOOD VESSELS DILATE

more blood to skin
surface→increased heat
loss from skin by-
RADIATION   (Cannot
CONVECTION   occur if air
CONDUCTION   temperature
                 is above
                 body's)
Increased by
voluntary ingestion of
cold foods and fluids
and by use of fans.

SWEAT GLANDS SECRETE
Increased heat loss by
evaporation from skin
surface (unless atmosphere
is already water saturated
as e.g. in Tropics)

DIMINISHED HEAT
INSULATION
by voluntary reduction
of CLOTHING worn

DIMINISHED HEAT
PRODUCTION
SKELETAL MUSCLE 'tone'
reduced - and often
voluntary relaxation
→ less work done →
less heat produced

REDUCTION of 'ENERGY INTAKE'
by voluntary restriction of
PROTEIN in DIET

[The increase in activity during the day
probably accounts for the gradual Physiological
rise in body temperature from about 96·5°F
(35·8°C) in the early morning to about 99·2°F
(37·3°C) in the late afternoon.

Unless exercise is very strenuous or environ-
ment is very hot and humid these measures→RESTORE BODY TEMPERATURE
to NORMAL

Fig. 6-6. Maintenance of body temperature. (McNaught, A., and Callander, R.: Illustrated Physiology. Edinburgh, E. & S. Livingstone, Ltd.)

ing and anywhere from 1500 to 3000 ml for heavy to severe sweating when playing football on a hot, humid day. A football player may lose 3 to 4 g of salt in addition to other electrolytes daily, under hot, humid playing conditions, that must be replaced to establish electrolyte balance. Many electrolyte replacement solutions available commercially are too concentrated to be beneficial. They need dilution by 1 part electrolyte solution to 2 parts of water. The temperature of the fluid offsets the rate of absorption and therefore, its effectiveness; cooler is better.

Heat Stress. Coaches, trainers, and team physicians must be able to train their athletes to become acclimatized to high temperatures and humidity; they must be able to recognize and cope with conditions of heat stress when they occur.

No one can study the deaths from heat stress as correlated with the climatic conditions for the time and place and type of activity involved without the firm belief that 98% of all such reactions are avoidable. A heat stroke is not a chance proposition like being struck by lightning. It is a predictable phenomenon.

HEAT STROKE. Heat stroke is an acute medical emergency, the onset of which may be sudden or delayed. It requires heroic emergency measures once it appears.

Excessive heat is produced in the body by exercises that cause the body temperature to rise. If a heat balance cannot be obtained by loss of heat to the surroundings because of atmospheric or other reasons, the hypothalamus becomes excessively heated by the rise in blood temperature (Fig. 6–6). The heat-regulating ability of this structure becomes depressed and sweating is diminished.

The athlete may develop an abnormally high rectal temperature (105° to 110° F). Characteristically, he does not sweat despite the high environmental temperature. His face is flushed and his skin is dry and hot because of capillary dilatation. His pulse is elevated and strong, but his breathing is increased and labored. He may complain of weakness, headaches, nausea, and dizziness, and experience convulsions, projectile vomiting, and shock. The absence of sweating despite exposure to high environmental temperature should make one suspect heat stroke rather than heat exhaustion.

Emergency measures designed to reduce the athlete's temperature must be undertaken while preparations are made to transport him to the hospital. Place him in a shady and cool spot. Strip him of all clothing and apply cold compresses to his head. Give him cold sponge baths or place him in a tub of water with ice. Vigorous skin massage of trunk and limbs helps to dissipate body heat. Frequent sips of cool liquid are recommended. However, do not waste time playing doctor on the field or in the dressing room. Get him to a hospital where he can have an air conditioned room, hypothermic blankets, intravenous therapy (intravenous saline solution drip containing 50 mg chlorpromazine repeated every 20 to 30 minutes up to a maximum of 200 mg daily), and a laboratory work-up as quickly as possible.

HEAT EXHAUSTION. In this condition, there is excessive sweating and associated loss of salt in the sweat. Because cell membranes are freely permeable to water and there is constant to-and-fro filtration between compartments (Fig. 6–4), equilibrium is quickly established between the extracellular and intracellular fluids when some of the intracellular water passes into the extracellular by osmosis. However, if there is not adequate fluid and salt replacement, the osmotic pressure of the extracellular fluid is lowered, causing it to flow into the intracellular compartment. This leads to diminished extracellular volume, including plasma volume, and results in a decreased circulating blood volume, decreased venous return, tachycardia, and poor cardiac output leading to a state of shock.

Clinically the athlete complains of fatigue, headache, muscle weakness, and muscle cramps. His face is pale and perspiring; his mouth is dry; the skin of his limbs is cold and clammy; he has absent or collapsing peripheral pulses. The urinary volume is low, as are the sodium and chloride concentrations. Strangely enough, thirst is frequently absent. This condition may go on to nausea, vomiting, diarrhea, and even fainting. Treatment is directed to the replacement of water and electrolytes, especially sodium, to increase the osmotic pressure of the extracellular fluids. Water replacement alone only aggravates the sodium loss. In marked exhaustion, get the athlete to the hospital as soon as possible for clinical and laboratory control.

Athletes, coaches, trainers, and physicians are well aware of the necessity of taking electrolyte supplements during physical activity and liberally salting meals during meal times. Obviously, water replacement alone in the face of mineral depletion would aggravate the latter by further diluting the mineral content of the blood. The need for a proper proportion of minerals and fluids in the form of a drink has become an accepted conclusion. There are a number of broad-spectrum mineral drinks with a relatively high potassium content, along with sodium, chloride, magnesium, zinc, and calcium available.

HEAT CRAMPS. Heat cramps are painful contractions of the voluntary muscles characterized by twitching, cramps, and spasms of the arms, legs, and abdomen. They are caused by a loss of salt and possibly potassium through heavy sweating. High external temperatures are not necessary for their occurrence; any prolonged period of sweating without replacing essential electrolytes, especially salt, might cause them.

Treatment consists of resting and replacing electrolytes, especially sodium chloride and potassium, with an oral solution. Even salt tablets taken orally with water can be irritating to many people, but they are used even though they lack some of the other minerals, particularly potassium. Severe cases might require hospitalization and intravenous administration of normal saline solution. Salt tablets are contraindicated on the field. They are likely to cause undesirable fluid shifts unless taken with appropriate amounts of free water. Heat cramps might be prevented by prior acclimatization, liberal intake of salt with foods, and proper use of an electrolyte solution during activity.

Prevention of Heat Stress. Warm weather, heavy uniforms, and prolonged play without a prior period of acclimatization may lead not only to a loss of weight, but to a loss of life. This is especially true in September football, when all these variables are mixed together indiscriminately. Warm weather induces perspiration, which is further augmented by physical activity. An athlete working out in temperatures of 65° F or less in light gear sweats little if there is little humidity. However, with humidity up to 70% he will perspire much and even chill. If the external temperature goes over 70° F and the humidity remains high, he will sweat significantly. A coach must be watchful in early season workouts when the temperature is above 80° F and the humidity is 50% or more. Prolonged workouts in moderate heat cause excessive perspiration and electrolyte loss. When the water loss is about 2% of the body weight, the athlete develops a thirst. When an athlete loses 6% of his body weight in water loss daily, he develops a marked thirst, dry mouth, and oliguria, and is on the way to heat exhaustion if not promptly treated appropriately with water and electrolytes. Higher percentages of weight loss with accompanying physical weakness, fatigue, mental changes, and others will lead to heat strokes and eventually death, if immediate steps are not taken. These conditions can be prevented if adequate water and electrolytes are available and consumed.

Although the coach is unable to control the weather, he must be able to handle such variables as scheduling and type of workouts, clothing, gear, climate-controlled housing and play areas, and food and drink. In hot weather, the coach must acclimatize his athletes to the heat, to avoid heat stress reactions. Acclimatization, or heat training, causes the following changes in the body:

1. Increased circulation to the skin and dilatation of the blood vessels in the skin.
2. Increased extracellular fluid volume.
3. Increased ability to produce large volumes of dilute sweat. The same degree of exertion produces less of a rise in body temperature and pulse rate compared to the unacclimatized individual.

Acclimatization requires that the athlete work out in the heat, perhaps for an hour the first day, gradually increasing the length and the severity of the practice. Adequate electrolyte and fluid replacement must be maintained. In this manner, an athlete is almost fully acclimatized after 5 to 7 days; full acclimatization occurs after 2 weeks of training. It must be remembered, however, that 50% of this acclimatization may be lost after 1 week if exercise in the heat is stopped, and it disappears completely after 2 weeks without exercise, requiring complete retraining to prevent illness.

Interscholastic and intercollegiate football practices are mandated to practice specified periods of time in early season football to acclimatize the athlete and avoid heat stress reactions. Football players should start off in hot weather with shorts and T shirts only. In hot weather, it may be advisable to schedule practice sessions during the cooler morning and early evening hours. Coaches should be liberal with rest periods, water, and electrolytes during hot weather. While thirst is a good guide for the replacement of fluids for athletes, weight loss per unit of time is more exact.

The coach and trainer should regulate and adjust practices when the temperature and humidity are so great that practicing is dangerous. Two methods have now been developed to determine levels of heat and humidity. A Wet-Bulb Globe Temperature Index (WBGTI), developed by the United States Marine Corps, is calculated from three thermometer readings: (1) a wet bulb thermometer; (2) a dry bulb thermometer, and (3) a black globe thermometer. An apparatus containing these three devices may easily be built, and is placed on the playing field.

The wet bulb is a standard thermometer with the bulb wrapped in a gauze wick that is in contact with a water reservoir. Temperatures recorded by this thermometer reflect the moisture content of the air. A low external moisture content allows evaporation of water from the wick, which lowers the thermometer reading. The dry bulb measures air temperature without being affected by the humidity. The black globe thermometer consists of a standard thermometer with the bulb encased in a copper tank float ball that has been painted with nonreflective flat black paint. This measures the radiant heat from the sun, which may be considerable even on cloudy days.

The heat index (HI) represents the sum of 70% of the wet bulb reading, plus 10% of the dry bulb reading, plus 20% of the black globe reading. For example:

Wet Bulb Reading	$75° \times 0.7 = 52.5$
Dry Bulb Reading	$88° \times 0.1 = 8.8$
Black Globe Reading	$111° \times 0.2 = 22.2$
Heat Index	83.5

The HI may be adapted to guiding football practice as follows:

HI	Precaution
Below 80	None necessary
80 to 85	Cancel drills in full uniform during first weeks of practice (practice in shorts and T-shirts instead). Limited drills in full uniform after heat acclimatization is complete.
85 to 90	Cancel all drills in full uniform. During first week of practice, use indoor sessions.
Above 90	Stop all training. Skull sessions and demonstrations.

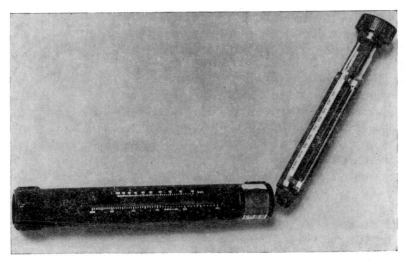

Fig. 6-7. A sling psychrometer. (Courtesy of Cramer Products Inc., Gardner, Kansas)

Calculations of indoor heat are made from 70% of the wet bulb reading plus 30% of the dry bulb reading; the black globe is not used.

The sling psychrometer (Fig. 6–7) is an instrument containing both wet and dry bulb thermometers in a rotating arm attached to a handle; the handle has a built-in slide ruler that correlates the two temperature readings to give the percentage of relative humidity. The rotating arm containing the thermometers is twirled to allow air circulation around the wet bulb thermometer. If over 60° F, the coach should insist that electrolytes and water be available. Below this temperature, use weight loss as a guide as previously determined under similar conditions so that fluids and electrolytes may be replaced accordingly. The following recommendations have been made in reference to football players:

Wet Bulb Temperature	Precautions
Under 60° F	None necessary.
61° to 65° F	Alert observations of all squad members, particularly those who lose considerable weight.
66° to 70° F	Insist that salt and water be given on field.
71° to 75° F	Alter practice schedule to provide rest period every 30 minutes in addition to above precautions.
76° F and higher	Practice postponed or conducted in shorts.

(Whenever the relative humidity is 95% or higher, great precautions should be taken.)

Coaches should use the daily weight of their athletes to prevent heat-stress reactions. For a 188-pound athlete, temperature and humidity could induce a 3% weight loss, which would be over 5 pounds, the upper limit of safety. The athlete would have a 5% weight loss (9 pounds) if he is suffering from frank heat exhaustion, so coaches and trainers take heed.

Overseeing the training program of athletes could be done more scientifically if various laboratory procedures, such as urinalysis, blood volume, electrolytes, and a host of others, could be done on the field. However, on the field and in the gym, the coach, trainer, and team doctor must depend on what they know about the weather, strenuousness of play, and clinical appearance of the athlete to guide them in the training program as well as the prevention of untoward mishaps of heat cramps, heat exhaustion, heat stroke, and water exhaustion. Although the body is fortified with homeostatic regulators, such as antidiuretic hormone and aldosterone as well as electrolyte balances, the athlete himself may undo inborn protective mechanisms and expose himself to a serious disturbance.

On the intercollegiate level with full-time trainers, the Wet Bulb-Globe Temperature Index (WBGTI) is used. The sling psychrometer is also useful for the same purpose at a much lesser expense. When neither the WBGTI nor a sling psychrometer are part of the equipment, the coach should call the local weather station for the humidity index reading. Some locales even have radio stations that give this information in the public interest.

Keeping and Interpreting Weight Charts. The daily use of a training-room scale before and after a workout, and the recording of these weights on a weekly chart marked "in" and "out" for each day will help a coach and his staff to note weight fluctuations and to follow the progress of an athlete's conditioning. Weight charts may also be used to prevent immediate or delayed clinical states of water loss, heat exhaustion, and heat stroke. Also noted daily on the weight chart should be the daily environmental temperature, humidity, and the severity of the workout.

On the first day of practice, the coach instructs the members of the team to record their weight daily before and after a workout wearing the same attire—a genital supporter is sufficient. Systematic, honest recording of weight gain and loss should be done by a trainer or manager if such help is available.

The athlete's daily weight loss will be greatest early in a training program, ranging from 2 to 8 pounds, with the average around 5 pounds. Most of this is water. As the program continues, foodstuffs are oxidized, contributing to the loss of body protein, carbohydrates, and fat depots. A balanced diet provides the athlete with necessary operating calories. The water loss is replaced daily. Eventually, the daily fluctuations on the athlete's weight chart start to level off; at this point he has reached his best weight for maximal efficiency. However, he may still continue to show a daily weight loss owing to sweating, but this weight is regained overnight. The less physically fit an athlete's body is, the longer it takes for him to reach his best playing weight. Obese athletes may take longer than a thin person to reach a satisfactory plateau.

Interpretation of weight records as an index to the level of conditioning requires judgment, experience, and training. If an athlete continues to lose weight beyond his expected leveling-off period, the physician should be suspicious of illness, inadequate diet, emotional problems, drug use, lack of sleep, or other problems. It could also indicate a state of being overtrained, or "stale." The reason should be found and appropriate remedies instituted. In the case of staleness, a vacation or break from the monotony of training for one or two periods is especially therapeutic.

The objective of getting into condition is to achieve maximal physical efficiency for a sport. This entails a loss of excess weight and the development of firm, elastic muscles. If the athlete is overweight, it is necessary to eliminate layers and rolls of fat that result from overeating. This demands hard work and self-discipline. The body gives up stored fats slowly and reluctantly, and this type of weight is the hardest to lose.

A persistent, continuous reduction of an athlete's weight within 1 or 2 weeks by use of a "crash" diet, steam baths, and drugs is easily discernible on a weight chart. Boxers and wrestlers frequently resort to these measures in order to participate in a lighter weight class. It is a dangerous procedure. The use of diuretics by an athlete may have serious consequences. The faking of a weight-loss record when in fact no obvious weight changes appear in the athlete's build is inexcusable. The coach must act quickly to stop these practices. When a squad of players continues to lose weight or displays symptoms such as irritability, sleepiness, nausea, cramps, and cardiac palpitation, the coach may be driving his men too hard or is overemphasizing a game or games. Such coaching practices need review and modification because they are not in the best interest of the team.

The training-room scale is a simple and important mechanical aid that can impart valuable information if used daily and honestly by the athlete and if the coach correlates his knowledge of the athlete and the external factors of the training program. Conclusions drawn from the daily weight record may help prevent fatalities arising from water and electrolyte imbalances. Under no circumstances should a coach or trainer make a medical judgment based on weight-chart records. They should call in the team physician whenever there is any suspicion of an irregularity noted on the weight chart or impending stress to the athlete as a result of the training program, especially when the athlete is subjected to heat stress. Although this is a valuable parameter for athlete surveillance, an institution needs a large staff to implement for effectiveness.

Football

Preseason Conditioning. Many sports allow ample time for proper conditioning after school opens. In football, however, the time available for preliminary training and conditioning is woefully short. Each day taken to develop strength (ruggedness), endurance, and speed reduces the available time for teaching the fundamentals and complexities of the sport. No less than 6 to 8 weeks of conscientious hard work are required to get an athlete into tiptop shape for intensive football competition.

Therefore, the football player must follow a carefully planned program of training that includes spring football when possible, and that is followed during the summer. This enables him to report at the opening of the playing season in good physical trim, and prepares him sufficiently to participate in the strenuous work necessary to develop fundamentals and teamwork within a week after the opening of the training season. A summer exercise and conditioning program will aid in heat acclimatization, so that heat-stress reactions are less likely to occur as the training becomes intensified during the regular season. The more graduated, intensive, and persistent the training routine, the more efficiently the body responds to the increased demands upon it. Preseason conditioning is now being stressed as an absolute necessity to lessen the frequency of serious injuries. It is practically indispensable in football.

Coaching Instructions. As we mentioned in the beginning of this section, running provides an excellent means of building general strength and endurance in order to avoid injuries early in the season that could affect the player for the entire season. Football squads should get extensive practice in running during the early season. Moreover, all participants in contact sports should learn techniques of falling, rolling, and changing speed and direction. Since most shoulder and arm injuries occur when a player falls and strikes the arm or shoulder, football players in particular should learn to fall when tackled by tensing themselves, bringing their arms in close to their bodies, and flexing their heads and bodies into a fetal position.

Most adolescents tend to be "awkward" when they first participate in contact sports in high school. Therefore, they should receive instruction in tumbling, agility, and leg action during preseason practice and throughout the season. Learning proper running techniques helps a player to avoid over-reaching on pivot plays or plays that require abrupt changes in direction. All these methods help to improve coordination, equilibrium, and prevent joint, muscle, and ligament injuries.

At the end of spring football practice, the coach should call a meeting of the varsity players and newcomers to talk about the importance of the team's reporting in good condition at the opening of the following season. He may emphasize the fact that players who do not take time to stay in good condition might have to take time out—i.e., if they go stale or become disabled with injuries—and that their chances of making the team are bettered or worsened by their physical fitness. The coach may also point out that the athletic life of a youth is a rather short one and that he may as well make the most of the span.

Before the departure of the athletes, the coach should obtain their summer addresses. As the summer progresses, the coach should drop them occasional "reminders" (postcards or personal letters) covering pointers noted below. (See Appendix, pp. 301 to 305.)

Helpful Suggestions for Summer Conditioning*

1. Use electrolyte solutions before, during, and after workouts.
2. Loosen up well before doing sprints; stretch the leg muscles.
3. Take good care of your feet. Use plenty of foot powder. Use two pairs of socks; cotton socks next to the skin and a pair of wool socks over these. If you feel a hot spot on your foot, apply petroleum jelly over the area between the two pairs of socks.
4. Do not wait until the last moment to start a balanced diet.
5. Strengthen the muscles of the thigh and foreleg for knee and ankle problems, respectively.
6. Take short sprints to develop speed. Do distance running to develop endurance. Run in circles and figure-eight's to strengthen ankles, knees, hips, and back.
7. Exercise 15 to 30 minutes, depending on your physical condition.
8. Do a general toning up of all muscles with special emphasis on those muscles important in your sport. Do not perform violent or excessive exercises.
9. Take a short rest period between exercises.
10. Do not exercise immediately after a meal or when fatigued.

Players should be warned against going to extremes. Some youngsters are so anxious to make a good showing that they report too "fine," so that the coach has a problem keeping them from going stale when the strenuous workouts start.

Preseason Conditioning Program. This program is designed to get an athlete in excellent physical condition for the practice sessions and the season ahead. Speed, strength, endurance, flexibility, agility, balance, and neuromuscular coordination must be developed.

Most athletes do not know how to condition themselves when they

*To be sent to athletes along with prescribed exercises.

are on their own. The following conditioning program is for high school or college football prospects. This program can be done 6 days a week during the month of July; in August, the tempo should be increased.

The following exercises are included in the preseason program:

Hurdle Position. Sit in hurdle position with left leg forward. Bend trunk forward and touch left foot with both hands. Repeat 10 to 15 times; then extend right leg and repeat 10 to 15 times. This is a great exercise for stretching hamstring muscles; however, it may pose some problems for a heavily muscled linesman.

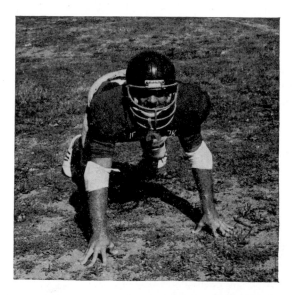

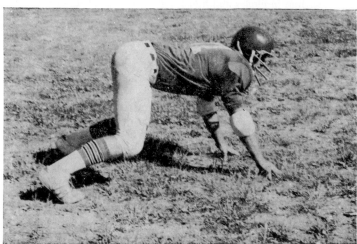

Fig. 6-8.   A, B. Crab position, front and side views.

REACTION DRILLS IN CRAB POSITION. Face down, weight on hands and feet. Move crab-like on command in a forward, backward, and sideward maneuver rapidly about 10 yards. This exercise not only quickens reflex reaction to changing football situations, but enhances agility. It also stretches groin muscles (Fig. 6–8 A,B).

ROCKING CHAIR POSITION. Lie flat on back, bring knees to chest, place hands around shins and rock back and forth 20 times. This exercise stretches the back muscles.

PUSH-UPS. Lie flat on stomach with hands on the ground at sides and near shoulders. Legs are extended and toes pointed. Push down with hands and push body off the ground. Do a series of five pushups in less than 5 seconds. Relax for a couple of seconds and repeat four additional series, totalling five series. This exercise strengthens arm, abdomen, chest, and leg muscles. Two additional series of five pushups can be done using finger tips as support. This latter exercise strengthens the fingers and hands.

CHIN-UPS. Grasp a chinning bar, a cross bar, top of door or a tree limb. Pull your body upward until chin passes bar. Lower your body to complete extension of the arms and repeat six times. This is a good therapeutic exercise following shoulder injuries.

STOMACH DRILL POSITION. Lie flat on back with hands on chest, legs straight together, and toes pointed. Raise feet slowly with a slow count of 10 until the legs are perpendicular to the ground, then lower legs slowly counting from 10 to 1. When the number 1 is reached, the feet should be about 6 inches above the ground. Hold position for the count of 10. Repeat 10 times. This is a good exercise for the abdominal muscles.

CALF-RAISES. Performed on a 2-inch board with toes pointed and heels placed on the ground.

Preseason Football Conditioning Program

Activity	Amount
FIRST WEEK (DAILY)	
1. Rope skipping	5 minutes
2. 440-yard lap (walk, trot, stride)	1
3. Stretch/flexibility exercises	8 to 10 minutes
4. Reaction drills in crab position	8
5. Rocking chair drills	20
6. 25-yard dashes (¾ relaxed running speed)	4
7. 50-yard dashes (¾ relaxed running speed)	3
8. Push-ups (series of 5)	5
9. Chin-ups	6
10. Stomach drills	10
11. 440-yard run	1

SECOND WEEK (DAILY)

1.	Rope skipping	10 minutes
2.	440-yard lap (walk, trot, stride)	1
3.	Stretch/flexibility exercises	8 to 10 minutes
4.	Reaction drills in crab position	10
5.	Rocking chair drills	20
6.	25-yard dashes (¾ speed)	6
7.	50-yard strides (¾ speed)	4
8.	100-yard strides (¾ speed)	1
9.	Push-ups (series of 10 quickly)	3 to 4 reps
10.	Push-ups on finger tips	10
11.	Chin-ups	8
12.	Stomach drills	15
13.	Bench presses at maximal weight (series of 6)	3 reps
14.	Cleans with maximal weight (series of 6)	3 reps
15.	Calf-raises with maximal weight (series of 6)	3 reps
16.	½-mile run (easy ¾ relaxed striding; walk and jog ½ mile to cool down afterwards)	1

THIRD WEEK AND FOURTH WEEK (DAILY)

1.	Rope skipping	15 minutes
2.	660-yard lap (trot, stride, no walking)	1
3.	Stretch/flexibility exercises	8 to 10 minutes
4.	Reaction drills in crab position	15
5.	Rocking chair drills	25
6.	25-yard dashes (¾ speed)*	6
7.	50-yard dashes (¾ speed)*	3
8.	100-yard dash (¾ speed)*	1
9.	Push-ups (series of 10 quickly)	5 reps
10.	Chin-ups	12
11.	Stomach drills	25
12.	Bench presses with maximal weight (series of 6)	3 reps
13.	Cleans with maximal weight (series of 6)	3 reps
14.	Calf-raises with maximal weight (series of 6)	3 reps
15.	Two-hand presses with maximal weight (series of 6)	3 reps
16.	Half-squats with maximal weights resting on shoulders (series of 6)†	3 reps
17.	Power rack exercises, at varying heights and weights	10 to 15 minutes
18.	Weight training exercises	On alternate days
19.	40-yard sprints at maximum speed done 10 times. The interval between sprints is the time to walk 40 yards. Backs are expected to achieve each run within 4 to 5 seconds; linemen, between 4.5 to 5.5 seconds.	1

*May be run with weight spats about the feet.
†Between each series of six half-squats with weights, a series of half-squats without weights are done to help pump the blood out of the legs.

Most running in the games consists of quick, short bursts, and the athlete must condition himself for these. The 20-yard burst is really important, and the first three steps are crucial. The entire preseason program should be repeated until the season begins.

The football player who fails to condition himself during the summer is at a distinct disadvantage when he reports for the season's opening. He soon realizes that he has wasted valuable time that not only impedes his progress, but also makes him vulnerable to injuries. The coach does not have time to wait for the athlete to get into physical condition after reporting for practice or to recuperate if he is injured because he is not in shape. The time between the season's opening and the first game is generally short. The athlete who reports in good physical condition will find that the game of football can be beneficial if he has prepared himself properly for the coming season.

The best criterion for coaches is how fast you can run 40 yards with full uniform. Timing for speed is big with coaches. There is no substitute for speed and power.

Practice Sessions. Because there is no short cut to experience, every practice session counts. In most secondary schools and colleges, there are only 3 to 4 weeks of practice time between the opening of the season and the first game. In this short period, the football coach has the herculean task of getting his team into peak physical condition and teaching them fundamentals, skills, strategies of offense and defense, and protective maneuvers. He must build up a high morale and esprit de corps among his athletes. He knows that although each player has received a written set of exercise instructions to be followed during the summer, the athletes will come back in different states of conditioning, requiring individual attention.

Since early sessions are usually held twice a day until the first game, the coach and his staff must check out each athlete's condition of readiness for the season's rigors by questionnaire and interview. Only in this manner can the coach avoid overtaxing his players, which would set them back and seriously hamper their conditioning program. It is in the early days of the season when the temperature is hot and the players are not yet in shape that coaches can wreck their athletes by being overzealous. Although muscle soreness is to be expected following the first days of practice, working an athlete too hard during the first days may result in a major problem that may seriously hamper the progress of a team, particularly if key players are slowed down by it. Although most athletes usually recover in a few days, valuable time has been lost and their activities limited. Muscle pulls, particularly in the groin and hamstring areas, are also quite frequent among athletes during early season practice; efforts must be made to avoid these troublesome injuries.

As already mentioned, the coach should schedule the practice sessions in the cool hours of the early morning or late afternoon to avoid the hottest hours of the day. Practicing at these times helps to prevent heat-stress reactions and fatigue states, provided the athletes take salt and water as needed. When an athlete tires, the reaction time of his reflexes is slowed down and he is more prone to injuries. Twice-a-day practice sessions should be spaced as far apart as possible. This interval allows the athlete to rest and recuperate, so necessary when maximal efforts are expended. Be liberal with rest periods during a practice session.

Each practice session should begin with 10 minutes of stretch/flexibility and/or agility drills designed to warm up all the major muscle groups and stretch ligaments. Coaches are now relying more heavily on agility drills such as crabouts, carioca drills, monkey rolls, and others of this nature than old-fashioned calisthenics. However, the coach must not overdo or dwell too long on this phase of the program; it hardens muscles and helps to prevent injuries, but does not teach the players anything about football. After the warmup sessions, the athletes should go to their respective groups where specialty coaches teach them football and give them exercises designed to strengthen the muscles associated with their respective positions in the lineup.

Off-season Conditioning. Training is not only a seasonal affair; it should be carried on throughout the year. After the season is over, the athlete should continue exercising to keep his body in good condition. Since he has worked hard to attain top physical condition, he should not stop suddenly. He should follow a program of exercises designed to keep his muscles toned and provide recreation simultaneously. The following activities are good to accomplish such a purpose: badminton, basketball, bicycle riding, bowling, touch football, golf, handball, cross-country running, squash, racquet ball, roller skating, paddleball, swimming, tennis, and just plain walking several miles daily. Weight training is the most important off-season activity; boxing, handball, squash, and tennis are the best agility activities.

Basketball*

Basketball is a team sport with a great deal of body contact. Rule changes have speeded up the game offensively, and increasing emphasis is being placed on using tall, large-sized athletes. These aspects have made the sport increasingly more rugged. Today's well-muscled basketball players move with almost incredible speed and agility and are constantly running into, bumping, pushing, and elbowing their opponents voluntarily and involuntarily. Consequently, basketball players are subjected to tremendous pounding and roughness during a game. The athlete must trim down excess weight and harden flabby muscles to withstand these hazards. A tall player without sufficient muscle mass may not be able to stand the rigors of this sport.

Basketball players are continually running, interspersed with abrupt stops and starts. Basketball is similar to track, in that only by running

*We gratefully acknowledge the assistance of Ernest Vandeweghe—former All-American and "Knick" professional basketball player and presently a pediatrician.

can strong legs and adequate cardiorespiratory endurance be developed. The heart and lungs must reach a degree of efficiency to supply sufficiently oxygenated blood to meet muscular demands and remove waste metabolites. The player with sufficient cardiovascular reserve may be able to put on enough extra pressure in the last 5 minutes of a game to win a close one or ice a near-win. Unless the basketball player does a lot of preseason running conscientiously, he will fatigue easily during the season. Basketball players should follow a running program to aid preseason conditioning. They should run up hills, multiple short sprints including running backwards and angular run to three spots at 10-yard intervals at top speed with another person pointing to the next designated spot is a variation of a running pattern to assist in fitness for basketball. This can be followed by 20 minutes of stretch/flexibility training. Weight spats or sneakers with lead in the soles have been used in running programs in the past.

Spectacular jump shots and rebound efforts place a tremendous strain on the antigravity muscles of the back, hips, and legs. Well-conditioned basketball players exhibit great muscle elasticity and joint flexibility. Jumping ability can be increased by mechanical resistance equipment, but they should be used only under expert supervision. A simple and revolutionary method to improve jumping ability is by jumping in shoulder-height water dipping below the water and exploding straight up in sudden violent contraction without the resistance of weights (water buoyancy). Repeat 10 times in rapid succession. Wrist weights to increase the strength of the arms have been used in the past. The amount of weights can only be determined by experience and experimentation.

Basketball conditioning starts in earnest with the beginning of the fall season, and the player should be thoroughly conditioned when the season opens officially in October. A combination of the following constitutes a sound basis for basketball conditioning program:
1. Running
2. Conditioning drills
3. Flexibility
4. Weight training

The summer conditioning and the preseason exercise programs mentioned for football may also be used by basketball players. Great athletes work on their sport 12 months a year.

Boxing*

Fighting is a natural sport of man. Boxing is an individualistic combative sport that requires courage and skills not possessed by average

*Both Angelo Dundee and Cus D'Amato were consulted in the preparation of this section.

men in the general population. Thus, a thorough toughening process is necessary; boxers spend years hardening their bodies. Blows do not affect them as they would an unprepared male, who no doubt would be easily battered and bruised.

A fighter's legs, along with his endurance, enable him to avoid and to withstand the rigors of this rough sport. His legs must be agile and quite strong; maneuverability helps him to avoid being hit and brings him to his target at the appropriate time. The boxer's legs must be strong enough to "stand up"—in the boxing ring, there are no substitutions or doors. As Joe Louis, former heavyweight champion of the world, once said, "In the ring you can run but you can't hide."

Every muscle from head to toe is developed in the training and conditioning of a boxer. Every fighter needs a different training routine tailored to his particular physical and emotional needs. However, some basic requirements of training are expected of all fighters to prepare them properly for the rugged career they have chosen. Boxing, gym work, roadwork, and mental discipline are essential. Three rounds of boxing are equivalent to ten rounds of gym work. Gym work encompasses small and heavy bag punching, rope jumping, calisthenics, shadow boxing, and wall weight pulleys. Angelo Dundee, trainer of many world champions, doesn't use wall-weight pulleys for his boxers. Cus D'Amato, trainer of two world champions, recommends them, if used properly, because they use muscles used in boxing. However, they are obsolete in most gyms. Generally a boxer must train per day a minimum of double the number of rounds he is scheduled to box.

Punching the small bag aids in speed, rhythm, timing, and coordination of the hands and eyes. The heavy bag helps a fighter to develop leverage to get the most effect from his punches. He practices his various maneuvers and develops muscle control on the bags. A relaxed arm does not hurt anyone; snap, shoulder movements, swiveling of hips, and turning of feet are responsible for the strength of a punch, and these skills can be developed with light- and heavy-bag punching.

To become an excellent boxer, one does not just wake up one morning and decide to be a champ. Boxing is an art that takes years to master. A boxer must be toughened up from childhood, eating simple, nutritious foods, leading a clean, wholesome life, and getting sufficient rest and sleep. To be a boxer, you cannot burn the candle at both ends —you must maintain physical fitness at all times through various types of exercises and calisthenics designed to build the stamina and endurance needed to move in, out, and around your adversary. It is most important to box often in competition before large crowds. A "boxer" might box well in a gym, but get "stage fright" when he hears the roar of a crowd and sees the ring lights, and may lose control of his boxing ability. All the gym work in the world cannot supplant actual boxing.

A workout starts with limbering and loosening up exercises, to get the kinks and stiffness out of the muscles and joints. This takes about two to three rounds. All parts of the musculoskeletal system are put through their ranges of motion, especially the neck, shoulders, trunk, upper and lower extremities. The head and neck are rolled around several times, first in a clockwise and then in a counter-clockwise direction. The shoulder ridge muscles are shrugged and the shoulder joints are put through a range of motion. A few deep knee bends are done. The trunk is rotated in all planes, including a few toe touches and alternate toe touches. The boxer jumps and bounces around in small circles with his hands and arms held high. From this position he throws a few punches as if he were shadow boxing, and then he goes into the shadow boxing routine.

Shadow boxing is done for two to three rounds before a body-size mirror or in the ring. Offensive and defensive moves are planned and executed against an imaginary opponent. Following the shadow boxing, the fighter boxes with a sparring partner for an appropriate number of rounds. Boxers need sparring practice while training. The frequency and number of rounds depends on his state of conditioning. Every new punch or maneuver must be practiced in shadow boxing and with sparring partners. Boxing often with different partners also acquaints the fighters with various styles of boxing and adversaries. Instruction is usually given during round breaks, but occasionally the bout may be stopped to emphasize a point.

The sparring is followed first by heavy-bag punching for a minimum of two rounds to develop leverage, strength, and execution of maneuvers. This is followed with two to three rounds of little-bag punching to develop speed, rhythm, timing, and strength to keep the hands high. Rope skipping is done for about three rounds to develop footwork, coordination, strength and flexibility of arms, wrist, and legs. This exercise keeps the muscles from stiffening up and assists in developing cardiovascular-respiratory endurance. The training session is concluded by floorwork (calisthenics) consisting of exercises to strengthen the abdominal muscles (sit-ups), the neck (bridging), and the legs (bicycling). Dundee eliminates shoulder pushups for his charges. The boxer then dries off and gets a rubdown.

Massages and rubdowns are still an important part of the training program. Massage varies with the size and physique of the fighter, but the rubdown must not be done too vigorously, or else the muscles may go into spasm. Massage reaches those muscles that some exercises miss and loosens up those muscles that may become sore or tighten up from exercise. Heat liniment can be used for some areas, as well as infrared lamps. Each trainer prefers a particular brand or mixture of rubdown material, which ranges from Omega oil, wintergreen, and alcohol to various combinations of these ingredients. These help evaporate the water from the skin giving a cooling effect. Dundee doesn't believe in massages for his young boxers. He says "everything natural is better."

Roadwork helps develop stamina and endurance; it "cleans out the lungs." It is essential for all boxers from the 3-round amateurs to the 15-round professionals. The amount of roadwork depends on the number of rounds of the upcoming bout as well as the importance of the match. Some fighters jog the entire distance. Some fighters break up the roadwork with footwork moving the hands and trunk simultaneously. Roadwork is the best single conditioner in the training program for boxers. This, of course, depends on the boxer's needs and what helps him most.

If a boxer is overweight, water and caloric intake must be counted. He should dress in heavy clothing and be encouraged to sweat. Thin boxers should be dressed in light clothing. The boxer must be weighed every day before and after his workout, to enable the trainer to assess the degree of conditioning. The trainer must keep the boxer at the weight at which he achieves a competitive edge and at which he functions best. The trainer must be able to dry out the fighter without weakening him. Approximately 2 to 3 pounds daily can be lost in the drying-out process. However, if the fighter becomes too drawn or tight, he may be on the verge of going stale, i.e., reaching a state of boredom. At this point, eliminate a day of running or boxing. Two days before a contest, all training is stopped except for light roadwork.

Fight Camps. Many boxers who compete in main events and championship bouts do their training in a fight camp. Although this is the ideal place to train for a bout, fight camps are losing their importance because most fighters cannot afford them. Training starts 4 to 6 weeks before the contest, depending upon when the boxer had his last bout or training period and his state of conditioning. The fighter starts his day by arising between 6:00 and 6:30 A.M. and does 2 to 3 miles of roadwork, which includes sprints, jogging, and various forms of footwork. It is best to run with company.

Following the roadwork, the fighter lies down and rests for 1 to 2 hours until he is completely sweated out. Some trainers rub their fighters down at this time. At 10:00 A.M. he has breakfast, consisting of cereal, three eggs (usually poached), toast, and tea with lemon. He then walks for one half mile and rests again until the afternoon.

Fighters usually do not have lunch. The gym routine starts between 2:00 and 3:00 P.M. The boxer weighs in, and starts with a few rounds of shadow boxing. Six rounds of boxing are done with three fresh sparring partners. If enough sparring partners are not available, the amount of heavy-bag punching is increased. He skips rope for three rounds, followed by a complete floorwork routine. The boxer takes a hot shower, follows with a cold shower, weighs himself, and gets a rub-down by his trainer.

The boxer lies around until dinner time—about 6:00 P.M. Steak, chicken, or lamb chops make up the main fare. Salad and tea with lemon complete the meal. Water and caloric intake is watched if he has to make a certain weight. Following dinner, he takes a walk in the woods or on the road for about 1 hour. He may then write letters, play cards, or see a movie. He goes to bed about 10:00 P.M. The time-honored traditions of wood chopping and sawing have proven too strenuous for modern fighters, and are not even shown today for publicity purposes.

Soccer

Soccer is truly an international sport, being played before crowds of 100,000 and more in stadiums in Latin America, Europe, Asia, Africa, and Australia.

Its international popularity has influenced the tremendous growth of this sport in the United States. This is especially true with the establishment of the North American Soccer League, established in 1971 with international stars such as American-born Kyle Rote, Jr. Over 70,000 people have come to see the Cosmos at Giant Stadium in the Meadowlands with such famous names as Pele, Franz Beckenbauer, Giorgio Chinaglia, and others. The inherent physical, mental, and social factors that have made the game so popular throughout the world have inspired physical educators to include soccer in the physical education curriculum and in interscholastic programs from the grade-school level up through college.

The conditioning of the soccer athlete is similar to that for an athlete who participates in other contact sports that require running, speed, agility, neuromuscular coordination, and endurance. In addition, soccer players must develop the ability to accelerate instantly in forward, backward, and lateral directions. Therefore, the soccer player must develop especially strong legs, ankles, feet, abdominal and neck muscles. Running, running, and more running is necessary. The strong, "educated" feet of a soccer player can only be developed by coordinating the kicking and running skills of the athlete.

The soccer field, stadium, and cross-country terrain may be used to develop the strong legs necessary for soccer players. A practice session starts with 10 minutes of loosening up. This is followed by 10 to 15 minutes of sprint drills on the soccer field. The athletes are encouraged to run around the field any number of times, depending on the condition they are in. Jogging once around the field is followed by an all-out sprint of 30, maximum 50 yards, with and without the ball. Training with the ball should be emphasized. This is followed by a ¾ sprint for

50 yards, another jog, an all-out sprint for 50 yards, and another jog. To avoid the boredom of always sprinting about a soccer field, cross-country running for 2½ to 3 miles, accelerating up the hills and coasting downhill, is substituted. All-out sprinting is encouraged on the flat. Alternate jogging and sprinting may also be done on a large, flat field.

Strength and power in the muscles of the legs can be gained by running up rows of stadium seats in sneakers. The athlete runs up a complete level of about 100 feet at full speed, walks down and runs up again. This exercise is done on a progressive basis until ten ascents can be done. Instant acceleration is also developed by this type of running. Running is done 6 days a week.

Piggy-back races in 25-yard relays aid in developing leg strength. Hurdling 8 to 12 hurdles that are 3 ft., 6 in high aids in agility, stretches back, hip and leg muscles, and develops endurance. Daily bridging and twisting exercises for the neck are necessary to improve heading techniques. Daily exercises for the abdomen are also stressed, such as sit-ups with the soles of the feet flat on the ground.

When practicing, a soccer player should not only run in a forward direction, but must also practice running in reverse and lateral directions. This helps him to recover his position if beaten to it by his opponent; recovery is essential, since failure can be to the opposition's advantage.

Individual skills and game situations are developed next. Work on the weak-side extremities is stressed. Goalies also need training in gymnastics, in addition to the usual skills of soccer players.

Before the start of each game, the players should run onto the field and do short wind sprints in all directions, alternated with jogging, with or without the ball. These should take place in an area of 5 to 10 yards. The timing of the wind sprints and jogging should be approximately 2 to 5 minutes. After this, the players should do "stretch-out" exercises. For example, the player spreads his legs and touches his toes, both in an erect and supine position, turns his head in different directions and jumps up and down, and moves his head up and down practicing head balls. Fifteen minutes of kicking and heading should be practiced before each game. The player should work up a light perspiration just before the start of the game.

The day following the game, relaxing exercises with no physical contact are encouraged, such as groups of four players practicing head balls, trapping the ball, and so forth.

In the winter season, indoor running and exercise should be done at least every other day. Dribbling with short passes should be practiced during these months. Indoor swimming is recommended to increase vital capacity. During the summer, running on sandy shores, hiking, and mountaineering are useful in building up stamina.

The regularity of exercises and running is the key to building of stamina. This sort of intensive program develops agility, speed, strength, neuromuscular coordination and instant acceleration, which are so important for a soccer player.

Swimming

As a sport, swimming provides fun, health, and fitness. It is an excellent therapeutic modality for many musculoskeletal injuries. It also develops a feeling of security in handling oneself in water. Few sports contribute as much as swimming to total-body conditioning by means of strengthening the cardiovascular system, stretching, and coordination techniques. Swimming can build muscular strength, power, and endurance.

During the summer months, the athlete should work on long-distance swimming and exercise in a well-planned and supervised program that will help build arm strength, leg strength, neuromuscular coordination, and increase lung volume.

Cross-country running and the preseason condition guide given for football players may also be recommended for swimmers. It is suggested that the swimmer work on weights during the season to develop his shoulder, arm, and leg strength. Recreational swimming at the beach during the summer months is not sufficient for competitive swimmers, who should train in pools. When the season begins, the athlete should be in such top physical condition for competitive swimming that he could participate in a race if necessary.

General Swimming Training Program*

(This program can be done all through the season.)

A. *Calisthenics*
  1. 55 days
  2. 30-minute sessions
  3. 5 days weekly
B. *Weight Training*
  1. 55 days (Mini-Gym)
  2. 30-minute sessions (Nautilus)
  3. 5 days weekly (Nautilus)
C. *Pulley Work (Light Weights with Repetition)*
  1. From beginning of school to December 1
  2. 15-minute sessions
  3. 3 days weekly
D. *Pull-ups (Chinning)*
  1. 55 days
  2. Maximum each time
  3. 3 times per week
  These should be done about 90% of the time with an overgrasp to bring the back of the neck to the bar. This is done to develop the triceps. The other

*Adapted from the programs used by Dick Steadman, Head Swimming, Diving, and Water Polo Coach, Monmouth College, N.J.

ten per cent of the time, an undergrasp is used to bring the chin to rest on the bar. This develops the biceps.

E. *Running*
   1. 1 month
   2. 1 mile distance
   3. 3 times per week

F. *Water Work (Swimming, Kicking, and Pulling)*
   1. From beginning of school to December 1
   2. 1 hour daily
   3. 5 days practice per week

G. *Workout Procedures*
   1. Swim all distances with repeated swims at varied intervals of 25, 50, 75, 100, 125, 200, 500, 1,000 and 1,650 yards.
   2. General guidelines for total distance per daily workout are as follows:
      Sprinters—4,000 to 6,000 yards daily
      Middle distance—6,000 to 8,000 yards daily
      Distance—10,000 to 12,000 yards daily

These are done in two sessions. The swimmer sets up his own daily schedule and uses those distances that suit him best, varying them daily to improve his performance. Success is spelled w-o-r-k. Whenever in doubt, swim more distances.

Tennis*

Tennis has always appealed to both sexes, both young and old. Although it is more of a participant's sport than a spectator's sport, it is an exciting game to watch when played by top-ranking performers.

The conditioning of the athlete is similar to that of an athlete who participates in any other sport that requires running. Speed, agility, neuromuscular coordination, and endurance must be developed to play a good game of tennis. One must have strong legs; cross-country running and bicycle riding are excellent ways to condition the leg muscles. Special attention in performing calisthenic exercises should be placed on strengthening the ankle, knee, wrist, arm, and shoulder joints.

In order to keep the feet from getting sore and blistering, the player should wear two pairs of socks, especially when playing on hard courts such as asphalt, cement, composition, or wood. Playing during the summer months is an ideal way to condition the body and improve the tennis game.

Track and Field

Since the publication of the first edition of this book, the most significant change in track is the increasing number of females going into these events as competitors and coaches, the use of the coordinated staff of coaches and the change from the English to the metric system. Traditionally, men coached male and female track athletes, although there have always been a number of female coaches who coached fe-

*More information about tennis appears in Chapter 9.

male athletes. However, with increasing numbers of women going into coaching, the philosophy of the coordinated staff is now being employed; here the coach, regardless of gender, will coach athletes of both sexes depending, of course, on what specific talent the coach has to offer. This is an efficient way of utilizing coaching talents maximally for the benefit of the athlete. Although female athletes have traditionally accepted male coaches, the reverse is not true, but attitudes are changing. More time is necessary to effect this change. Therefore, it behooves coaches who train female athletes to be conversant with those problems attendant with the breast, menarche, and conception. Although the coach must be able to speak with some degree of understanding about these matters, the right of privacy of the athlete must always be respected, and the coach must be able to refer the troubled athlete to the proper physician.

Track and field is a demanding sport that requires speed, endurance, and strength. This requires strict adherence to a training and conditioning program so a constant output of energy over a certain period of time can be generated and maintained. Such conditioning requires that the athlete progressively push his body to the limits of exhaustion and fatigue, learn to tolerate the pain and discomfort resulting from such training to a safe level, and expect full recovery when the event is over. Conditioning is essential because events can be won and lost as a result of it.

In track, the athletes must be in the right frame of mind for the task ahead. Above all, athletes must believe in themselves and in the coach and trainer and be willing to pay the price to get into proper condition through the vigorous training schedule outlined.

The coach and trainer must understand and be aware that their athlete will be nervous before the meet and especially the event. Applying the right motivation is crucial for a coach in readying the athlete for an event. The wrong motivation can be as unrewarding as lack of proper conditioning. The coach and trainer must know the individual personalities of their athletes, which comes only from experience with athletes. The coach must also be patient.

Most of the general training and conditioning techniques stated in the first edition of this book are still valid. For instance, the first few weeks of practice employ conditioning techniques such as cross-country running, easy jogging, interval training, and warm-up including stretching/flexibility exercises that relax the ankle, knee, and hip joints, and the adjoining musculature. During the first month, endurance, speed, and distance are progressively increased. By this time, exercises should include rhythmic jumping on both feet to develop flexor and extensor muscles that control bending of the hips, knees, and ankles. Every athlete should have some background in distance work.

It will serve him well in competition. In distance work, endurance and stamina are developed with distance rather than speed.

The following are applicable for sprinters, hurdlers, and middle-distance runners:

1. *Jogging.* Jogging is important in beginning warm-ups and conditioning. Mixing striding and walking over a distance is better than jogging all the way.
2. *Warm-Up.* Warm-up is important before practice and before participation in different competitive track events. A runner is not ready for hard work until the athlete has thoroughly warmed-up.
3. *Starts.* In similar, although augmented fashion, reaction time and training are essential to good starting. The start is the most important part of racing.
   a. "On your marks." Starting blocks should be used for all sprint starts. The runner takes a place on the starting line. Before the runner gets on his mark, he should take three deep breaths and think of reaching the finish line first. The runner must be completely relaxed when the command "On your marks" is given.
   b. "Get set." The hips are elevated according to which start is used. This position should make the back level and thrust the weight forward. The runner is now ready for the gun. A faster reaction to the gun will be made if the runner reacts to the gun automatically.
   c. "Go." The runner should aim for quick action of the right foot (keep it as close to the ground as possible), fast hand and arm movements, and tremendous push from the left foot. The runner should keep in mind that the legs will go only as fast as the arms. Therefore, the sooner the arms get going, the faster the legs will go. The focus of the eyes rises to a point further down the track. The runner must strengthen up gradually as the runner races down the track.
   d. The Finish. The body should be pressed forward. The head should be well forward. The eyes should be kept straight ahead. Maintain proper running form. Keep the speed until 5 yards beyond the finish line and slow down gradually after passing the finish line.

General Fall Conditioning Program for Track*

Sprinters and Hurdlers†

Activity	Amount
MONDAY	
1. Cross country‡	4–5 miles
2. 400 meters at intervals	¾ speed, 3 minutes, 3 times
TUESDAY	
1. Cross country	
2. Weight-training program for legs and arms	¾ hour

*This program was adapted from the program used by Jay Dakelman, Head Football and Track Coach, Highland Park High School, Highland Park, New Jersey, voted no. 1 in both of these coaching categories in 1977.

†All athletes must record body weight daily before and after practice.

‡Where straight runs of any considerable distance are outlined, hurdlers may incorporate a hurdling technique with interval training rather than a long run. All hurdlers' workouts are preceded with a warm-up period including stretching/flexibility exercises.

WEDNESDAY

1. 400 meters at intervals   ¾ speed, 5 times
2. 100 meters at intervals   ⅞ speed, 6 times,
                                                             preferably on grass

3. Rest period for 5 minutes
4. Ten starts

THURSDAY

1. Cross country
2. 100 meters at intervals, running almost at   5 times
   maximum speed
3. 75 meters at full speed   5 times
4. 55 meters at intervals   ¾ speed, 5 times
5. If time is available, some additional workout on
   weights

FRIDAY

1. Fartlek running (run, walk, and jog for fun)   20 minutes
2. Baton passing, preferably on grass   20 minutes
3. 400 meters at intervals, 3 minutes rest   3 times
4. Sprinters will do their straight away running;
   hurdlers need only do 200 meters

SATURDAY

1. Cross country
2. 300 meters at intervals   3-minute intervals,
                                                             5 times
3. 150 meters at intervals   3 times
4. 100 meters at intervals   3 times
5. Work on 6–8 starts (hurdler's work on starts is
   to his first hurdle). It is important for the hurdler to use precisely the exact number of steps to
   get to his hurdle. His steps, and the number of
   them, are very important to his performance.

SUNDAY

1. Cross country

All cross-country runs are from 4 to 5 miles and the routes are of the athlete's own choosing. They are varied to keep the workout from becoming boring, dull, and monotonous and are usually done after school.

Weight-training programs vary with the philosophy of the coach and the available equipment. Some coaches do it daily, others on alternate days, but generally, arms and legs are done on different days. Regardless of the philosophy of the coach, weight training must be done throughout the season if the athletes are to benefit from it.

Middle-Distance Runners

MONDAY

1. Cross country   4–5 miles
2. 600 meter at intervals   ⅞ speed, 2 times,
                                                             3-minute intervals
3. 200 meter   ⅞ speed, 3 times,
                                                             3-minute intervals
4. Weight training

TUESDAY
1. Cross country   4–5 miles
2. Weight training

WEDNESDAY
1. Repeat Monday's schedule
2. 100 meters at intervals at top speed   4 times

THURSDAY
1. Cross country
2. 500 meters at intervals at full speed   3 times
3. 200 meters   ¾ speed, 3 times

FRIDAY
1. 500 meters at intervals   ¾ speed for form,
                                                            5 times
2. 800 meters   ¾ speed
3. Cross country   4–5 miles

SATURDAY
1. 300 meters at intervals   ¾ speed, 6 times
2. 3 interval runs with 3 minutes rest then a 10-
   minute rest period; follow up with 3 more interval runs

SUNDAY
1. Cross country on your own

*Preseason Conditioning for Competitive Distance Runners Including
Cross Country, 3000 and 5000 meters*

MONDAY
1. Easy over distance depends on condition of   6–10 miles
   athlete
2. Upper-body weight training

TUESDAY
1. Repeat 800 meters   ¾ speed,
                                                            10 times
2. 100 meter easy striding   10 times
3. 800 meter jog to warm down   1 time
4. Lower body-abdomen weight training

WEDNESDAY
1. Over distance with change of pace every 800   8 miles
   meters; go slow to fast, fast to slow
2. Repeat 100 meters with acceleration   10 times
3. Upper-body weight training

THURSDAY
1. Repeat 3000 meters with 10-minute rest period   5 times
   between
2. Striding 100 meters   12 times
3. Lower-body weight training

FRIDAY
1. Easy over distance   6–10 miles
2. Upper-body weight training

SATURDAY   (Hard workout)
1. Repeat Tuesday

SUNDAY
1. Easy 4-mile cross-country run

Shot Put and Discus*
MONDAY

1. Jog	4 laps
2. Exercise-warmup	½ hour
3. 55-meter dash, 55-meter sprints	20–30 minutes
4. Throw shot or discus from place in succession	8 throws
5. Toss shot or discus—using techniques	20–30 minutes
6. Weight lifting for shoulders, arms, legs	

TUESDAY
1 through 5. Same as Monday
6. Practice turning in the circle with the shot or discus in hand for technique (strap discus to hand)
7. Weight lifting

WEDNESDAY
1 through 6. Same as Monday

THURSDAY
1 through 7. Same as Tuesday

FRIDAY
1. Throw shot for distance
2. Work on turns in circle
3. Weight lifting for shoulders, arms, and legs

SATURDAY
1. Work on movement in the circle
2. Practice for distance

Long Jumpers
MONDAY

1. Jog	2 laps
2. Warmup exercises	½ hour
3. Run wind sprints, 100 and 300 meters	15 minutes
4. Jump hurdles for height practice	
5. Practice high jump	
6. Jog to warm down	2 laps
7. Weight training	

TUESDAY
1 through 7. Same as Monday

WEDNESDAY
1 through 6. Same as Monday
7. Work on measurements of steps

THURSDAY

1. Practice on runway with hurdles at the beginning of the jump pit	
2. Run sprints 100 meters	6–8 times

FRIDAY
1. Compete with other long jumpers

SATURDAY
1. Practice steps
2. Practice height with hurdle

High Jumpers

MONDAY

1. Jog		2 laps
2. Warmup exercises		15 minutes
3. Practice jumping exercises		10 minutes
4. 400 meters		1 lap
5. Practice on high-jump bar		
6. Weight training		

TUESDAY

1   through   6.   Same as Monday

WEDNESDAY

1   through   6.   Same as Monday
7. Measure steps

THURSDAY

1. Warm up		
2. Practice for height		
3. 400-meter dash		1 lap

FRIDAY

1. Compete with other high jumpers

SATURDAY

1. Practice the actual jump
2. Measure steps
3. Weight training

Pole Vaulters

MONDAY

1. Jog		1 lap
2. Exercise		½ hour
3. 100-meter dashes, keeping knees raised high, sprint		1 time
4. Practice hand-stands		
5. Practice jumping a hurdle and the high-jump bar		
6. Pull-ups		until exhausted
7. Swimming and diving		
8. Wrestling, rope climbing stunts, and tumbling		
9. Rebound tumbling		
10. Stair-climbing on hands		
11. Trampoline		
12. Run with pole in hand		1 lap
13. Weight training		

TUESDAY

1   through   12.   Same as Monday

WEDNESDAY

1   through   12.   Same as Monday
13. Get steps on approach

THURSDAY

1   through   13.   Same as Wednesday

FRIDAY

1. Work with other vaulters over bar		
2. Run with pole in hand		1 lap

SATURDAY

1. Work on steps to the bar with pole in hand		
2. Run with pole in hand		1 lap

Since the first edition, the progress made by our female track-and-field athletes has been extraordinary and bodes well for future international competition. Women should be encouraged to wear supportive, custom-made bras as well as other appropriate, protective equipment for the sport.

When a female athlete complains of menstrual pain, menstrual irregularity, or other gynecologic symptoms, the coach should refer the athlete to her personal physician (see Chap. 1).

Baseball*

When winter is on the wane and the baseball season is not far off, an urge to play baseball grips many athletes. Professionals go off to training camps conducted by the major league clubs; here they train vigorously for 6 to 8 weeks to get into condition for a rigorous season of approximately 200 ball games of which 162 are regulation. The sunny climes of Florida, California, and Arizona are a welcome relief from the wet, cold, snowy weather of winter and are conducive to getting in shape.

The majority of the baseball aspirants in high school and college are not blessed with such ideal training weather and have a much shorter time to get in condition for 15 to 30 games of the season, which generally begin in early April and finish in May or early June. Regardless of the sponsorship and the variations accorded to players by virtue of the position they play, certain fundamental training and conditioning practices are used by most managers, coaches, and trainers for all baseball athletes. Notwithstanding the tremendous press coverage devoted to the throwing arms of pitchers, catchers, and fielders, and to the batting power of hitters, strengthening the legs, developing flexibility, aerobic and anaerobic power have primary importance in the conditioning program. As veteran managers and coaches state it, "get the legs and lungs in shape and the arms will come around." Conditioning also improves agility, timing, speed of foot, reflexive movements, and eye-hand-ball coordination.

The foundation upon which conditioning in baseball is built is running; this applies to all baseball players regardless of the position they play. It is best accomplished by running a prescribed number of laps as well as by wind sprints of varying lengths in the early weeks of training. Some managers run their athletes up to 2½ and perhaps 3 miles daily. As part of the running program, fielders shag flies in the outfield, participate in infield drills, run and slide into bases. A conditioned young ballplayer should be able to run from home plate to first base in about four seconds. As the ballplayer ages, it may take him 5 or 5½ seconds to run the same distance.

*We gratefully acknowledge the assistance of Willie Klein, Sports Editor, *Newark Star Ledger*, in the preparation of this section.

During the competitive season, most of the ballplayers, except the pitchers, get enough daily work to keep them in condition. It is between seasons that many ballplayers get woefully out of shape. If a baseball player can run a specified distance either cross-country, in a gymnasium, or in a park, he could keep some balance of condition. Swimming and bicycle riding would benefit him as well. If he could also play some handball, volleyball, squash, racquetball, and basketball, he could arrive at training camp reasonably physically fit. A surprisingly large number of professional players conduct their winter fitness programs and report to training camp in near "ready-to-go" condition. To do otherwise, they would risk their jobs. On the other hand, there are just as many top baseball players who go on "rubber-chicken" circuit.

In addition to running, the surest and most reliable method of getting these muscles in condition is static stretching exercises. These exercises are performed to stretch the ligaments and adjoining muscles of the larger joints, such as the shoulder, back, hips, knees, and ankles, in an effort to make the ballplayer supple and loose. Emphasis is then placed on those special exercise routines that stress bending of the trunk, throwing, and running. These are necessary physical attributes of a successful ballplayer who moves frequently in quick, graceful, fluid motion. One has only to bring to mind a spectacular fielding of a sharply hit ground ball by the shortstop as he flips or throws the ball for a double play or a put-out. Many of these activities are done in a manner to simulate actual baseball moves. These bending and stretching routines are best done in a group for 15 minutes at the beginning of each practice session and are varied to prevent monotony and boredom. They are continued until the player is quite loose and limber, and his stamina is improved. Usually the player enjoys increased physical well being. The feeling of suppleness can be maintained by engaging in games of pepper.

Players generally combine flexibility and conditioning exercises, and light throwing from the start of training. As the player's muscles become stronger and his stamina improves, he progressively throws the ball harder. After a ballplayer has reached a maximal level of conditioning, he should throw the baseball hard only after his arm has been sufficiently warmed up. The length of the warmup varies with each player. Although the optimum warmup time is still a matter of research, we know empirically that some ballplayers require just a few pitches and some may need as much as 10 to 15 minutes at varying paces. Each player knows when he is ready, usually when his arms and shoulders feel loose.

Weight work has now become an accepted method of preparing players for a season of baseball. For years, professional baseball pitchers have strengthened the muscles of forearms, wrists, hands, and fingers by squeezing hard rubber balls on and off the field. Babe Ruth developed calluses on his hands by gripping the handle of his bat as hard as he could in an effort to hit home runs. He said, "When I am after a homer I try to make mush of this solid ash handle." His calluses explain his home-run records. Most hitters now wear hand gloves to prevent calluses. Now more scientific methods are used to develop muscle strength (isokinetic apparatuses are the most popular).

The time devoted to baseball is divided into a preseason and competitive season. The preseason weather of March in most locales is hardly fit for outdoor training for high school and college teams, so the program begins in a gymnasium with the athletes wearing sneakers. Indoor sessions should last no more than 1 and 1½ hours and should be evenly divided between running exercises, light throwing exercises, light batting with a hard rubber ball and/or batting machines, infield drills, and teaching of skills. Running should include a prescribed number of laps around the gym floor and 10- and 20-yard sprints. Some weight work can also be incorporated in the preseason conditioning program.

As soon as the weather permits, the baseball aspirants are taken outdoors, where the same fundamental conditioning practices are continued. However, more time is devoted to batting. Playing pepper makes the players bend and become more agile and sharpens their reflexes. Fielders shag flies in the outfield, run and slide into bases. Infield drills are continued. Players become conditioned by gradually increasing the amount of play associated with their position. Athletes who have used sneakers in the gym must now change over to spikes; this should be a gradual process to get the feet and legs accustomed to the change and to prevent blisters. Drills for teaching fundamentals of the various positions may be modified to assist in achieving top condition, e.g., drills that stress running for pitchers and outfielders are used. A specific number of laps around the field as well as some wind sprints ranging from home to first base; first to second; first to third, and from second base to home plate. Pitchers should do their running near the end of the practice session. The other ballplayers may do their running at the beginning, during, or at the end of the practice.

The Pitcher. The conditioning and care of the pitcher's arm differs from the care extended to other ballplayers. Since the effectiveness of a pitcher may amount to 60 to 70% of his team's defense, it is understandable why pitchers merit more attention than other ballplayers. In a professional baseball game, the pitcher is physically the most active man on the team. He delivers as many as 150 or more pitches during the course of a game, and perhaps 50 to 70 in warming up. One has only to watch a pitcher to appreciate the tremendous total bodily effort that goes into each delivery; he may lose up to 9 pounds in a game. In the early days of the live ball, the pitcher was at a disadvantage against hitters like Babe Ruth, Lou Gehrig, Ted Williams, Johnny Mize, Mickey Mantle, Hank Aaron, and others; he had to bear down on each pitch in an effort to get it past the batter. Today the pitcher is better able to control the aggressive efforts of the batters such as Reggie Jackson, Chris Chambliss, Rod Carew, Pete Rose, Mike Schmidt, Carl Yastremski, George Brett, or Craig Nettles. The pitchers are coming up with more no-hitters, shut-outs, and generally reducing the batting averages and home run records of the baseball players. They do it with blazing fast balls, curves, screw balls, sliders, and other breaking stuff at their command. These unnatural motions in pitching, plus the tremendous braking forces to the momentum of the follow-through, put great strain on the shoulder, arm, and elbow and may cause abnormal clinical conditions at these sites.

Differences in training begin in the preseason program. In professional baseball, the pitchers and catchers go to camp about 5 to 10 days before the regular squad. This gives the pitchers an opportunity to get their legs and arms in condition before the remainder of the squad arrives. While the legs are getting into shape, the pitchers are gradually strengthening their arms, at first by light throwing to the catchers. As the arms unlimber from a winter sleep, they can throw harder or spin depending on the individual's progress. Premature spinning of the ball can injure an arm unless it is in excellent shape; it takes a minimum of 2 weeks of conditioning to reach this stage. Many trainers with professional baseball clubs like to stretch the muscles of the shoulders, arms, back, and legs of the pitchers before they go on the field and start throwing so they can more easliy bend down and follow through. These parts of the body must be made strong as well as loose. In some camps, the same result is accomplished by 15 minutes of calisthenics at the beginning of each session. Some of these exercises simulate game situations. Pitchers then follow up with pepper to improve bending, agility, and reflex action. After the remainder of the squad shows up, the pitcher is called on to pitch in batting practice.

Although a certain amount of stiffness, soreness, and discomfort is expected before the arm is fully conditioned, hard throwing in the early days of camp will lead to an unusual amount of pain and soreness that will not respond to rest, heat, massage, or gentle passive stretching. A pitcher must be cautioned against allowing this to happen since it may also lead to tight, sore arms and shoulders. If it does happen, the following procedure is recommended: The sore arm to above the shoulder is placed in a whirlpool bath at 105 to 110° F for 5 minutes. After the arm is removed, a cold wet towel is placed about it, and the arm is massaged through the towel for one minute. The athlete is then placed on the table on his back. The wrist of the affected arm is grasped by the trainer and the player's arm is flexed forward in the anterior sagittal plane from 0° to 180°. Slow, steady traction is exerted by the trainer's hand. The trainer then takes his other hand and places it on the upper edge of the scapula; his fingers grip the shoulder-ridge muscles and extend to the supraclavicular area. The elevated arm is then drawn to the side of the thorax while a slow, steady pull is still exerted on the arm. Some trainers combine these exercises with adduction of the arm across the body towards the other shoulder and with rotary movements of the arm at the shoulder. This procedure passively stretches and relaxes the tight muscles about the arm, shoulder, and shoulder blade. The maneuver is applied for 1 minute and usually causes these muscles to relax. If the trainer feels a point of resistance accompanied by pain during this manipulation, additional traction with a quick jerk of the arm is applied. This usually releases the tightness. Then the arm is returned to its neutral position. If relief (looseness or loss of kink) is accomplished, the maneuver need not be repeated; if only some relief is afforded, it may be repeated 2 or 3 times. Catfish Hunter's shoulder was salvaged into a winning season after manipulation under general anesthesia by Dr. Maurice Cowan, former Yankee baseball team doctor.

When a player is scheduled to pitch, the trainer should immerse the pitcher's arm to above the shoulder in a whirlpool at 105–110° F for 5 minutes a half hour before game time. Following removal from the whirlpool, a cold wet towel is placed about the entire arm to close the pores, and the arm is massaged with the towel in place for about one minute. The athlete puts on his uniform to maintain the heat and protect the arm and shoulder from the cold. This kind of pregame care improves the muscle tone of the arm and makes arm movements easier and more effective. A pitcher must be warmed up well and feel loose before a pitching stint. The importance of keeping a pitcher's arm warm when he is not using it cannot be overemphasized. It may seem old-fashioned to expect the pitcher to wear a long-sleeved undershirt and jacket between innings or when he gets on base, especially in hot or warm weather, but it is an effective practice, necessary to protect his arm from cool or cold air.

If a pitcher has warmed up sufficiently to become loose and perspire, but is not going to be the game pitcher, he should change to a dry sweat shirt. After pitching, it is good to sit around the dressing room and cool off in a dry sweat shirt. Some pitchers like to have their arm "milked" after a game: the arm is held elevated and the blood is drained from the finger tips towards the shoulder. The trainer facilitates this drainage by "milking" the arm with his hands; this increases the venous and lymphatic circulation and reduces swelling. It is also recommended that the trainer ice massage the pitching arm for 15 minutes prior to showering. This technique rids the pitcher of the heavy feeling in his arm following a pitching stint, although some pitchers and trainers prefer only a massage following a game.

Most ballplayers, managers, coaches, physicians, and trainers agree that a conditioning program based on the general outlines discussed here will ready all ballplayers for a season of play and prevent sore or pulled muscles.

Wrestling

Although great muscular strength is desirable in a wrestler, he must also develop cardiovascular and respiratory endurance, as well as timing, balance, agility, flexibility, and coordination. A wrestler can reach top condition by strictly adhering to a program that includes running, calisthenics, weight training, fundamental wrestling techniques, and actual competitive wrestling. Proper nutrition and diet play a significant part in this program. Superb physical condition is absolutely essential for success in wrestling.

A coach should begin training under the assumption that no one on his squad has worked out since the final wrestling practice of the preceding year. Wrestlers should not be hurried in the first few weeks of formal practice. Some coaches make the mistake of starting the first practice sessions as though the athletes are well-conditioned—this causes pain, pulled muscles, and other injuries that may plague a wrestler for much of the season.

The conditioning program should be a gradual one. The early practice sessions should be adequate to challenge those who are going to participate, yet not so strenuous that the athletes suffer extreme exhaustion and contemplate leaving the squad. Many fine, potential wrestlers are lost in this "washing out" period before they have an opportunity to develop their abilities. The first few weeks should be devoted to conditioning the cardiovascular and respiratory systems and developing muscle strength, flexibility, balance, timing, agility, and coordination. The practice session should be long enough to include a warmup period of stretching, calisthenics, conditioning drills, instructional period, drilling of moves, and actual competitive wrestling. Of course, the routine should be changed occasionally to allow a change of pace, which will renew the team's interest in the conditioning program.

Daily running is necessary to strengthen the wrestler's cardiovascular and respiratory endurance. Running distances range from one-half to one mile during the first and second weeks of training. If a track is available, the athlete runs one lap at top speed and jogs one lap at half speed. The running distance is increased to two miles or more depending on the athlete's response and the coach's conditioning practices. Usually, if the athlete experiences some difficulty, he continues on the one-half to one mile course until he can run it easily. Some coaches recommend running for 15 minutes before practice without regard to the number of laps circled. Whether or not daily running is encouraged depends on the training program established by the coach. We recommend daily running throughout the wrestling season because it maintains the condition of the athlete and keeps the legs strong. Running up and down stairwells during inclement weather provides an alternative and serves the purpose of developing wind along with leg strength. Running keeps the body loose, but coaches recommend that the athletes loosen up before running to avoid muscle pulls.

The development of strength in the muscles of the neck, shoulders, chest, arms, back, trunk, abdomen, hips, thighs, and legs is important in the training and conditioning of a wrestler. This can be achieved by overloading the muscles of these regions by conventional, buddy, and other types of exercises, either done individually or as part of a circuit drill. Eight to 12 of these exercises are done daily for 35 to 45 minutes during the first month of the season. As the conditioning program progresses, these muscles are progressively overloaded by increasing the number and severity of the exercises. Conventional exercises, such as front and back neck bridging and sit-ups for abdominal and hip muscles, push-ups for chest and shoulder muscles, and back-jacks for back muscles, are all excellent muscle strengtheners. In addition, stretch exercises are designed to loosen up the muscles of the limbs, trunk, back, groin, and abdomen; they are extremely important and must be stressed because they prevent muscle pulls. Many wrestlers are lost for a good portion of the season because of neck injuries or pulled hamstring or back muscles, which could have been prevented with proper training and conditioning. Some buddy exercises include floating, in which each wrestler floats with a partner in each position usually for 1 or more minutes; and two-man stand-ups, in which a partner is draped over the shoulders of his buddy.

When the wrestlers are fairly well-conditioned, many coaches reduce the calisthenics' period to about 20 minutes. Ten minutes of stretching and calisthenics seem to be the ideal combination to prepare for practice once the season gets underway. These exercises should not cause strain or tiring and should be organized to work several muscles at one time. Calisthenics should help build agility, conditioning, and endurance. Exercise drills should produce coordination, balance, timing, and precision in the execution of holds. Spinning, floating, and other innovations of the coach may be used at this time.

Calisthenics should be followed by an instructional period, in which experienced wrestlers assist the neophytes with holds and moves. This

5

is the testing period before actual competition. In actual competition, some coaches usually have a wrestler go 9 minutes. However, some prefer multiple short shots of wrestling, in which the wrestlers start from a referee's position and wrestle hard for periods of 10 to 15 seconds with a 2- to 3-minute interval, with the wrestlers changing positions at the end of each wrestling period. The number of competitive periods depends upon the time element, available space, and level of conditioning sought. Before securing the wrestling room for the evening, the wrestlers should have a final round of calisthenics and some running. A coach should change the practice routine occasionally to avoid team boredom.

The workouts should be challenging even to the most conditioned wrestler on the squad. The workout the day before a wrestling meet should be one that will get the wrestlers loose and break a sweat. It should not be long and tedious; we have found that wrestlers do not operate effectively the next day in a varsity match if they have had a grueling weight-losing session the previous day.

The coach should discourage excessive weight reduction. Most physicians recommend a maximal weight loss of 5%. Many wrestlers believe that the lower the weight class in which they participate, the better their chances for success. This might be true in some cases; however, the athlete can lose too much weight, suffer illness, and lose strength.

The coach should check the weight of his wrestlers daily before and after practice. If one of his wrestlers is several pounds over his weight class the day of the match, he should not be permitted to lose the excess weight in the gym, during study halls, or physical education classes. In many cases, a wrestler who loses 4 pounds between 9:30 A.M. and 4:00 P.M. is weak and will not perform up to his ability. Most wrestlers normally lose 1 to 2 pounds during the day in calorie metabolism and the natural process of elimination.

Once the season is over, many wrestlers gain too much weight. The athletes should be encouraged to participate in other sports, e.g., football, cross-country, track, and soccer. This helps keep their weight down and provides conditioning. Those who participate only in wrestling should be encouraged to work out on their own in the off-season. Weight training and running should be encouraged, and the coach should assist in establishing a positive weight program. For example, the athlete could lift weights on Monday, Wednesday, and Friday, and run, play basketball or handball on Tuesday and Thursday. However, some time must be taken off. A holiday away from home base will break the monotony, but at the end of the holiday the athlete must return to his workout program.

It takes a well-conditioned wrestler to perform effectively. Proper dieting, social activities, and conditioning programs are imperative.

Athletes find it difficult to be successful without the proper programs and guidance from the coach. Success is measured in the win/loss column, and the success of the season depends on the training program and instructions formulated by the coach.

JUDO*

Traditional jujitsu, the precursor of judo, has its roots in ancient Japan where it is difficult to separate fact from legend. Judo was first introduced into the United States by Jigoro Kano, a Japanese professor of physical education who came here on a lecture-demonstration tour in 1938 following a trip to Cairo, where he attended an International Olympic Committee meeting. Kano changed the ancient martial art of jujitsu by eliminating some of the dangerous techniques and retaining some of jujitsu's best techniques. He combined these with some of his own ideas, improvements, and improvisations and developed a modern martial art now known as kokodan judo, which is the type of judo practiced in our country. Kano developed a sport that not only was a system of self-defense, physical fitness, and self-discipline but also a spiritual experience in which one's opponent was held in high regard. In judo, the body and mind are trained together to attain a moral goal for modern life. A major principle of judo is embodied in the expression "gentle way."

Judo pupils and experts are ranked by the color of their belts: one starts with a white belt and moves upwards to green, brown, and finally, the coveted black belt, which has its own various degrees. Higher rankings are earned by five dans. Beyond these five dans, there are five more that are purely ceremonial.

Judo is now one of the fastest growing sports in the United States and includes male and female participants. Judo was a subcommittee of the Wrestling Committee of the Amateur Athletic Union until 1953, when it became an independent AAU Committee. In 1981, in accordance with the recent law enacted by Congress giving each sport separate jurisdiction over its own affairs, judo left the AAU and formed United States Judo, Incorporated, which is the sport's national governing body. In 1974, the United States won its first Olympic medal when a Plainfield, New Jersey, athlete won a bronze in the heavyweight classification.

The judoka (judo player) aspirant should join a club with a good coach who will initiate the athlete into the world of judo; self-taught judo is poor at best and lacks the spirit of the sport. The coach will start with the basics, for mastering the basics will protect the athlete from injuries.

*We gratefully acknowledge the assistance of Thomas J. Lynch, and Rolando L. Cheng, M.D., in the preparation of this chapter.

TRAINING AND CONDITIONING

All judo players must start with a warm-up including stretching, flexibility, and joint-loosening exercises. The judo player moves his head and neck and all the major joints of the upper and lower extremities including the back and foot. The participant does a number of stretching exercises for the various joints. Fifteen minutes is usually sufficient for the warm-up.

The judo instructor places great stress on *ukemi* (breakfalls) as a means of limiting the potential of injuries, such as fractures, sprains, strains, and cerebral concussions. The following is a list of ukemi:

1. Sidefall.
2. Backfall.
3. Frontfall.
4. Forward roll.

The neck is particularly vulnerable to injury because of its proximity to the spinal cord. Fracture-dislocations of the neck can be catastrophic. The neck is protected by flexing the head and neck forward and then the judo players roll over onto the mat. Exposed joints such as the shoulders, elbow, and knees can be protected by the judo player landing on the overlying soft-muscle mass. The object is to land on the side of the body and thighs to protect the knees.

In backward breakfalls, slap the mat with the arms and forearms to absorb some of the energy when hitting the mat. To prevent the head from striking the floor, bend the neck directly forward so that the eye can focus on the knot of the belt. Coaching and mastering the protective mechanisms does not take long. This is done for about 5 minutes before the player proceeds to other techniques.

A student must be proficient in ukemi before he can proceed to *randori* (free exercise), which consists of free movement around the mat while working with a partner under the conditions of an actual contest, and *kata* (form), which is a formal system of prearranged exercises designed to teach and perfect the techniques, or *waza*.

The following waza are used in training and practice:

I. Nage-Waza (throwing)
    A. Tachi-Waza (from a standing position)
        1. Te-Waza (hand throws)
           Tai-Otoshi (body drops)
        2. Koshi-Waza (hip throws)
           Ogoshi (major hip throws)
        3. Ashi-Waza (foot or leg throws)
           Osoto-Gari (major outer reaping throws)
    B. Sutemi-Waza (from lying down on back)
        1. Masutemi-Waza (with back on mat)
           Tomoe-Nage (stomach throw)

  2. Yokosutemi-Waza (from lying down on side)
      Yoko-Gurums (side wheel)
 II. Katame-Waza (grappling, or frequently called "Ne-Waza," mat work)*
     A. Osae-Waza (hold downs)
         1. Kesa-Gatame (scarf hold)
     B. Shime-Waza (chokes)
         1. Okuri-Eri-Jime (sliding collar choke)
     C. Kansetsu-Waza (joint locks)
III. Ate-Waza (striking techniques)†
     A. Ude (hand)
     B. Foot

In judo, your opponent's strength is used to defeat him through speed, movement, and feinting. Three elements make up throws: breaking balance (kuzushi); getting yourself in position (tsukuri); and throwing (kake).

In choking, the hands use the opponent's collar in a pulling, twisting motion that somewhat resembles the motion of wringing out a towel. Choking (as used in judo) is accomplished by pressure of the forearm radius bone against the carotid artery in the neck, shutting off blood to the brain. It has nothing to do with air passages to the lungs.

Careful rules set up the procedures for chokes and arm bars; great care is exercised to ensure that these rules are learned and followed explicitly to guard against injury. The loser must tap the mat without delay. With choking techniques, unconsciousness comes with surprising suddenness. In a good choke, the loser simply "goes to sleep." In arm locks, great care must be taken by all concerned; the loser should tap the mat, and the winner must watch constantly.

In judo mat techniques, fairly frequently the winner may be at the bottom and seem to be losing.

COMPETITION

All judo players who desire to achieve any degree of proficiency should compete against different clubs and participate frequently in tournaments. This is an entire daily program of roughly 2 hours 3 times weekly; however, many clubs meet twice a week for about a 2-hour workout.

COMMON INJURIES

In addition to contusions and abrasions of the face, trunk, upper and lower extremities, judo players sustain a wide assortment of orthopedic

---

*For safety, arm locks are allowed only to advanced judo players; none are allowed to players below brown belt.
†Ate-waza is used in self defense only; striking techniques are prohibited in judo.

injuries, including sprains of all the major joints and especially of the shoulders, knee, and ankle. Dislocations of the shoulder, elbow, and patella, and fractures of the clavicle, ribs, humerus, forearm bones, and wrist are not uncommon. Strains of muscles and of the groin are also encountered. All of these injuries are treated by conventional methods.

ICE HOCKEY*

Scottish settlers in Canada brought a version of field hockey to the New World and called it "Shinty." Their children changed the name of the game to "Shinny" and began hitting stones with broomsticks on ice-covered ponds, lakes, and other waterways. Thus, Canada is the birthplace of this exciting sport.

Because of its popularity, ice hockey became a major organized sport by 1855 in Kingston, Ontario, although sport historians claim it was already well established in cities such as Halifax, Montreal, and other Canadian cities. By 1893, Lord Stanley, then Governor-General of Canada, established the Stanley Cup for the best amateur ice-hockey team. Since the turn of the century, this coveted ice-hockey trophy goes to the best professional ice-hockey team.

Ice hockey soon achieved popularity beyond its national borders. American universities such as Yale and Johns Hopkins fielded ice-hockey teams and the sport spread quickly to many other colleges and universities. The first American amateur hockey league was formed in New York in 1896, and soon a Baltimore hockey league was formed. In 1920, ice hockey became an official sport at the Amsterdam Olympics, where Canada won the first Olympic Ice Hockey Gold Medal; they continued to dominate the sport in the 1924, 1928, and 1932 Olympics. At the 1936 Olympics, however, Great Britain's team ended the Canadian winning streak. The Russian team claimed Gold Medals in the 1956, 1964, 1968, 1972, and 1976 Olympics (the streak was interrupted in 1960 by the American team). An American team triumphed over the highly favored Russians in the 1980 Olympics Games in Lake Placid.

Ice hockey is a violent, exciting, hard-hitting collision sport that requires speed, agility, endurance, balance, maneuverability, and neuromuscular coordination. It is an aggressive sport in which players are constantly running, bumping, elbowing, and pushing their opponents voluntarily and involuntarily. They body-check their opponents and are frequently slammed into the boards that line the rink. Players must harden their bodies to withstand the physical shock of this forceful contact. They must also develop and use carefully coordinated skills such as skating, controlling a puck at the end of the blade of a stick by dribbling it, passing quickly and accurately on the move to teammates,

*We gratefully acknowledge the assistance of Peter M. Maniscalco, Ed Purdy, and Vincent McInerney, M.D., in the preparation of this section.

and scoring on the move. Eye-hand-stick coordination as well as co-ordinated movements of the upper and lower extremities and the trunk are also essential. Hockey blends individual skills and teamwork.

Hockey players skate in abrupt starts and stops. Occasionally, players are able to break away from opponents and pass the puck to a moving teammate or shoot the puck at speeds up to 100 mph for a goal. Speed and agility are most important especially in breakaway situations. Because ice hockey is essentially a stick-and-ball (puck) game with the players on skates, the skaters must be able to change direction quickly and faultlessly. They must feel comfortable on skates and possess full body control for balance and movement. This necessitates strong legs, ankles, and feet.

Ice hockey is a team sport that requires many skills. Because these skills take years to master, it is best for the hockey player to start training early and progressively to perfect the various skills. Those young-sters who start before the age of 8 are called "mites"; ages 8 to 10, "squirts"; ages 11 to 12, "pee wees"; ages 13 to 14, "bantams"; ages 15 to 16, "midgets"; ages 17 to 20, "juniors"; and the rest, "seniors." The sooner the hockey aspirant starts, the better the opportunity to advance and develop skills. The player must develop power, speed, endurance, and mobility on skates and be able to stop, turn, cut to left and right, and skate backwards. Pushing off forcefully helps develop speed.

Coaches have a difficult time trying to incorporate all of the many basic techniques and advanced components of a training and conditioning program for a hockey player. A regimen would include:

1. Warmups.
2. Individual skills and tactics.
3. Small group skills and tactics.
4. Total team strategy and tactics.
5. Aerobic or anaerobic conditioning or training.

Some of these must be accomplished by players practicing on their own under the previous direction of the coach. In order to save *ice time*, each coach should instruct his players to engage in the following activities 6 to 8 weeks before team assemblage.

OFF-ICE TRAINING

Off-ice training activities should include stretching and flexibility warm-ups for about 10 minutes, and interval or circuit training to build up the athlete's cardiovascular-respiratory status (endurance). Interval training should be composed of all-out sprinting for about 2 minutes, followed by 25 calisthenic exercises as prescribed. Take a 1-minute rest and repeat the entire interval training cycle and exercises.

The time for this is approximately 1 hour. This is done 3 times weekly. On alternate days, the athlete engages in about 1 hour of weight training. This will build up maximal muscular strength and endurance.

ON-ICE TRAINING

All training sessions begin with 15- to 20-minute warm-ups. These warm-ups include flexibility/stretching exercises; leg-drags while skating for groin, hamstring, and heel stretching; sit-ups; push-ups; knee pull and knee bends for knee- and leg-muscle balance; windmills to loosen up neck, shoulders, back, and abdomen; and power-skating drills.

The warm-up is followed by *agility* and *skating drills*. The agility drills require the player to do leg kicks with the hockey stick held horizontally at shoulder level with alternate toe touches while skating; alternate knee touches while skating; jump over obstacles; forward rolls; and dive to ice and recover.

Skating drills to develop endurance and skating skills should last for 10 to 15 minutes and include the following: long strides with knees apart, body leaning forward and half squats; sprinting in both circular and straight fashion at coach's whistle; power-skating drills to enhance endurance and performance in backward and forward motions; and simple puck and stick drills to enhance passing and shooting skills, using wrist shots, slap shots, and backhand shots.

Some coaches eliminate pucks during the first week to encourage players to develop skating skills. As the season progresses and the player becomes better conditioned, the warm-ups are decreased to 10 minutes.

The second week is for simple stick-and-puck drills. Stick-handling and passing drills are emphasized. Toward the end of the second week, the forwards perform stick-handling and puck drills against defensive players. As the stick-handling becomes more advanced, passing drills are practiced under simulated game conditions. Players are taught to react automatically and appropriately to constantly changing game situations.

During the third week and thereafter, the skills of skating, stick-handling, shooting, and checking are integrated for offensive and defensive strategies. These skills are applied to simulated and actual game situations. At the end of the third week, a controlled scrimmage is held for the coaches to correct any problems that have become evident during the pressure of a game situation.

In the fourth and fifth weeks, the team continues to practice with more emphasis on coordinated skills such as the various shots and body-checks. Advanced passing and skating drills are started and gradually integrated into the practice schedule prior to scrimmages with outside clubs.

In the sixth week, the team should be conditioned and trained for an outside schedule.

Special techniques are required for face-offs, power plays, and penalty-killing situations. Goal-tending is a key position requiring a great deal of agility, coordination, flexibility, strength, maneuverability, and courage. Protective equipment, especially the face mask, is very important to the goal-tender.

This is a suggested training and conditioning program that can be modified or augmented depending on the coach's philosophy and the players' age and experience.

The following minimal protective equipment is essential and must fit properly and comfortably:

For Skaters

1. Skates that are comfortable yet close-fitting when laced correctly over one pair of socks.
2. Shin guards with knee pads.
3. Pants to provide protection for thighs, hips, and ribs.
4. Shoulder and elbow pads.
5. Gloves to protect against bruising and slashing.
6. Helmet.
7. Mouthpiece.
8. Genitalia cup.

For Goalies

1. Helmets with a cage-type face mask, throat protector and internal mouthpiece.
2. Chest protector.
3. One-piece shoulder and upper-extremity pad.
4. Leg pads.
5. Heavily padded pants.
6. Catching glove and waffle-shaped pad (on stick hand used to deflect puck).
7. Genitalia cup.
8. Specially padded skates.

All of the goalie's equipment is heavily padded in order to withstand the impact of the puck. His stick must be of proper length and lie.

All equipment, including skate blades, should be aired and dried after every use.

The ice hockey injuries listed on page 122 are common.

Head

1. Facial lacerations and eye injuries.
2. Loss of teeth.

Shoulder

1. Acromioclavicular separations (separated shoulders).
2. Shoulder dislocations and subluxations.
3. Rotator cuff tears in older players.

Upper Extremities

1. Elbow: Olecranon bursitis.
2. Forearm: Contusions and fractures.
3. Wrists and Hands: Sprains and fractures, especially of the carpal navicular bones.

Trunk

1. Rib fractures.
2. Contusions and strains.
3. Low-back sprains and strains.
4. Hip pointer (iliac crest contusion).

Lower Extremities

1. Groin strain.
2. Hip and thigh contusion and myositis ossificans.
3. Knee sprains and internal derangements.
4. Lower leg contusions.
5. Ankle sprains and fractures.
6. Ingrown toe nails.
7. Fractures of the feet, especially metatarsals.

REFERENCES

American College of Sports Medicine (ed.): Guidelines for Graded Exercise Testing and Exercise Prescription. 2nd Ed. Philadelphia, Lea & Febiger, 1980.

Apple, D.F., and Cantwell, J.D.: Medicine for Sport. Chicago, Year Book Medical Publishers, 1979.

Asuma, T.: Judo—Encyclopedia of Sports Sciences and Medicine. New York, Macmillan Company, 1971.

Balakian, G., et al.: Helping your athlete stay in shape. Patient Care, *10–20*: 100–115, 1976.

Bartlett, E.G.: Judo and Self Defense. New York, Arco Publishing Co., 1962.

Dominy, E.: Judo—Beginner to Black Belt. London, W. Foulshan & Co., 1958.

Drucker, T.: Personal communication, 1982.

Elliot, J.: Hockey, seemingly so vigorous, brutal, turns out to be a physiologic cakewalk. Medical News. Vol. 2, No. 1. Jan. 9, 1978, p. 19.

Feigenbaum, H.: Echocardiography. 3rd Ed. Philadelphia, Lea & Febiger, 1981.

Galbraith, R.F.: Safety in hockey. Minnesota Medicine, Nov. 1981: 671–673.

Goldberger, E.: A Primer of Water, Electrolyte and Acid-Base Syndromes. 6th Ed. Philadelphia, Lea & Febiger, 1980.

Guyton, A.C.: Textbook of Medical Physiology. 6th Ed. Philadelphia, W.B. Saunders, 1981.

Harrison, E.J.: Manual of Judo. London, W. Foulshan & Co., 1952.

Haycock, E.: Sports Medicine for the Athletic Female. New York, Van Nostrand Reinhold, 1980.

Hollering, B.L., and Simpson, D.: The effect of three types of training programs upon skating speed of college ice hockey players. Journal of Sports Medicine, 17:335–340, 1977.

Hyman, A.S., et al. (eds.): Encyclopedia of Sports Sciences and Medicine. New York, Macmillan, 1973.

Ikai, J.M.: Judo—Encyclopedia of Sports Sciences and Medicine. New York, Macmillan Company, 1971.

Jensen, C.R., and Fisher, A.G.: Scientific Basis of Athletic Conditioning. 2nd Ed. Philadelphia, Lea & Febiger, 1979.

Jokl, P.: What is Sports Medicine? Springfield, Charles C Thomas, 1964.

Katz, J., and Brunning, N.P.: Swimming for Total Fitness: A Progressive Aerobic Program. Garden City, Doubleday, 1981.

The Kodokan: Illustrated Kodokan Judo, Tokyo, Kodansha, 1955.

————: Kodokan Judo. Tokyo, Kodansha, 1963.

Koizumi, G.: My Study of Judo. New York, Cornerstone Library, 1960.

Kotani, S., Osawa, Y., and Hirose, Y.: Kata of Kodokan Judo Revised. Kobe, Japan, Koyano, Bussan, Kaisha, Ltd., 1968.

Leggett, T.P., and Watanabe, K.: Championship Judo, Tai-Otoshi and O-Uchi-Gari Attacks. London, W. Foulshan & Co., 1964.

Mack, R.: Ice hockey injuries. Sports Medicine Digest, 3, no. 1:1981.

MacLean, N.: The high school hockey room. In Sports Trail. Kendall Co. Sports, Division 27, 1972, pp. 4–7.

————, Willner, B., and Hoerner, E.: Soviet Sports Exercise Program. London, Drake Publishers, 1977.

Mangi, R., Jokl, P., and Dayton, O.W.: The Runner's Complete Medical Guide. New York, Summit Books, 1979.

Masking the pain in hockey. Medical World News, October 11:41–44, 1974.

McArdle, W.D., Katch, F.I., and Katch, V.L.: Exercise Physiology: Energy, Nutrition, and Human Performance. Philadelphia, Lea & Febiger, 1980.

Medical News: Hockey leaves its marks on players. J.A.M.A., 235, no. 23:2465, 2468, 1976.

Medical News: Masks could reduce hockey's toll on eyes. J.A.M.A., 235, no. 23: 2464, 1976.

Michaelson, M.: Today's Health. Feb. 1968, pp. 31–37, 80–82.

Mifune, K.: Canon of Judo. Translated by K. Sugai. Tokyo, Seibundo-Shinkosha Publishing Co., 1958.

Muckle, D.S.: Injuries in Sport. Chicago, Year Book Medical Publishers, 1978.

Mulvoy, M., and Editors of Sports Illustrated: Ice Hockey. Philadelphia, J.B. Lippincott, 1971.

Nakabayashi, S., Uchida, Y., and Uchida, G.: Fundamentals of Judo. New York, Ronald Press Company, 1964.

Novich, M.M.: Olympic boxing. In 1980 Yearbook of Sports Medicine. Chicago, Year Book Medical Publishers, 1981.

————: What really happens in boxing. The Physician and Sportsmedicine, 2: 28–32, 1974.

————: Prefight physical examination for amateur boxers. JAMA, 223:1048, 1973.

————: Physiologic basis of training and conditioning of athletes. J. Med. Soc. N.J., 69:841–845, 1972.

————: The physiological responses and requirements of participation in boxing. In Encyclopedia of Sports Medicine. New York, Macmillan, 1971, pp. 323–325.

————: Clinical examination necessary prior to participation in boxing. In Encyclopedia of Sports Medicine. New York, Macmillan, 1971, pp. 435–437.

————: A.A.U. boxing physician reports contest on Soviet Union. Medicine in Sports Newsletter, 10:3, 1970.

————: Boxing program for youngsters. N.Y. State J. Med., 70:1300–1305, 1970.

Parker, W.: Varsity hockey team evaluated for "health" conditioning criteria. Medical Tribune, *21,* no. 9: 1980.

Schwartz, R., and Novich, M.M.: The athlete's mouthpiece. Am. J. Sports Med., 8:357–359, 1980.

Smith, D.: Face-Off. New York, Sadia Sports Publishing, 1973.

Smith, M.A.: Agility Training for Young Hockey Players. U.S. Hockey/Arean Biz, 1977, pp. 28–31.

Smith, M.A.: The Application of a Soviet Conditioning Technique-Circuit Training to Hockey. Report of Lecture at a Hockey Clinic, Long Island, Feb., 1974.

Spackman, R.R.: Conditioning for Ice Hockey. Carbondale, Ill. Hillcrest House, 1973.

Strauss, R.H. (ed.): Sports Medicine and Physiology. Philadelphia, W.B. Saunders, 1979.

Tennis elbow: who's most likely to get it and how. Round table: The Physician and Sportsmedicine, 3:43–57, 1975.

Tetu, R.G.: "Tennis Elbow: An Epidemic?" Master's thesis. University of Illinois, 1977.

Vandeweghe, E.M., and Flynn, G.L.: Growing with Sports: A Parent's Guide to the Young Athlete. Englewood Cliffs, Prentice-Hall, 1979.

Watt, T.: How to Play Hockey. Toronto, Coles Publishing, 1980.

William, T.G., and Sperryn, P.N.: Sports Medicine. 2nd Ed. Baltimore, Williams & Wilkins, 1976.

7

Nutrition of Athletes*

INTRODUCTION
The body is in its most literal sense the product of its nutrition. Nutrition is a process that begins with the ingestion of foodstuffs and ends in the functioning of the living body. Neuromotor skills are only as effective as the physical fitness of the athlete; the four main features of a course in physical training for an athlete are diet, adequate sleep, use of the physiologic overload principle for the muscular, cardiovascular, and respiratory systems, and the absence of all drugs not used for therapy.

Food provides the following:
1. Energy for various physical and mental activities.
2. Materials for the building or repair of tissues.
3. Energy storage depots.
4. Body heat.
5. Insulation.
6. Regulating substances, such as vitamins and minerals, necessary to carry out complex body functions.
7. Gross tissue mass.
8. Normal acid-base balance.
9. Normal blood-sugar level.
10. Body fluids.
11. Satiation of hunger.
12. Satisfaction of appetite.

Obviously, the coach and trainer must show as much interest in the diet of their athletes as they do in their conditioning program. They must understand the physiology of the gastrointestinal tract and its preparation of foodstuffs for absorption and assimilation into body tissues and fluids. They must have a working knowledge of which foods are best converted into body substance for growth, tissue repair,

*We gratefully acknowledge the assistance of Robert R. Gross, Ph.D., Milton Singer, M.D., and Nathan J. Smith, M.D., in preparation of this chapter.

maintenance, and energy. They must have an excellent understanding of body fluids and electrolyte balance (p. 76). They must know the approximate number of calories required for different athletic activities, and how to supply the necessary foods in balanced, appetizing meals.

GASTROINTESTINAL PHYSIOLOGY

Gastrointestinal physiology is concerned with the conversion of food substances into body substances. This is done by mechanically and chemically altering ingested food into simpler units that can be absorbed and assimilated by the body. The process starts with chewing (mastication), which mixes the food with the saliva. The more thorough the chewing of the food, the greater the ease with which it is rolled up into a soft bolus and swallowed. The presence of sufficient digestive enzymes, gastrointestinal motility, neural and hormonal regulators, appetizing and palatable foods, and an anxiety-free environment are conducive to maximal digestion.

Liquids and semisolid foods pass through the stomach and into the small intestine in a relatively short time by peristaltic contractions of the stomach. Passage of these foods proceeds normally in the absence of gravity, and they may reach the pyloric sphincter in 1 to 5 minutes. When solid food enters the stomach, it accumulates near the cardiac end; it may take 3 to 5 hours before the last part of a solid meal leaves the stomach. Proteins leave the stomach more slowly than carbohydrates, and fats more slowly than proteins.

Digestive secretions from the liver, gallbladder, pancreas, and intestinal mucosa enter the small intestine. Here the most important processes of digestion take place, resulting in basic substances that are absorbed by the bloodstream and assimilated by body tissues. Certain substances such as vitamins and bile, speed the absorption of fats and other nutrients by the bloodstream.

The first part of a solid meal may reach the ileocecal valve in 4½ hours and be in the cecum in 5½ hours.

Although the large intestine does not play a major role in actual digestion, it allows rapid absorption of fluid and electrolytes which is necessary for digestive processes. The residues of undigested food are excreted in 12 to 24 hours in most people.

NUTRITIONAL REQUIREMENTS OF ATHLETES

The principles of good nutrition are the same for athletes as for nonathletes, except that athletes must consume additional calories to compensate for their greater energy expenditure. To balance the increased output of energy, a high caloric diet—5,000 to 6,000 calories for football and crew and a lesser amount for hockey, track and baseball—is accepted as standard fare. However, great differences of opinion exist among coaches and trainers as to the best diets for track and field athletes before their competition.

What an athlete should eat immediately preceding a game is still unsettled. What is the best pre-event food for swimmers? Does the ingestion of steaks and other high-protein pregame foods affect an athlete's performance? What is the status of the pregame liquid meals? The following discussion shows how the athlete can get the most out of nutritionally selective food to benefit his health and athletic performance.

Carbohydrates. The optimal range of carbohydrate apportionment in a person's total daily caloric need has never been scientifically established. Current opinion recommends a 50% carbohydrate allowance for total energy requirements. However, Thorndike reported 44% carbohydrate allowance at a football training table where an average of 5,600 calories were consumed daily. The amount of carbohydrates consumed is not fixed by hard and fast rules. It should be flexible enough to vary with locale, climate, and individual food preferences and customs.

Carbohydrates are more swiftly metabolized into energy by the body than is fat. Even though carbohydrates yield only half as many calories per gram as fat, there is a 10% higher caloric output when a given amount of oxygen is used to burn carbohydrates than when used to burn fat or protein. Under certain competitive conditions, this difference can be advantageous. Athletes on high carbohydrate diets performing in sports of endurance and prolonged activities show a slightly increased efficiency—a minimum of 5%—as compared with those on high fat diets. Carbohydrates that are ingested in excess of tissue needs and glycogen storage capacity are converted into fat and stored as adipose tissue.

Although there is no proof that exercises of short duration, such as 100-yard swims, are benefited by a carbohydrate pregame meal, many nutritionists and coaches still recommend a high carbohydrate meal preceding the event. Carbohydrate reserves may be augmented by performing tapering-off exercises about 48 hours before a game and offering a high carbohydrate meal, particularly complexed carbohydrates such as pasta and cereals, immediately preceding the event.

Fats. Fats provide the following in the diet:
1. Reserve fuel.
2. Essential unsaturated fatty acids.
3. Absorption of fat-soluble vitamins.
4. Palatability, flavor, and aroma.

After the available stores of carbohydrates are used, the body breaks down tissue fat and protein to provide additional energy. The glycerol component of the oxidized fat is used as a carbohydrate, releasing heat and energy. Enough fat and carbohydrate should be available in the diet to prevent the breakdown of body protein to provide energy.

The fat proportion of the daily caloric intake for the average person in the United States and Canada ranges from 35 to 44%. Depending upon the activity of the athlete, the fat allowance ranges from 20 to 35%. Fat is the most concentrated source of energy reserve and produces twice as many calories per gram as do carbohydrates or proteins; however, it releases this energy quite slowly. Therefore, carbohydrate is the preferred food for quick and prolonged energy expenditures. Fortunately, there is a close reciprocal relationship between fats and carbohydrates as sources of energy. Although fat is the only food that can be stored in significant quantities, endurance is impaired by a high fat diet. In sports of light-energy expenditure interspersed with periods of rest, diets dominant in fat or carbohydrate do equally well. In athletic activities of light or strenuous nature unrelieved by rest, carbohydrate meals are best.

Fat lends palatability to a meal; most people require its presence to make a meal acceptable. Its presence in meat is an index of tenderness.

Table 7.*

KEY NUTRIENTS†	SOME REASONS WHY YOU NEED THEM	IMPORTANT SOURCES
Protein	Builds and repairs all tissues; helps form antibodies to fight infection; supplies energy	Meat, fish, poultry, eggs, cheese, milk; dried beans and peas, peanut butter; cereals and breads
Fat	Supplies large amount of energy in small amount of food; helps keep skin healthy by supplying essential fatty acids	Butter and cream, whole milk; salad oils and dressings; cooking fats; fat meats
Carbohydrate (Sugars and Starches)	Supplies energy; carries other nutrients present in foods	Breads and cereals; potatoes and corn; dried fruits and sweetened fruits; sugar, jelly, syrup, honey
Minerals Calcium	Helps build bones and teeth; helps blood clot; helps muscles and nerves react normally; helps tired muscles recover and delays fatigue	Milk, cheese, ice cream; turnip and mustard greens, collards, kale, and broccoli

Table 7.* (*continued*)

Key Nutrients†	Some Reasons Why You Need Them	Important Sources
Iron	Combines with protein to make hemoglobin, the red substance in blood that carries oxygen to cells	Meat, especially liver; eggs; dried beans; green leafy vegetables; some dried fruits—as raisins, prunes
Vitamins Vitamin A	Helps keep skin clear and smooth; helps keep mucous membranes healthy and resistant to infection; helps prevent night blindness; helps control bone growth	Liver; deep yellow fruits; dark green and yellow vegetables; butter, cream, ice cream, whole milk, yellow cheese
Thiamine (Vitamin B_1)	Helps promote normal appetite and digestion; helps keep nervous system healthy and prevent irritability; helps body release energy from food	All meats, especially pork; fish; poultry; eggs; enriched and whole grain breads and cereals; milk; white potatoes
Riboflavin (Vitamin B_2)	Helps cells use oxygen; helps keep vision clear; helps keep skin and tongue smooth and prevent scaly, greasy skin around mouth and nose	Milk, cheese, ice cream; meats, especially liver; fish; poultry; eggs
Vitamin B_6, Vitamin B_{12}, and Folacin	Helps prevent anemia; helps enzyme and other biochemical systems function normally	Vitamin B_6—Meats, potatoes, dark green leafy vegetables, whole grains and dry beans Vitamin B_{12}—Milk, cheese eggs, and meats Folacin—Green vegetables, whole grains and dry beans
Ascorbic Acid (Vitamin C)	Helps to make cementing materials that hold cells together; strengthens walls of blood vessels; helps resist infection; helps prevent fatigue; helps heal wounds and broken bones	Citrus fruits as orange, grapefruit, lemon; strawberries and cantaloupe; tomatoes; broccoli and green pepper, raw cabbage, white potatoes
Vitamin D	Helps the body absorb calcium from the digestive tract and build calcium and phosphorus into bones	Vitamin D milk; fish liver oils; sunshine on skin (not a food)

*Adapted from Gregg, W. H.: A Boy and His Physique. Chicago, National Dairy Council, 1970.
†When you eat the foods that supply enough of these nutrients you also supply others which your body needs in smaller amounts. Water is also essential, although we may not think of it as a food.

Many of the substances that enhance the flavor and aroma of food are associated with fat in the diet. Fat-containing meals also have a high satiety value because they "stick to the ribs." The fat in the meal delays stomach emptying time and decreases intestinal motility; this delays the onset of hunger.

Protein. Coaches have traditionally stressed the need for consuming large amounts of meat, especially beef, in the mistaken belief that it replaces muscle protein losses resulting from heavy muscular activity in athletics. Steak plays an honored role in these diets. Refuted scientifically many times, the practice still continues. Actually, the protein needs of the body are governed by its rate of growth rather than its activities. Therefore, additional protein sources, such as milk, eggs, meat, fish, and cheese, are indicated only for growing boys, such as high school athletes, and for athletes who are making muscle mass. Wide variations of protein intake do not seem to influence performance. A well-balanced diet that includes a protein intake of 10 to 15% of the total daily caloric needs should supply protein sufficient for growth, defense mechanisms, tissue repair, and maintenance.

Because water is required for excretion of nitrogenous waste resulting from protein metabolism, an increased fluid intake makes additional toilet trips necessary. For this reason, protein intake should be reduced to a minimum at the pregame meal.

Vitamins. Vitamins are neither body building nor energy giving, but they are key nutrients in that they are important links in metabolism. Vitamins cannot be substituted for one another. They are involved in normal growth, resistance to infection, health, and well-being. Only the highlights of the vitamins important in athletics are mentioned here; the reader is directed to other sources for more comprehensive information.

Fat-soluble Vitamins. 1. Vitamin A. For function and sources, see Table 7. Deficiency leads to ocular disturbances, night blindness, skin disorders, retarded growth, proneness to infection, intestinal disorders, impairment of epiphyseal bone formation.

2. Vitamin D. For function and sources, see Table 7. Deficiency leads to rickets in children, osteomalacia in adults, enamel and cementum disorders of teeth, loss of skeletal muscle tone, retarded growth, and lack of vigor.

3. Vitamin K. Essential for synthesis of several prothrombin related proteins and the normal clotting of blood. Sources are leafy vegetables, spinach, cabbage, fish meal, egg yolk, hempseed. Deficiency leads to prolonged clotting time, hypoprothrombinemia, multiple hemorrhages.

Water-Soluble Vitamins. 1. Vitamin B_1 (Thiamine). For function and sources, see Table 7. Deficiency leads to marked retardation of growth, beriberi, polyneuritis, loss of appetite, nausea, and vomiting.

2. VITAMIN B₂ (RIBOFLAVIN). For function and sources, see Table 7. Deficiency leads to ocular difficulties, atrophy of skin, stomatitis (lesions on lips and mucocutaneous junction, corner of mouth), inflammation of tongue (glossitis), cessation of growth in young. In the absence of riboflavin, minor injuries become aggravated.

3. VITAMIN C (ASCORBIC ACID). For function and sources, see Table 7. Deficiency leads to scurvy, delayed healing of wounds, failure of osteoblasts to form osteoid tissue; odontoblasts (dentition and enamel of teeth).

Minerals. Many minerals are required for optimal nutrition; these are interrelated and kept in balance with each other in carrying out certain body functions. The role of calcium in the formation of bone and teeth is commonly known. However, calcium also regulates the heart beat and exerts a balance between potassium and sodium in maintaining muscle tone. A low blood calcium level may result in impaired muscle action and coordination or in muscle and nerve hyperirritability leading to tetany. Calcium is necessary for acid-base equilibrium. Under normal conditions, it catalyzes the conversion of chemical energy into meaningful muscular contractions.

Salt and Fluids. Sodium chloride, or salt, is vital to the maintenance of life. Sodium helps to regulate fluid balance, as demonstrated by the high proportion of sodium ions in the blood (normal level—138 to 142 mEq Na^+/L serum). Sodium, calcium, and potassium ions are important in the maintenance of acid-base equilibrium. In addition to its biochemical role, salt has a distinctive flavor, which is a pleasant additive in seasoning food.

The average daily adult intake of sodium chloride is 10 to 15 g. An intake of 30 g or more may result in edema, because it disturbs water balance through the extracellular deposition of sodium chloride in body fluids. Ninety per cent of sodium is excreted by way of the kidney as sodium chloride or sodium phosphate. Sodium chloride is also excreted in perspiration; thus, salt requirements are increased when an athlete performs excessively or in hot humid weather, i.e., 85° F or higher (see pp. 77 and 78). Athletes may suffer heat stroke or heat exhaustion from fluid and salt depletion if they perform in this kind of weather without a period of acclimatization or replacement of fluid and salt losses. Preventive measures should be taken, especially in hot and humid weather. Despite some studies by reputable investigators that extra salt may not be necessarily reliable, traditions suggest that salt with water should be replaced, to aid absorption, sugar should also be given. Gatorade is a satisfactory replacement. Potassium loss is usually not a problem. An athlete should take an additional 6 g of salt or its equivalent throughout the day by liberally salting his food compatible to his taste and by taking salt tablets at each meal and practice session. In hot weather, he should take two 1-g enteric coated salt tablets before practice and one after practice. Salt may also be replaced with a solution made by adding about 20 g of salt tablets to 1 quart of water. (This comes out to slightly more than 0.1% solution [0.14%]). Including some lemon juice and sugar masks the taste of the salt and makes the drink more palatable; it may be given before and after a contest.

Fluids for the body are ingested in prepared foods, fruit juices, soft drinks, and water. Most people need 4 to 8 glasses (1 to 2 quarts) of fluids daily. One or more glasses of water at a meal aids digestion. Usually, the sensation of thirst compels an individual to drink water or its equivalent; under normal conditions, this is a satisfactory guide to proper fluid balance. In athletics, because of increased muscular activity and perspiration, the body requires 7 to 14 ounces of water for every 30 minutes of strenuous play. Additional supplements of water are necessary if the activity is performed in hot, humid weather.

Under conditions of excessive sweating or extreme heat, as many as 5 to 10 pounds of body weight may be lost by an athlete in a single workout; this loss is largely water. The sensation of thirst may not keep pace with actual water requirements, and large additional intakes of water and salt may be necessary. Free use of water should be allowed on the playing field, but the athlete should be encouraged to rinse his mouth, take small sips of water, and not to "drown" himself or produce a distended stomach. The use of small paper cups, plastic squeeze bottles, or portable water fountains by which the athletes squirt water into their mouths, help discourage excessive drinking. The taboo on the use of ice water because it supposedly causes stomach cramps is not justified by scientific evidence; ice water and other cold drinks may be consumed by athletes when they are thirsty. However, the fluid intake and loss must be carefully watched, since a disturbance of the fluids may cause an alteration in the electrolyte balance. Water needs are best monitored by frequent nude weighings. Although prescribed amounts of water and electrolyte replacement have been mentioned, the body via the kidney and other systems is the best monitor for homeostasis.

THE BEST PLAYING WEIGHT

Being in condition includes achieving one's best playing weight. When athletes report for a playing season, they are frequently not at their best playing weight. Some athletes are overweight, although not necessarily obese. Some may even find it necessary to gain weight. For sports such as boxing, judo, wrestling, and others, making a specific weight in a proper class is a decided help. In football, lacrosse, soccer, and hockey, where the emphasis is on heft, being a trifle overweight appears useful.

The athlete in many situations can decide for himself at which weight he participates best by using the scale, tape measure, performance, fatigue, and his age as guidelines. This athlete carries no excess weight to consume needlessly the energy necessary for participation. Through long hours of hard play and some food and fluid restriction, he reaches a state of being "in condition," wherein he performs maximally.

Loss of Weight. Nutrient calories in excess of the daily caloric requirements for maintenance, growth, repair, and energy are converted into fat and stored in adipose tissue. The objective of losing excess fat is to reduce the energy cost of moving about additional poundage, which results in an associated reduction of body reserves. Thus, weight loss helps achieve a body weight conducive to maximal physical efficiency and optimal health.

Loss of weight can be accomplished in two ways. The safest way is through oxidation of fat depots. Because the body gives up its stored fats slowly, loss of depot fat is best accomplished by restricting total calorie intake. However, this reduction must take place at a slow, even rate to prevent acidosis. A loss of 3 to 4 pounds weekly is the maximal loss of weight permitted until the stored fats are utilized.

Loss of weight may be accomplished quite rapidly by removing body fluids. This is a dangerous method that carries the risk of losing enough electrolytes to cause a disturbance of the finely balanced concentration of electrolytes in the body fluids. As stated previously, this delicate balance is vital for normal body physiology. Rapid or prolonged dehydration upsets this balance, leading to weakness, muscular incoordination, and neurologic disturbances.

If the coaching staff and the athlete were more aware of food composition, calories, and the energies needed to burn up ingested foods, the athlete could spend more time perfecting his athletic skills instead of being concerned with losing excess poundage that depletes energy and body reserves.

Approximate energy expenditure (calorie costs) with relation to different sports are:

Sport	Calories per Minute
Volleyball	3.5
Golf	5.0
Tennis	7.1
Skiing	9.9
Cross-country	10.6
Swimming—crawl (55 yds/min)	14.6

Table 8.   Energy Equivalents of Food Calories Expressed in Minutes of Activity.

		ACTIVITY			
FOOD	CALORIES	Walking*	Riding bicycle†	Swim-ming‡	Run-ning#	Reclin-ing¶
		min.	min.	min.	min.	min.
Apple, large	101	19	12	9	5	78
Bacon, 2 strips	96	18	12	9	5	74
Banana, small	88	17	11	8	4	68
Beans, green, 1 c	27	5	3	2	1	21
Beer, 1 glass	114	22	14	10	6	88
Bread and butter	78	15	10	7	4	60
Cake, 1/12, 2-layer	356	68	43	32	18	274
Carbonated beverage, 1 glass	106	20	13	9	5	82
Carrot, raw	42	3	5	4	2	32
Cereal, dry, ½ c, with milk and sugar	200	38	24	18	10	154
Cheese, cottage, 1 Tbsp	27	5	3	2	1	21
Cheese, Cheddar, 1 oz	111	21	14	10	6	85
Chicken, fried, ½ breast	232	45	28	21	12	178
Chicken, "TV" dinner	542	104	66	48	28	417
Cookie, plain, 148/lb	15	3	2	1	1	12
Cookie, chocolate chip	51	10	6	5	3	39
Doughnut	151	29	18	13	8	116
Egg, fried	110	21	13	10	6	85
Egg, boiled	77	15	9	7	4	59
French dressing, 1 Tbsp	59	11	7	5	3	45
Halibut steak, ¼ lb	205	39	25	18	11	158
Ham, 2 slices	167	32	20	15	9	128
Ice cream, ⅙ qt	193	37	24	17	10	148
Ice cream soda	255	49	31	23	13	196
Ice milk, ⅙ qt	144	28	18	13	7	111
Gelatin, with cream	117	23	14	10	6	90
Malted milk shake	502	97	61	45	26	386
Mayonnaise, 1 Tbsp	92	18	11	8	5	71
Milk, 1 glass	166	32	20	15	9	128
Milk, skim, 1 glass	81	16	10	7	4	62
Milk shake	421	81	51	38	22	324
Orange, medium	68	13	8	6	4	52
Orange juice, 1 glass	120	23	15	11	6	92
Pancake with sirup	124	24	15	11	6	95
Peach, medium	46	9	6	4	2	35
Peas, green, ½ c	56	11	7	5	3	43
Pie, apple, ⅙	377	73	46	34	19	290
Pie, raisin, ⅙	437	84	53	39	23	336
Pizza, cheese, ⅛	180	35	22	16	9	138
Pork chop, loin	314	60	38	28	16	242
Potato chips, 1 serving	108	21	13	10	6	83
Sandwiches						
Club	590	113	72	53	30	454
Hamburger	350	67	43	31	18	269
Roast beef with gravy	430	83	52	38	22	331
Tuna fish salad	278	53	34	25	14	214
Sherbet, ⅙ qt	177	34	22	16	9	136

Table 8.   Energy Equivalents of Food Calories
Expressed in Minutes of Activity. (*continued*)

			ACTIVITY			
FOOD	CALORIES	*Walking*°	*Riding bicycle*†	*Swimming*‡	*Running*#	*Reclining*¶
Shrimp, French fried	180	35	22	16	9	138
Spaghetti, 1 serving	396	76	48	35	20	305
Steak, T-bone	235	45	29	21	12	181
Strawberry shortcake	400	77	49	36	21	308

° Energy cost of walking for 70-kg individual = 5.2 calories per minute at 3.5 mph.
† Energy cost of riding bicycle = 8.2 calories per minute.
‡ Energy cost of swimming = 11.2 calories per minute.
# Energy cost of running = 19.4 calories per minute.
¶ Energy cost of reclining = 1.3 calories per minute.
(From Konishi, F. J.:   J. Amer. Diet. Assoc.)

Table 8 graphically demonstrates the activities required to burn up calories from foods chosen at random.

The interpretation and keeping of weight charts by the coach and trainer are discussed more fully on pages 84 to 86. The team physician should be consulted if any problems arise concerning the weight of an athlete.

PLANNING THE DIET

Since athletic activities require more energy than is needed for the daily routine of living, a great amount of energy-producing food must be consumed. Each athlete has his own requirements depending upon his particular nutritional assessment. During the early part of the training program, the caloric intake varies as to his specific needs for losing or gaining weight. As soon as he gets into condition and has reached his best playing weight the caloric intake must balance the output.

The minerals, vitamins, and water requirements must not be neglected when diets are being planned; these also share in the athlete's daily nutritional needs. Supervised diets usually include enough of these nutrients for the daily needs. Lack of supervision may lead to clinical conditions that interfere with the skills of an athlete.

In planning a suitable diet for an athlete with allowances for individual differences, a coach and his staff should take the following into consideration:

1. Age: High school athletes between the ages of 15 and 19 (a period of growth and development) require more protein than older players.

2. Season or climate: Although energy intake varies with the athletic activity, the locale and climate have a bearing upon the amount of carbohydrates and fats that need to be consumed. Less is needed when the temperature is relatively high; more when it is low.

3. Physique of the individual: A quarterback weighing 125 pounds should not eat as much as a lineman weighing 190 pounds.

Foods. Foodstuffs may be grouped in the following manner:

1. *Milk Group.* Two servings with substitutions of cheese or ice cream. Milk supplies protein, calcium, riboflavin, niacin, and vitamin A. Fortified milk also supplies vitamin D. For adolescents, the milk group supplies about 80% of the body calcium; for adults, it supplies 75% of the calcium.

2. *Meat Group.* Two or more servings daily. Fresh, canned, or frozen meat, fish, poultry, and eggs. Alternates such as dried beans, peas, nuts, and peanut butter also supply protein for growth and repair of body tissues, iron and vitamins such as thiamine, riboflavin, and niacin.

3. *Vegetable-Fruit Group.* Four or more servings daily. Include a citrus or other fruit, e.g., cantaloupe, and a vegetable like cabbage or tomatoes to provide ascorbic acid (vitamin C). Dark green and deep yellow vegetables such as broccoli, green peppers, spinach, carrots, and sweet potatoes are good sources of vitamin A.

4. *Bread and Cereal Group.* Four or more servings daily. Includes all breads. Cereals are nourishing and provide carbohydrates, protein, iron, and the vitamin B complex.

In planning a suitable diet, good nutrition may be provided by many different combinations of food. From these basic four groups of foods, an athlete can select and consume a variety of appetizing and nourishing foods of sufficient calories to balance the daily expenditure of his athletic energies. The diet must be adequate and flexible enough for body growth, maintenance, and repair, provide sources and reserves of available energy, and aid the athlete to reach his best playing weight.

Meal Patterns. Juggling calories should not include missing meals. Meal regularity aids digestion, morale, and discipline as well as the efficient utilization of nutrients. Most mature athletes require a minimum of 3 complete meals a day. For protracted and exhausting sports, some athletes may require 5 lighter meals. Adolescent athletes may need a midafternoon and evening snack. Whatever eating patterns have been established at home, the athlete in training must be made to understand that his proper nutrition means long-term diet regulation. Any athlete who depends solely upon the pregame meal to get ready for a contest is as deluded as one who thinks that contests are won on natural endowment without the benefit of training and conditioning.

Athletic skills and their neuromotor coordination are the result primarily of natural endowment, conditioning, training, and motivation. Performance cannot be improved by the addition of ergogenic aids such as special foods, vitamin supplements, or drugs. Nor is performance improved with amphetamines, despite the myth that has surrounded them (see pp. 146 to 147). However, a faulty or inadequate diet may impair performance. In the Roaring Twenties, the adage in boxing was that one had to be hungry to become a champion. However, in our present affluent society, "hunger"—or motivation—has to be instilled into the athlete.

Breakfast should and can be a welcome meal. The digestive and nutritional states of the body are at their lowest upon awakening in the morning. and need replenishing for the day's activities. Breakfast is even more pleasant and enjoyable when one works for it by doing some roadwork or calisthenics before eating. In addition to a generous supply of milk and eggs, a serving of bacon or ham periodically should not be overlooked. Carbohydrates are supplied by fruit juices, fruits, jellies, jams, breads, and cereals. Hot coffee gives some adults a real lift. The cereal and grain industries have developed an array of cereals, especially dry ones, that will meet any and every athlete's preference. Each brand varies in its protein, carbohydrate, fat, mineral, and vitamin content, which are listed on the container. These cereals are ready sources of energy. In the fall and winter, cooked cereals may be used.

Lunch and dinner meals usually are selected from the same basic food groupings, and slight differences between these meals depend on personal preferences. Both meals are built around a serving of meat, poultry, or fish that may be preceded by an appetizer of fruit, vegetable juice, or soup. Beef is not necessarily the best and only meat recommended; various cuts of lamb, pork, and veal are just as good. The entrée may be served with at least two vegetables of different colors, one preferably deep green or yellow, with a serving of potatoes periodically. The raw vegetables in a salad may be regarded as one of the required vegetables. Traditionally, desserts consist of cooked, preserved, dried, or raw fruits, puddings, cookies, Jello, or ice cream. Milk and other beverages may be consumed with or between meals.

Before the afternoon practice session, the main serving at lunch should be an easily digestible food such as lean meat, fish, or eggs, accompanied by milk, fruits, and breads. Such a meal prepares the athlete for the afternoon practice session, which should take place 3 to 5 hours afterwards. This allows sufficient time for digestion, absorption, and conversion of the foods so that the blood needed for the process is shunted from the gastrointestinal tract to the musculature of the trunk and extremities.

After practice sessions, the athlete should not eat until his body has reverted to its normal prepractice physiologic condition, which may take as much as 1 hour. The size of the servings varies with the athlete. He must discipline himself to satisfy wisely his appetite and hunger. In the case of the high school or college student, satisfying a ravenous appetite may cause him to fall asleep soon after his meal and his studies may suffer as a result. Much versatility must be shown by those who prepare and serve these meals to provide top quality nutrition while preventing the meals from becoming boring and monotonous.

Importance of Milk. Milk or substitutes for the ingredients contained in milk should play a role in the diet of an athlete. These are important and necessary because of their unique nutritional combination of protein, carbohydrate, fat, and minerals, especially calcium and phosphorus, and of vitamins, especially A, D, niacin equivalents, and riboflavin. These foods contribute to the overall needs of the body. It would be difficult to meet recommended standards for daily intake of calcium and riboflavin without including milk or certain milk products in the diet. The important role of calcium has already been discussed. However, some coaches have eliminated milk from the athlete's diet during the training season or from the pregame meal because of unfounded beliefs that milk cuts down the athlete's wind and endurance, increases mucous secretions in the respiratory tract, causes "cotton mouth" and reduces respiratory effort. None of these beliefs has a basis in scientific fact. Experiments have shown that milk consumed during a pregame meal had no adverse effects either on performance or production of gastrointestinal disturbances.

Special Considerations. As the day of the contest approaches, it is commonplace for the athlete to become tense, excited, and anxious. These symptoms build up into greater and greater proportions until they are released in muscular activity by the start of the game. Some of these impulses are somaticized into abdominal cramps, nausea, vomiting, urinating, and diarrhea. Digestion of the pregame meal is disturbed, causing a delay in stomach emptying time with a resultant delay and impairment of absorption. The amount of energy available for musculoskeletal activity is consequently reduced.

A training table supervised by a dietitian is a decided asset for an athletic team. Not only are food requirements met scientifically, but individual differences are satisfied. Professional and college teams are favored with such luxury, but, unfortunately, this is not the lot of growing, immature, adolescent high school athletes, who may be beset by many complicating social, financial, and emotional problems.

The high school athlete's lunch is usually inadequate, too frequently consisting of hamburgers, hot dogs, french fries, and pizza pies, usually accompanied by a soft drink. These foods are popular because they are readily available and more quickly served and eaten than a full-course meal. He may occasionally treat himself to a sandwich of fried eggs, fried ham, or roast beef. Although these foods are appetizing, they are not nutritively adequate for growing adolescents who face a tough practice session the same afternoon. Most school cafeterias offer a well-planned meal that includes meat, milk, salad, and fruit, but it is often ignored by the athlete. Home-cooked meals may be nourishing, but many mothers work and are not at home to supervise lunch, or the students cannot travel the distance home for lunch. The coach or a member of his staff should communicate and interpret to the athlete's mother or other members of the family some of the nutritional needs of the growing teenager who is participating in sports.

Food preferences are important to the athlete and should be just as important to the coaching staff. "What is meat for one is poison for another." A player knows from personal experience the specific foods that seem to disagree with him and therefore should be avoided.

Food allergies are best handled by the team physician. The coach should not hesitate to call for medical help when there is a fluid or food problem; certainly, all gastrointestinal disturbances are the proper concern of the physician. Qualified nutritionists make excellent consultants for both physicians and coaches.

Except for a greater quantity of calories, the athlete's diet differs little from that of any other healthy person. It includes fluids, salt, vitamins, and minerals, and in addition to satisfying nutritional, biochemical, and physiologic requirements, should be tasty, look attractive, and satisfy appetite. Variety makes eating more interesting.

REFERENCES

American Dietetic Association: Handbook of Clinical Dietetics. New Haven, Yale University Press, 1981.

Goodhart, R.S., and Shils, M.E.: Modern Nutrition in Health and Disease. 6th Ed. Philadelphia, Lea & Febiger, 1980.

McArdle, W.D., Katch, F.I., and Katch, V.L.: Exercise Physiology: Energy, Nutrition, and Human Performance. Philadelphia, Lea & Febiger, 1980.

American Dietetic Association: Nutrition and physical fitness, 7615:437–443, 1980.

Novich, M.M., and Kaufman, T.: The High-Energy Diet for Dynamic Living. New York, Grosset & Dunlop, 1976.

Serfass, R.C.: Nutrition for the athlete. N.Y. State J. Med.: 78–11, 1824–1825.

Smith, N.J.: Food for Sport. Palo Alto, Bull Publishing, 1976.

Wilmore, J.H.: Proper nutrition for exercise and sport. *In* The Wilmore Fitness Program. New York, Simon & Schuster, 1981, pp. 193–209.

8

Drugs in Sports

INTRODUCTION

In order to understand why athletes use drugs in the hope of improving their performance, it is worthwhile to examine the genesis of this practice, which certainly exists on all levels of modern athletic activity. The psychophysical development of today's athlete is qualitatively no different than that of his predecessors. Aggression, hostility and competitiveness in a child are normal, instinctive drives to achieve growth, maturity, and recognition. The child uses athletic activities as a play outlet to reach these goals. For most normal children, winning is very important because it gives them personal satisfaction and the approval of parents, friends, and spectators. This desire extends into adolescent and adult life.

The athlete prepares for his sport by training and conditioning. His natural physical endowments, skills, training, and degrees of aggression, hostility, competitiveness and motivation determine the effort he puts into an athletic activity in an attempt to win. Jim Tatum once said, "Winning isn't everything; it's the only thing." Winning remains the goal of athletic competition, despite the high-sounding phrases of the Olympic Creed, which states that "the most important thing in the Olympic Games is not to win but to take part. . . ." Any athlete worth his salt does not participate without wanting to win.

The athlete's desire to win becomes associated—consciously and unconsciously—with personal tensions, stresses, and pressures. The further an athlete advances in his sport, the tougher the competition becomes; the champion or athlete on the first team is always being challenged for his spot. He must work harder to overcome the competition and keep in first place, and this subjects him to tremendous psychophysicial stresses that produce anxieties. When an athlete makes it to the top, whether as pro or amateur, he has advanced to a pressure-boiler type of life complicated by the risks and hazards inherent in his sport.

Where their athletic prowess is concerned, many athletes tend to be narcissistic, superstitious, impressionable, faddish, gullible, and even hypochondriacal. This may be due to either inherent or developmental psychologic deficits—characteristics that an athlete is motivated to overcome through excellence in sports. Because of these weaknesses, athletes are prepared to try special diets, drugs, and physical and mechanical body-building aids in an effort to enhance their performance and assure their superiority in athletics. This is more true now than ever because the competition is keener and the rewards greater. Athletes base their beliefs in these aids on hearsay, misconceptions, exaggerated claims, half-truths, inconclusively documented experiments, and advertising.

Examples of Drug Use in Modern Athletics. *Boxing.* The early days of modern athletics saw little or no controlled basic research to determine the physiologic effects of drugs on athletic performance. Thus, a variety of concoctions were taken by athletes on an empirical basis, not only in the hope of improving performance, but in some instances just to prolong performance. As a result, some colorful if not dangerous situations resulted.

Prizefighters of yesteryear were given strychnine tablets, sips of dilute solution of aromatic spirits of ammonia, drinks of honey combined with brandy, or brandy alone before and during a fight. Honey and brandy were frequently given veteran fighters between rounds, especially toward the latter part of a bout. Some fighters had their head, face, and neck sponged with champagne between rounds to pep them up, and occasionally some of this sparkling fluid found its way into the fighter's mouth as well. In any event, in small doses this might have had a stimulating effect temporarily, although primarily psychologic.

Strychnine, an established central nervous system stimulant, was used in professional boxing to energize a boxer who was showing signs of weariness. However, it had to be given in nearly toxic doses to produce the desired "hopping" effect. Another method of stimulating a groggy boxer was to apply a lighted match to his low back, which usually aroused him in a hurry. Strychnine and lighted flames are not used anymore in sports.

Some prizefighters had the face and body massaged with an ointment containing cocaine and cocoa butter prior to the bout. This afforded some surface anesthesia to nullify the effect of the blows, and also provided some illusory and imaginary recuperative strength as the fight wore on. Cocaine acts on the central nervous system to allay sensations of fatigue, resulting in an increased capacity for work. However, cocaine is considered a narcotic, and dependence on it is not only injurious to health, but its possession and use without a doctor's prescription are illegal.

In 1910 James J. Jeffries, after being kayoed in the sixteenth round by Jack Johnson, claimed his "tea was drugged" the day of the fight. This allegation was never proven. In 1955, Harold Johnson, following his early knock-out by Julio Mederos, claimed he was "doped by a poisoned orange"—this allegation was proved correct. Barbiturates were detected in blood and urine tests performed immediately after the bout, providing sufficient proof for the Pennsylvania State Athletic Commission that Harold Johnson was in fact under the influence of a depressant drug during the fight. The method of administration was never discovered. Because barbiturates and other central nervous system depressants were accidentally or purposely dropped into a prize-fighter's water bottle, a trainer was specially assigned to watch this bottle. The opening of the bottle was taped or corked before and during the course of a bout. These precautions considerably reduced the opportunity for drugging a fighter.

Cycling. Professional cyclists comprised one of the hardiest breeds of athletes ever developed—they had to be, to keep up with the tremendous physical toll that this sport demands. For instance, a 100-kilometer (62½ miles) motorpaced bicycle race was cycled in an average time of 1½ hours. Unfortunately, the youth of today are not privileged to witness such sensational and spectacular sport events, which characteristically brought out tremendous feats of strength, stamina, and endurance. In "6-day" bicycle races, which have also disappeared from the sporting scene, cyclists pedaled over 2,000 miles in 142 hours. In 1914, Grenda and Goullet set a 6-day bike record of 2,759.2 miles, which still stands today. This was not only a grueling sport, but also bruising. Falls and tangled bicycles commonly occurred, accounting for many splinters, floor burns, fractures, dislocations and other acute trauma. Consequently, bike riders resorted to all sorts of drugs, secret brews, and concoctions purported to help them to withstand the fearful grind, rigors, fatigue, sleepiness, and injuries.

Most 6-day bike riders depended on black coffee, tea, narcotics, alcoholic beverages, and secret medical preparations. A Thermos bottle of black coffee with a few drops of peppermint flavoring and caffeine capsules was always handy when a cyclist needed a mouthful to stave off sleep and fatigue. Spiking the coffee with cocaine or strychnine was also a common practice, and made the rider less aware of fatigue. Some cyclists preferred tea mixed with brandy. However, it was the manner in which the coffee or tea was administered and the agent with which it was combined that determined whether the desired results would be produced. Cyclists would be served only coffee or tea for the first 3 days. Starting on the fourth day, the trainer combined the tea or coffee with such agents as an ounce of brandy or capsules of cocaine and continued this for the fifth and sixth days of the race. This method of administration increased the concentration of the stimulant to a maximal peak that was supposed to benefit the athlete most in the closing hours of the race.

Cocaine and heroin were frequently used by 6-day cyclists. Cocaine produced a marked stimulation by allaying sensations of fatigue, leading to a sense of euphoria, confidence, exhilaration, and an illusory feeling of an increased capacity for muscular activity. However, there is plenty of evidence of interference with judgment. Its effectiveness depended on the dosage and method of administration, which were usually the responsibility of the trainer. Cocaine was used orally in a capsule form combined with caffeine, or as flakes applied directly to the tongue. Cocaine snow was combined with cocaine butter in an ointment administered by a prostatic or body massage. Veteran cyclist trainers have stated that a fatigued 6-day bike rider could roar back into action after a cocaine administration. When a rider had a good concentration of cocaine in him, his eyes might shine like moons because of the markedly dilated pupils. This often leads to poor visual accommodation. In the 1972 Munich Olympics, one member of the Dutch bicycle team ran off the course and smashed his bike causing his entire team to be disqualified. Cocaine, like narcotics, is habit forming and can cause mental aberration.

Heroin acts by depressing certain parts of the brain as well as other parts of the nervous system. It provided 6-day bike riders with a temporary psychologic lift by dulling their awareness of the harsh realities of this sport. At the same time, the constant pain and discomfort associated with fatigue, sleepiness, and injuries were lessened by its analgesic properties. As the body became tolerant to the drug, larger doses became necessary to achieve the same effects. Heroin is habit forming and also highly toxic. The risk of addiction and the deleterious effects of narcotics are well known and too replete with documentation to repeat here. These are drugs that are best left alone.

Foreign bike riders talked openly about their stimulants, which supposedly possessed mystic powers and were contained in little black bottles. The French riders were fond of a preparation known as Caffeine Houdes (a trade name), which are also used by many French students while cramming for examinations. These are beige granules taken in teaspoonfuls. It was claimed that this drug acted as a tonic. Another French tonic was a 2-ml ampule that was poured into broth and orange juice. The Belgian riders were fond of sugar cubes wetted down with a few drops of ether. This sugar cube was held between the teeth and sucked during the race. One famous Canadian rider had a boxful of secret preparations—apart from his first-aid kit—which he used to stave off fatigue and sleepiness as well as to charge up his performance. American riders had their favorite agents as well. Unfortunately, we may never find out the exact contents of these colorful foreign and domestic preparations, but they included camphor, digitalis, insulin, trinitin, atropine, epinephrine, and vitamins, besides the other drugs mentioned. Many riders were wise enough to take advantage of every opportunity to sleep. Some even drank beer, brandy, or bourbon at the beginning of rest periods to make them sleepy. A well-known French rider slept his rest periods in an oxygen tent. Unfortunately, the body cannot store pure oxygen even when one sleeps in it; beneficial effect, if any, must be considered psychologic.

Nitroglycerin tablets taken before a mile and 5-mile cycle sprint diminished the intensity and duration of the dyspnea that so frequently followed these violent efforts. This drug relaxes the smooth muscles of the coronary blood vessels, relieving any ischemia due to excessive oxygen needs of the myocardium. However, taken by an athlete not used to its physiologic effects, nitroglycerin causes such side-effects as nausea, vomiting, pallor, cold sweat, flushed feeling in the head, severe headaches, and even fainting.

DRUGS USED BY ATHLETES

In athletics, a large variety of chemical agents have been consumed as foods, dietary supplements, or drugs to improve performance. These have produced a wide range of physiologic changes.

Dietary Supplements. Beyond the extent to which they are required for normal nutrition, different kinds of amino acids, carbohydrates, vitamins and minerals have been used in an effort to provide instant and reserve energy, increased work capacity, and to delay fatigue. No objections of unfair play are raised when dietary supplements are added to the training diet in an effort to improve performance, probably because in controlled experiments these substances have failed to be truly ergogenic. Athletes who consume sufficient amounts of milk and milk products, cereal and cereal products, meat and meat products, fruits and vegetables are supplied abundant amounts of vitamins and minerals. The common practice of giving pregame vitamin B_{12} injections to professional football and hockey players has no scientific justification. The same may be said of vitamin E, administered either by tablets or in cereals. Vitamin B_{12} is medically indicated for pernicious anemia, but vitamin E has no specific medical uses. Any benefits that athletes or their handlers claim for these vitamin supplements are either purely psychologic or based on misinformation. Nevertheless, they may be given without harm if the athlete feels he is definitely helped by them. However, injections must be given under strict aseptic conditions.

The use of protein or amino-acid supplements in the training diet or of sugar as a pre-event supplement have not fared any better scientifically than vitamins or minerals in improving athletic performance. Dietary supplements are not indicated except for athletes with special medical needs. Diabetic athletes may need insulin along with proper regulation of the carbohydrate intake.

Drugs Affecting the Nervous System. Another large and popular category of drugs has physiologic effects on selected sites of the central and autonomic nervous systems. This group includes alcohol, amphetamines, caffeine, cocaine, ephedrine, heroin, metrazol, nicotine, strychnine, and others. Amphetamines, ephedrine, and epinephrine are related chemically and have similar physiologic effects, with some important differences. They are known as sympathomimetic agents, because they elicit responses in the body similar to those induced by the sympathetic nervous system, such as raising the blood pressure, alerting the body for stress, and causing constriction of blood vessels.

Except for amphetamine, cocaine, heroin, and strychnine, the previously listed drugs were never popularly used in sports. Alcohol, popular both on and off the athletic scene, could never be considered a worthwhile ergogenic aid because of its depressant and other undesirable effects. Cocaine, which has a colorful past along with heroin and strychnine, has reappeared on the sports scene. Amphetamine, the controversial "pep pill," is still with us, wrecking athletes but not improving their performance.

Narcotics. Narcotics are those drugs that can produce stupor, complete insensibility or sleep. Their analgesic properties are well known and are used by physicians to eliminate pain and induce sleep in sick and injured patients. Prolonged use may cause dependence on the drug, which is injurious to health. Narcotics are divided into four groups.

1. Opiates—substances with an addiction-forming or sustaining liability similar to morphine or cocaine or whose derivatives have such a liability.
2. Coca leaves and derivatives.
3. Marijuana.
4. Meperidine (pethidine).

The use of narcotics in competition has increased, reflecting the excesses in today's drug-abusive society. Marijuana is a favorite with high school athletes who use it to get "high or stoned" for celebrating victory or combatting a letdown following defeat. Some youngsters experience more difficulty buying liquor than marijuana. Cocaine and heroin have been discussed with a past breed of athletes because of the ingenious ways they were administered. Actually, the use of narcotics by an athlete for other than post-injury pain can only lead to a reduction in performance, and it actually hastens the termination of his athletic career. These drugs are regulated under the Harrison and other federal nar-

6

cotic laws. Illegal possession of narcotics may jeopardize a person's career and social position with a police record.

Amphetamines. The commonly used amphetamines ("pep pills") are Benzedrine, Dexedrine, and Methedrine. Benzedrine and Dexedrine are commonly referred to as "bennies"; Methedrine is also known as "speed." In athletics, amphetamine may be referred to as "the magic pill." Amphetamine and its derivatives have had a colorful and varied past since their discovery in the twenties as powerful central nervous system stimulants. In the thirties, a Benzedrine inhaler was popular for head colds and stuffy noses. It also became popular among college students to reduce mental and physical fatigue by reducing or eliminating sleep requirements; this produces a state of wakefulness and alertness that enables one to study and cram for examinations. During World War II, soldiers used amphetamines to delay fatigue, improve the mood, increase confidence and to help accomplish feats of strength and courage needed on dangerous missions. Following the return of veterans to colleges and universities, amphetamine "pep pills" were commonly used by professional and intercollegiate athletes. High school coaches and their charges imitated the pros and amphetamines became popular even in interscholastic athletics. Currently, these drugs are also used to control appetite for weight reduction.

Clinicians, pharmacologists, and physiologists agree that amphetamine is a potent stimulant of the central nervous system that causes, among other things, stimulation of the cerebral cortex, excitation of the brain stem reticular activating and arousal mechanisms and facilitates mono- and polysynaptic transmission in the spinal cord. The respiratory center of the medulla is stimulated to increase the rate and depth of respiration.

Cardiac ouptut is increased by direct myocardial action and by peripheral constriction of the arterioles, much like the action of epinephrine. The person taking the drug feels a sense of exhilaration, well-being, and even euphoria. The drug user may state he feels "pepped up" (by reduction of fatigue) and able to exert greater energy than usual; he may manifest an increased physical activity, but there is little or no effect on basal metabolism. The use of amphetamines by an athlete may produce psychic stimulation, which can impair his judgment and give him a false impression that his athletic performance has been improved.

High dosage may result in undesirable side-effects, such as dizziness, nausea, headache, agitation, and anxiety. Gross overdosage may cause extreme restlessness, rapid pulse, hypertension, shallow respiration, pallor, and collapse.

In June, 1957, the House of Delegates of the American Medical Association had to consider a charge that the use of pep pills was widespread among athletes in an attempt to improve athletic performance. It was widely rumored in sports circles that the 12 record-breaking performances for the mile run, accomplished under 4 minutes at that time, were achieved with the help of "pep pills." This rumor was vigorously denied by the trackmen and their coaches.

Because there was such a welter of conflicting and confusing opinions regarding the exact effects of amphetamines on athletic performance, the Board of Trustees of the American Medical Association financed a research study at Harvard University by Beecher and Smith to determine these effects. They also provided some financial assistance to Karpovich at Springfield College, who already had such an experiment under way. These two studies remain the most widely cited, controlled experiments of their kind; however, they come to different conclusions.

In the Harvard study, improvement was noted in about 75% of the athletes who were given 14 to 21 mg of amphetamines per kg 2 to 3 hours before their running, swimming, or shot putting events. Notwithstanding this conclusion, these authors state that their findings do not prove that athletic performance would be helped by amphetamines in intercollegiate competition. Pierson did an in-depth analysis of the Harvard study, finding many scientific and statistical faults. He stated that the conclusions were not substantiated by the data. However, many of his criticisms were already noted by the experimenters themselves.

The Springfield study gave 10 to 20 mg amphetamine per athlete 10 to 30 minutes before running, swimming, and treadmill tests; Karpovich found improvement in only three out of 54 athletes. One athlete's performance was affected deleteriously. In a personal communication Karpovich stated "I am very pessimistic regarding all these ergogenic aids. In some additional experiments, I found that instead of increasing speed or endurance of trackmen it decreased. Golding and Bernard did an extensive study on use of amphetamines and athletic performance; they, too, found no beneficial effect. In response to my (M.N.) queries to a large cross section of team physicians, physiologists, coaches and trainers, the majority do not agree with the conclusion of the Harvard study.

The strong prohibition spearheaded by the medical profession induced a negative response by the athlete and his handler. As a consequence, an unsubstantiated myth has been established about the "magic power" of this drug. The fable of the amphetamine "pep pill" may take many years to dispel, and may be more difficult to eradicate than the myth of the "athletic heart."

Barbiturates. No one seriously objects when central nervous system depressants such as barbiturates, tranquilizers, or other sedatives are used to relax or produce sleep in anxious, agitated, tense athletes, particularly if insomnia is a problem. This is a common practice among professional football and hockey players, as well as amateur athletes. Barbiturates are the most popular of this group because of their sleep-producing properties. They reduce alertness and the capacity to function by dulling the senses and depressing the cardiac and respiratory centers. Skeletal muscular activity is reduced; reactions and responses are slowed. Coordination becomes impaired. Sufficient dosage gradually brings on sleep. Professional football and hockey players take barbiturates the night before a game to assure some sleep; some take the drug immediately after the game. Because barbiturates potentiate the action of analgesics, an athlete may also take them the night after the game along with an analgesic to enable him to get some rest for his weary, bruised, and injury-wracked body.

The athlete has a wide variety of barbiturates from which to choose and the list gets longer yearly. Barbiturate action may be short-acting and fast-starting, such as pentobarbital (Nembutal) and secobarbital (Seconal). Phenobarbital (Luminal) and amobarbital (Amytal) are long-acting and slow-starting. My (M. N.) favorite prescription for sleep is one 15 mg Dalmane capsule at bedtime, which in most cases affords a night of uninterrupted sleep. The short-acting barbiturates are called "goof-balls" or "yellow jackets" and are most frequently abused; the long-acting ones are called "red devils," "blue heavens," or "green dragons." Continual use of barbiturates can lead to dependency. Increased dosages are required to relax and calm the user and produce sleep. At this point a word of caution is necessary: one can easily take an accidental overdose of these drugs, because memory lapse following their use is not uncommon. Barbiturates are favorite agents for committing suicide.

Tranquilizers. Tranquilizers, another large group of psychotropic drugs, have the ability to sedate or calm an individual without causing sleep. These drugs can reduce anxiety, tension, and agitation without interfering with mental alertness and physical response. They also potentiate the effectiveness of analgesic medications. At least two tranquilizers are on the market that not only have psychotropic characteristics, but are also used clinically for relief of skeletal muscle spasm. Professional football players consume muscle relaxants by the handfuls. Although I (M. N.) use muscle relaxants clinically for muscle spasm, I am not prepared to state any conclusion about their ability to improve athletic performance; personally, I do not see how they can.

Caffeine. No one could seriously claim "doping" if an athlete is an avid drinker of coffee, tea, or cola drinks, which contain caffeine, an acknowledged central nervous system stimulant. These drinks are commonly used to allay fatigue and produce alertness, which results in an increased output of work. It may even cause some people to become restless and unable to sleep. Although the average cup of coffee may contain 100 to 150 mg of caffeine, this amount is too small to affect an athlete's performance. Several cups of coffee or tea might conceivably raise the caffeine in the blood to a level unacceptable to some medical committee of an athletic governing body. This could result in the disqualification of an athlete or his team. The disqualification of an athlete because of high concentrations of caffeine in his blood may sound farfetched, but liquids containing this compound are common items in the diet of the average U.S. athlete.

Alcohol. The use of alcoholic beverages—a common social phenomenon in the U.S.—is even more common in Europe, where it is customarily part of the training table. In European countries, beer and wine are consumed with meals much like coffee, tea, cola drinks, and soda pop are drunk in America. Nonetheless in the 1968 Mexico City Olympics, Sweden's Modern Pentathlon Team was disqualified and their Bronze Medal ordered returned to the International Committee when it was found that one of their pistol shooters was found to have used alcohol.

The regulations of the federation that governs the Modern Pentathlon specifically ban alcohol. This group asked the International Olympic Committee to check for and disqualify any Pentathlete found to have used alcohol. There is an old wives' tale that states that some drinks of beer can quiet the arm of pistol shooters.

It is generally acknowledged that alcohol, which is a known depressant, impairs coordination, judgment, and skilled performance. The athlete may develop a feeling of confidence and euphoria expressed in increased musculoskeletal activity as a result of lessening of the cerebral cortical inhibitory control. However, under no circumstances does alcohol improve or increase mental or physical ability, especially work requiring skill and attention.

Drugs Affecting the Circulatory System. Another group of drugs used by some athletes exerts physiologic effects on the circulatory system. In clinical medicine these drugs are most commonly used for the treatment of cardiac disease and peripheral vascular disorders. Because of their artery dilating properties and tonic effect on the heart muscle, they are very popular among cyclists, leading to the "Valley of the Dolls" for some and the morgue for others. Included in this group are beta-pyridylcarbinol, digitalis, nitroglycerin (see p. 144), and others.

Androgen-Anabolic Steroids. Endocrinologists during the past two decades have successfully used androgen-anabolic steroids to accelerate growth in children who were not developing physically as fast or as tall as expected. These steroids, by causing a retention of nitrogen, potassium, phosphorus, and increased endogenous growth-hormone level, bring on weight gain, increase in height, and a feeling of well-being. Unfortunately, drugs with these potentials intrigued wrestlers, weightlifters, football players, and field-event men, who started taking them in a wholesale manner. They reasoned illogically that the heavier they became, the stronger they would be.

When a physician treats a child with a pediatric disorder that can be helped by androgen-anabolic steroids, he is trained to adjust the dosage or stop the drug when adverse reactions such as priapism, hirsutism, edema, jaundice, gynecomastia (breast development), and other manifestations occur. Unfortunately, the healthy athlete who takes these drugs may not recognize an adverse reaction and allow irreversible damage to take place. It is unthinkable that any adult would give this drug to a prepubertal or pubertal male for the purpose of athletic participation. In the prepubertal person, these drugs in large amounts could cause premature closing of the epiphysis, leading to decreased height. In pubertal boys, a disturbance may occur in the production of testosterone by the testes, with irreversible cytoarchitecture damage.

Unlike the physician who understands the adverse physiologic effects of this drug, the athlete may be unaware that the increase in weight that occurs following use of the drug might be caused by salt and water retention (edema), which happens frequently with prolonged usage. Weightlifters who were proud of their pectoral-muscle development may have given Dianabol, the preferred androgen, undue credit for their conspicuous appearance. What appeared to the weightlifter as a hypertrophied pectoral muscle could in fact be the beginning of gynecomastia (breast development), another adverse reaction.

Many professional football players have taken this small, light blue tablet on the advice of their handlers without questioning what it does. It looks harmless enough. However, once they become aware of the dangers they discontinue its use because it can lead to testicular shrinkage, decreased libido, infertility, and liver damage, among other things.

Local Anesthetics. In 1934 Leriche popularized local procaine injections and early ambulation for knee and ankle sprains. The local anesthetic prevents afferent pain impulses that result in swelling and functional disturbance. Thus a vicious cycle is interrupted. Early joint motion prevents atrophy of the surrounding musculature. When Leriche postulated this method of treatment, it was directed not only toward the immediate relief of pain, but also toward reducing temporary and permanent disability. He surely did not have athletes in mind, and certainly not professional football players. This treatment worked well with sprains when the involved ligament was not lacerated or torn away with an avulsed piece of bone. This concept was further advanced by Steindler, who popularized procaine injections for painful, tender trigger-point areas of spastic muscles in low-back conditions, in which a similar vicious cycle of pain—muscle spasm—pain occurs, and functional loss results.

The use of local anesthesia with ethyl chloride spray and injections of procaine to eliminate pain in an injury site in order to allow an athlete to continue playing are common practices in professional and intercollegiate athletics. In high school, coaches and trainers use ethyl chloride for cooling down the pain of an injured area as well as to eliminate painful limitation of motion. This treatment has its hazards. For example, one coach in North Carolina dispensed with the services of a physician and did his own local anesthetic injections for sprained ankles for several of his football players. He was exposed when one of his athlete-patients did not respond to his method of treatment, which aggravated the condition. His actions are really not surprising since so much notoriety is given by the press about injections given to professional athletes so as to enable them to start or finish a game.

No physician should use any local block therapy for acute trauma to muscles or joints of a high school athlete unless he has first examined the injury. Following this examination, he may use ethyl chloride spray on a contused muscle or joint or joint sprain that is painful and causes painful restriction of motion, provided there is no fracture or tears of the myofascial, ligamentous and tendinous structures. The spray is effective by eliminating painful muscle spasm that results from local trauma. Ethyl chloride must not be used to reduce swelling through its chilling effect. To use ethyl chloride for this purpose is not only wrong, but could lead to using an amount so great that it causes various degrees of burn.

No physician should ever use procaine or other local agents to render an injured area analgesic in a high school athlete so that he can return to the game before sufficient healing has taken place. Elimination of pain gives the athlete a false sense of security, which could lead to further and perhaps irreparable damage. The chances for maximal restoration lessen with each recurrent injury. In high school athletes, the use of local anesthesia with or without a corticoid is indicated as specific treatment only for a painful ligament, tendon, or myofascial injury in which no significant tear exists and which has not responded to the usual, conservative treatment measures of cold, compression, heat, elevation, and immobilization. Return to participation depends on the response to treatment.

Most college athletes are young, emotionally immature and all too frequently imbued with a "do-or-die" school spirit. Therefore, the doctor must use his best judgment to protect the athlete from himself.

Although local injections have been used to eliminate pain in an acute joint or muscle injury to allow a college athlete to engage in sports, such practices may be undesirable. I know of an intercollegiate boxer who had a painful knuckle locally anesthetized before a bout. This could have led to a fracture, of which the boxer would have been unaware. If a young athlete has more than a mild sprain, he should not participate in athletic events. Participating in an athletic contest with an injured joint that has been locally blocked increases the opportunity for further damage and lessens the chances for complete healing; permanent residuals frequently result. In many instances, big-time intercollegiate football disregards the future health of athletes.

In professional football, the practice of injecting local anesthesia in knee, ankle sprains, muscle avulsion from the iliac crest, and stone bruises of the heel to enable an athlete to play or to be ready for a specific game is commonplace. Professional athletes are valuable to themselves and their teams only when they are playing. In most cases, the physician recommends this type of treatment only if he believes that the athlete can carry on effectively with a minimum of risk to himself. The doctor uses the following in making his medical decision:

1. Nature and extent of injury, and possible medical consequences.
2. Temperament, motivation and pain threshold of the athlete.
3. Game situation and circumstances.

This is never an easy decision for a doctor to make, since the player has placed complete confidence and trust in him. However, the annals of sport history are replete with the use of local anesthesia to permit an athlete to continue playing. Not too long ago a minor medical miracle was accomplished on a famous professional football quarterback who pulled the ligaments in his knee. These were injected with Novocaine and cortisone, which kept him going for the last half. Recently, a famous professional baseball pitcher had a painful ulcer on his toe injected with local anesthesia to enable him to pitch in a crucial World Series game. In earlier days, boxers had weak or glass jaws locally anesthetized prior to a bout. However, the anesthetic never warded off the effects of a K.O. punch that found its mark. One champion prizefighter I knew even had an aching tooth locally anesthetized before a bout.

ETHICAL AND MEDICAL ASPECTS OF DOPING

What is doping? In sports medicine literature, the use of drugs to improve athletic performance is referred to as doping. Historically, drugs have also been used to adversely affect an opponent's performance. Unfortunately, the use of the words "dope" and "doping" conjures images that are misleading medically, ethically, legally, and socially. The majority of drugs supposedly used to improve athletic performance are really not "dope" as the word is generally understood. A dictionary defines "dope" as "slang for a narcotic drug or a stimulant." The popular concept of dope and doping is usually associated with narcotics and other central nervous system depressants such as barbiturates, which not only produce sleep, stupor, and unconsciousness, but also many forms of erratic, irrational, and irresponsible behavior.

If it becomes known that an athlete has used pep pills or some other drug, a thunderous noise rolls out from all sorts of medical and athletic associations, claiming that this is doping, and that it is contrary to the ideals of amateur athletics to attempt to take unfair advantage of one's adversary. It is positively frustrating to hear or read self-righteous declarations on the topic of drug use by academicians, administrators, simon-pures, and physicians, many of whom have no contact with athletics in more than a passing manner. To most athletes these words fall on deaf ears. For example, one editorial on doping by the Comité International Olympique was not directed to the medical hazards and risks that can result from drug use, but was merely a moralistic discourse so emotionally charged that it revealed many unresolved conflicts of the author.

Some statements are sparsely written and ambiguous; others are verbose and ambiguous. Because of the arbitrariness and unrealistic manner of presentation, athletes seek out interpretive loopholes to circumvent the rules. For instance, the ten-clause policy statement of the British Association of Sports Medicine is too wordy, and is best interpreted by a lawyer, especially since it contains so much fine print. Stripped of all its wordiness, it states in essence that doping constitutes the taking of any chemical substance by an athlete which (1) is not present normally in the body during a period of competition, (2) does not play an essential or normal role in his health, and (3) is taken with the intention of improving performance. A chemical substance taken by a sick or injured athlete to cure or alleviate his disabling condition to improve his performance is also defined as doping. Not only are these statements cumbersome and unrealistic, but they produce as many questions as answers. Under these rules, merely taking an aspirin could make an athlete suspect.

The International Olympic Committee has listed the following as "dope": alcohol, pep pills, cocaine, vasodilators, opiates such as opium, morphine, heroin, pethidine, methadone, and hashish, and anabolic steroids. The positions taken by the International Amateur Athletic Federation and the Amateur Athletic Union are more reasonable and practical. To these governing sports bodies, doping is the employment of drugs with the intention of increasing athletic efficiency by their stimulating action upon muscles or nerves or by paralyzing the sense of fatigue. Using the latter rule, a boxer who takes a proteolytic enzyme, prior to a bout to minimize the swelling that will surely follow blows on his face and body would be secure from any charge of doping. This might not be the case with the position taken by the British Association of Sports Medicine. Habit-forming drugs are also prohibited by International Amateur Athletic Federation, Amateur Athletic Union rules.

In conclusion, we believe the entire problem of doping is being handled in an emotional and irrational manner rather than realistically. There has never been any proof that success in athletics was attributable to any single chemical substance, because so many factors are involved in the development of team or individual athletic performance. If a winner were found to have a "doping substance" in the urine, it might be interesting to perform urine tests on the losers, perhaps noting that they also have taken some forbidden chemical. Since in reality no secret chemical preparations or drugs exist that are not available to all athletes, what is the basis for the charge of unfairness that the sport-governing bodies keep harping about?

A more effective way of handling this drug problem would be to have physicians discuss with athletes the physiologic effects of these drugs and the psychologic needs that cause an athlete to use chemical substances in an illusory attempt to improve athletic performance. The team physician would explain in detail not only the physiologic actions of various drugs on the body, but also their adverse sequelae. He would also explode the myth regarding the ability of drugs to improve athletic performance. These discussions should be held with the entire team present, including the coaches, trainers, and managers. The initial lecture should be held at the beginning of the season, with additional meetings of this nature during competition as the need arises.

Since the users of such drugs have a propensity to develop a dependency on these aids, psychiatric orientation may also be indicated. A psychiatrist would be in a strategic position to help those athletes who find it necessary to resort to the use of pharmacologic agents in an attempt to improve their performance. Individual programs can be worked out, based on the above premises.

If a high school athlete becomes a user, despite this orientation and psychiatric help, the coach has no choice but to drop the player from the squad. The legal and medical responsibility is too much of a burden. A conference should be had with the parents and a physician before such a definitive action is taken. If the drug is being supplied by the trainer, manager, or even the coach, a severe penalty must be meted out to the offender. The same type of disciplinary action should be meted out to intercollegiate athletes and their handlers.

The problem is different with professional athletes. They are all adults, and playing sports is their profession. As long as all the hazards and risks are explained medically to these athletes, they make the choice fully aware of the risks and hazards. Under no circumstance does the team physician prescribe drugs for an athlete that are not indicated or not in his best interest. The physician must resist temptation to be the fall guy—to do otherwise only promotes disrespect and even contempt. Because the relationship is so close, the physician can act as a powerful restraining force on these unusually aggressive and powerful men. In the long run they will be better off medically and have a greater respect than if the doctor were to accede to their emotional and irrational appeal for illicit drugs.

If a physician prescribes medication for an indicated need, the athlete should be allowed to use it even during sport competition. Procurement of a drug for other than medically indicated needs is to be decried.

Because so much of this material is readily available in medical and lay literature, most athletes and their handlers are fully aware of the overall effects that can be expected when a specific drug is used. They are, however, not aware of or choose to ignore the side-effects and often dangerous sequelae that can result from large doses of drugs or their habitual use. If an athlete needs any convincing that it is extremely dangerous to get "hooked" on drugs, he need only read of the tragic death from heroin poisoning of the renowned veteran football tackle, Paul "Big Daddy" Lipscomb. In 1963, Billy Bello, a promising New York professional welterweight boxer, died from heroin poisoning. In 1959 an amateur cyclist during the famous Tour De France died in "acute cardiorespiratory insufficiency with a hyperthermic syndrome"; he had added eight tablets of an amphetamine to his flask of coffee. In 1967, the Tour De France claimed a British cyclist, Tom Simpson, who also died from an overdose of amphetamines. In 1960, a young Danish cyclist collapsed and died during an Olympic road race. Microscopic examination of autopsy findings showed a non-specific vascular congestion—his trainer, in an effort to increase the cyclist's peripheral circulation, gave him tablets of beta-pyridylcarbinol (Roniacol), a vasodilator that is used clinically for peripheral vascular disease. Another bike rider, Yves Mottin of France, died in 1968 apparently from an overdose of amphetamines. Not to be outdone by cyclists, Jean Louis Kquadri, an 18-year-old French soccer player, died in November, 1968, in Grenoble, France, from an overdose of amphetamines. The usual cause of death from amphetamines is cardiorespiratory collapse with hyperexia. Although no deaths have been reported from large doses or prolonged use of the androgen-anabolic steroids, a number of sequelae have occurred that are threats to an athlete's health. A rather ominous list of complications that can result from drug misuse has been presented. In a number of instances, these complications have resulted in death. The death of boxer Willie Classen on November 23, 1979, had overtones of drug involvement.

BLOOD DOPING

During the 1976 Olympics, a number of radio and TV sports announcers referred to blood doping for a number of days. It is presently only an experimental idea for athletes that was not used during the 1976 Olympics. Essentially, it is a transfusion of blood taken from an athlete while training and exercising on a treadmill. The red cells are separated out and stored. About a month later, another pint of blood is taken from the same athlete. Again the red cells are separated out and stored frozen. As much as three units may be removed for future transfusion to the same athlete. Approximately 5 weeks after the last unit is taken, the packed red cells are thawed and reinfused into the athlete. The benefits that may accrue from this innovative idea are small and the potential for serious problems is great. It is still too experimental to make any real judgment.

REFERENCES

Anel, G.: Residual effect of an anabolic steroid upon isotonic muscular force. J. Sports Med. Phys. Fitness, *14*:103, 1974.

DiPalma, J.R.: Drill's Pharmacology in Medicine. 4th Ed. New York, McGraw-Hill, 1971.

Fahey, T.D., and Brown, H.C.: The effects of an anabolic steroid on the strength, body composition, and endurance of a college male when accompanied by a weight-training program. Med. Sci. Sports, *5*:272, 1973.

Goodman, L.S., and Gilman, A.: Pharmacological Basis of Therapeutics. 6th Ed. New York, Macmillan, 1980.

Goth, A.: Medical Pharmacology: Principles and Concepts. 10th Ed. St. Louis, C.V. Mosby, 1981.

International Olympic Medical Commission. Rule 27. Olympic Charter, pp. 3–7.

Mofenson, H.C., et al.: Drugs in sports. Clin. Pediatr., *16.6*:501–502, 1977.

Novich, M.M.: Drug abuse in sports. N.Y. State J. Med., *73*:2597–2600, 1973.

Sperryn, P.N.: Ethics in sports medicine: The sports physician. Br. J. Sports Med., *14*:2–3, 84–89, 1980.

Williams, J.G.P., and Sperryn, P.N.: Doping. *In* Sports Medicine. 2nd Ed. Baltimore, Williams & Wilkins, 1976. pp. 233–242.

9

Diagnosis and Treatment of Athletic Injuries

INTRODUCTION

Injuries that result from athletics predominantly involve the musculo-skeletal system. Sprains, strains, contusions of joints and muscles, and fractures and dislocations of bones and joints make up the bulk of these injuries. Head, face, neck injuries and internal injuries of the thorax and abdomen statistically play a minor role, but they can be quite serious and even fatal. The attending physician must be aware of his limitations and should call in a consultant when an injury is beyond his training and experience.

Abrasions and lacerations of the skin and bruises of the subcutaneous tissue are so commonplace that they represent red and then black-and-blue status badges of body contact. These injuries present no great difficulty in treatment unless they become infected.

It is not within the scope of this book to discuss in detail the diagnosis and treatment of all the clinical conditions that result from athletic injuries. Only some basic principles can be noted for some of the more common injuries of the connecting and supporting structures of the body. The following discussions cover only that treatment that can be rendered up to and excluding surgical intervention or procedures requiring the use of an operating room.

Some of the terms used in this chapter to describe clinical conditions have been either discarded by the Advisory Panel on the Standard Nomenclature of Athletic Injuries of the Council on Scientific Affairs of the A.M.A. (e.g., "shoulder pointer" and "tennis elbow") or found unacceptable to the same committee (e.g., "pitcher's elbow" and "tennis leg"). We have retained these terms because, at the present stage in the development of athletic medicine, most coaches, trainers, and athletes are more familiar with these terms than with specific anatomic and pathologic terminology. The anatomy and pathology of these clinical conditions are explained in the text and in the glossary.

THE PSYCHOLOGY OF ATHLETIC PERFORMANCE

Any attempt to separate the psychologic from the physical in athletic performance is an artificial one. The two are inseparably and intrinsically entwined. It behooves the medical, coaching, and training staffs to be cognizant of this, because dealing with athletes depends on an understanding of this relationship.

Various personality types, which carry their own psychologic nuances, confront these professionals. These professionals must deal with the athlete; this task is best accomplished in caring for the athlete and is based on a mature understanding of both themselves and the athlete.

The varied personality types may be catalogued as they reflect the athlete's motivation and his response to pain. First, it cannot be emphasized too often that pain is nature's way of alerting the performer that something is wrong and needs attention. Though it is not the purpose of this chapter to classify the types of pain, it should be known that the athlete's personality will affect his perception of pain, particularly the degree to which he will accept or deny its presence. Then there are the psychologic factors, which will determine the athlete's perception of pain. For example, the excitement of the competition, the thrill of victory, the exhilaration of a good play, a winning score, an outstanding performance—all may contribute to the absent perception of pain in the heat of the contest. However courageous the athlete is, he must ultimately pay the piper in the various forms of injury or illness, if his pain is neither perceived by him nor detected by the medical and training staffs. Recent studies have also shown that within the excitement of the competition, the body may pour out its own natural pain antidotes, known as endorphins, which conceal the pain by the euphoria they bring about.

Thus, the team physician and trainer must appreciate that the peak-performing athlete may be razor-edge close to a state of injury or illness: One of the psychologic manifestations of peak performance is a certain euphoria or feeling of well-being, above and beyond the athlete's base-line personality mood. Conversely, signs of irritability, depression, and loss of interest should be detected, for these are signs of impending staleness, injury, or illness.

Whatever the status of the athlete, he must be treated as an equal. At the same time, it must be realized that each athlete is an individual and must be handled as such. The goal, therefore, of the physician and trainer now intertwine. The main goal should be prevention. How does one approach this?

In terms of prevention, the coach and trainer in getting the athletes ready, is also teaching certain lessons in life. Take for example, the warm-up. It is essential that the warm-up be adequate, for muscles that are literally warm and joints that are flexible are less liable to be injured. Here the lesson is that things must be worked at; you cannot obtain what you want immediately, and slow and steady often is what wins the race. The same is true of injury in a converse way in that you cannot always have your wish to be healed immediately. Injuries take time to heal, but what is necessary for proper healing is both a realistic and optimistic attitude. The trainer must assist the athlete, therefore, in using his time fruitfully during the range of time in which he cannot compete. It may be necessary to recommend an alternate form of conditioning during that lag period.

Though the trainer need not have any formal course in psychology, what is needed is a mature judgment on his part. He cannot let his own ego intrude, for if it did, he may be unrealistic either in getting the athlete back too soon, or may have unrealistic, even grandiose, conceptions of his influence. The trainer, hopefully, has gained the trust and rapport of his athlete so that he will freely come to him and tell him of pain, loss of interest, or any of the manifestations of impending danger as mentioned above. Total honesty on the part of the trainer, both in his dealings with his athletes and in his dealings with himself, is necessary to obtain the rapport which will not only prevent injuries, but provide the touch needed for the rapid and complete healing of injuries already sustained. This information is in time conveyed to the attending physician.

Finally, the athlete, coach, physician and trainer, must understand the principles of training and conditioning. This in turn involves the application of moderate amounts of stress for which the body compensates, making the person stronger and stronger. If the stress, however, is too much and the body cannot respond, injury and illness are the results. Stress comes not only in the form of measured stresses imposed by the athletic situation, but within the total stresses of everyday life. Awareness of this and of the athlete as an individual subject to the pressures of his everyday work, be it schoolwork and/or vocation, home life, or other personal stresses—all these contribute to the total need for adaptation on the part of the organism. This only underlines, therefore, the Athletic Advisory Personnel ability to know their athlete and have the rapport, trust, and understanding of him which is engendered by their own simple, honest, and open attitude.

THE USE OF ADHESIVE TAPE

Proper equipment is an important safeguard against injury in all sports. The athlete must be uniformed so that the vulnerable parts of his body are protected without unnecessarily limiting freedom of action. Each sport has special requirements for protective equipment. There are rules that prohibit the use of certain so called "protective" devices. The team physician, the coach, and the trainer should know about the fashioning and fit of protective pads, uniforms, and shoes. The use of protective and therapeutic wrapping and strapping affords some protection to the musculoskeletal system, which bears the brunt of athletic injuries. Because of anatomy and physiology, some parts of the musculoskeletal frame are better protected than others. Elastic bandages, nonelastic bandages, and adhesive tape are the materials used, but the latter is vastly superior to the other two in most circumstances providing they are used properly.

In athletics, the use of adhesive tape is a way of life. A trainer is not experienced unless he knows how to apply adhesive tape expertly. This requires not only manual skill, but also an understanding of the anatomy and the mechanism of injury in order to apply the tape for maximal preventive or therapeutic benefits. Thus, the application of adhesive tape is an art as well as a science, which can only be developed with considerable practice. Its primary function is to support ligaments and thereby prevent joint injury or reinjury. It can also be used therapeutically to reduce pain and discomfort, and to permit more rapid healing by pulling injured parts closer together and promoting repair. Adhesive tape is also used to hold protective pads and dressings in place. Once a trainer has learned the fundamentals of taping, he can determine the taping requirements best suited for the athlete and incorporate his own variations.

Some general rules for adhesive taping follow:

1. Clean the area with soap and water, shave and dry thoroughly. Oily or sweaty skin is difficult to tape.

2. Cover any laceration or abrasion with sterile dressing.

3. Spray area with a skin protectant such as tincture of benzoin or a similar agent. Such agents not only keep adhesive from slipping or becoming loose, but also reduce the incidence of tape dermatitis.

4. Place the part to be taped in the proper anatomic position for maximal benefits.

5. Select tape size that best conforms to the contours of the injured part.

6. Tape from roll.

7. A thin underwrap is also used preparatory to taping to prevent skin irritation.

8. Apply tape neatly and smoothly, molding with palm of hands. Avoid wrinkles.

9. Apply tape snugly, but never so tight that it causes constriction of the blood vessels.

10. Avoid circular taping when possible, since this may constrict and cause circulatory impairment. If it is used, circulation should be checked frequently.

11. Each strip of tape must overlap the preceding strip to avoid leaving exposed skin, which may cause skin irritation.

12. Following strapping, if movement of the part causes undue tension and/or pain, the strapping may have been incorrectly applied. Remove the tape and apply correctly.

13. Leave the tape in place long enough to promote healing; 5 days is sufficient. The strapping should then be removed, the skin cleansed with tape remover, alcohol, or ether, and the part retaped if indicated medically.

14. Do not retape an irritated area unless it is properly prepared.

15. If an athlete is sensitive to tape or to a skin protector, then an underwrap is necessary prior to taping.

16. Remove all circular strappings following a game or practice.

17. Remove all adhesive taping about a part if injury is suspected.

18. As much care should be exercised in removing the tape as was used in applying it. Never tear, rip or pull adhesive tape off the skin. Use a tape-cutter and gently push the skin away from the adhesive by exerting a little tension on the tape. Removal of ankle strapping is facilitated by vertical and horizontal cuts with bandage scissors previously coated lightly with a skin lubricant. Following removal, the area should be cleansed and a light bland oil massaged gently over the skin to replenish the natural oils and to stimulate circulation.

19. Avoid taping any area immediately after exposure to a whirlpool bath, hot shower, or other physiotherapeutic modality in which heat is emitted from the skin. If taping of this part is necessary, first apply a cold towel to reduce the dilatation of the skin vessels and close the pores; then apply the tape.

20. Adhesive tape is best stored in a dry, cool place with the container standing upright. If stored on its side, the rolls of tape may sag on their spindles and make it difficult to unwind upon application.

JOINT INJURIES

Contusions and sprains of joints constitute a large group of athletic injuries. Of the major articulations, the ankles, the knees, and the acromioclavicular joints—in that order—are injured most frequently. Although the majority of joint injuries involve ligamentous sprains, there also occur, to varying degrees, rupture of the blood vessels in the surrounding areolar tissue, the formation of hematomas, ecchymosis, and tears of muscles and tendons, depending on the severity of the trauma. These may also be complicated by injuries of the synovium, meniscus, and bursa. The degree of injury is revealed by pain, swelling, tenderness, ecchymosis, limitation of motion, and joint laxity.

Joint injuries present a greater challenge to the physician because of the anatomic and kinesthetic complexity of joints and their tendency to adhesions. Joint injuries may also lead to a late disabling osteoarthritis. Obtaining maximal restoration from treatment with a minimum of residuals requires a coordination of the skills and judgment of the physician and the trainer, the cooperation of the athlete, and the patience of the coach.

Sprains of joints result from a sudden twisting, wrenching, or external force applied to the bones that constitute a joint. This results in a mild ligamentous stretching or tearing, or a moderate to severe partial tearing or complete rupture of one or more ligaments. The joint may subluxate and reduce itself spontaneously if an isolated ligament ruptures. A joint dislocation occurs when more than one ligament and its capsule are ruptured. Sprains have been classified as first, second, and third degree, or mild, moderate, and severe, but there has never been any unanimity or wide acceptance of this classification.

Although this chapter is addressed to physicians, coaches, and trainers, we assume that, in most instances, the trainer is the first paramedical person on the scene to survey the injured athlete. After taking a history, the trainer performs a cursory examination and initiates the proper first-aid measures. He makes clinical notations of his observations of injured athletes in a permanent training-room record, which is available to the team physician at all times.

The appropriate first-aid measures for an athlete with an injured joint consist of applying a pressure bandage and cold compresses, resting and elevating the injured part, and administering analgesics. In fact, the trainer's first rules of action for most musculoskeletal injuries are set forth in the acronym ICE, which stands for (1) the application of ice, (2) the application of compression, and (3) elevation of the injured part, if possible. Cold compresses may be elastic bandages immersed in ice water, ice bags or towels containing finely cracked ice, or sponge rubber compression bandages wrapped about the injured part, which is then immersed in ice water. Another excellent method for cold compression is the use of towels and/or wash cloths previously frozen and stored in thermal picnic bags, which give a half hour of cold. Many commercial chemical cold packs are also on the market. When applying cold, avoid direct contact with the ice on skin. This can cause frostbite and burns. Compresses or compression reduces hemorrhage and edema about the joint. Although it is not necessary to make an accurate diagnosis immediately after the accident, one should be made before pain, swelling, and spasm of muscles surrounding an injured joint prevent a comprehensive examination. Abnormal motion at a joint due to a ligament tear or rupture is more easily diagnosed at the time of the accident, before muscle spasm prevents joint laxity.

Effective, definitive treatment must be started within 24 hours. This depends on the physician's analysis of the mechanism, nature and extent of injury. Supportive measures include giving analgesic and anti-inflammatory medication, strapping, heating, massaging, and exercising. These measures improve circulation, hasten healing, minimize adhesions, and return muscle tone and strength. Infrequently, hospitalization with surgery and/or cast application may be indicated.

Ankle Injuries

The ankle joint, despite its relatively small size, has the huge job of transmitting the body weight to the foot in standing, walking, and running. The ankle is subjected to frequent violent high-speed movements peculiar to athletics, which makes it the most frequently injured joint. Although its primary function is dorsiflexion and plantar flexion of the foot, the ankle is not the simple hinge joint that it is usually described to be. Actually, it is an arrangement of three joints that work in concert. The distal tibia, fibula, and talus, enclosed in a capsule supporting ligaments, tendons, and muscles, are connected at the ankle and form the tibiofibular, talotibial, and talofibular joints. As with all mechanisms having multiple moving parts, the ankle is vulnerable to injury when unusual forces are exerted on its structures, especially with sudden changes in body speed and direction, as in dodging an opponent, pivoting, or cutting away from or into an athletic situation. This is so because the ankle is largely a joint having hinge motion, and motions of the ankle-foot complex such as rotation, eversion, and inversion are considerably less. Because of the lack of "universality" of the ankle joint, tremendous mechanical stress is placed on it that may result in a sprain or other injury.

The ankle joint has connecting ligaments on all its surfaces. The ligament most commonly injured is the anterior tibiofibular; injury results from excessive external rotation of the foot on the leg or from internal rotation of the leg when the foot is fixed (Fig. 9–1).

The next most frequently injured ligament is the calcaneofibular portion of the lateral ligaments of the ankle. This injury occurs when there is a forcible inversion of the foot (turning the sole of the foot inward). If the foot is inverted while plantarflexed, the anterior talofibular ligament will sprain. Sprains from the reverse direction (turning the sole of the foot outward) involve the medial ligament (deltoid), and are infrequently seen. If this does occur, one should also suspect a fracture of the fibula and tear of the anterior tibiofibular ligament.

First-Aid Measures (First 24 Hours). *Step 1.* The trainer questions the athlete as to when, how, and where the accident occurred. Was the ankle ever hurt before? Did the athlete hear any snap, crack, or tear at the time of trauma? He carefully inspects the bony and visible soft-tissue landmarks about the foot and ankle, looking for deformity, swelling, and ecchymosis and carefully testing range of motion. He ques-

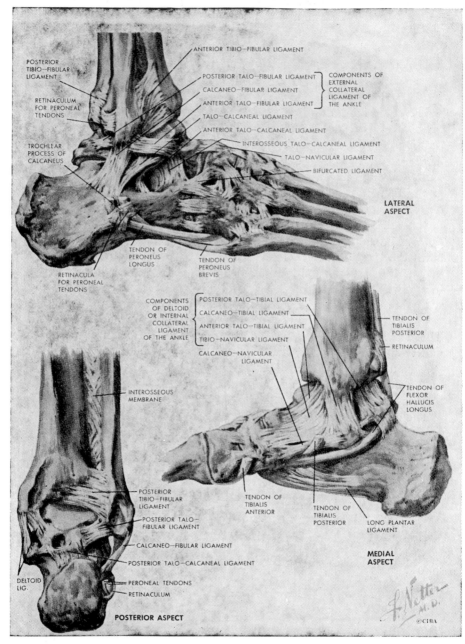

Fig. 9-1.   Ligaments of the ankle and foot.

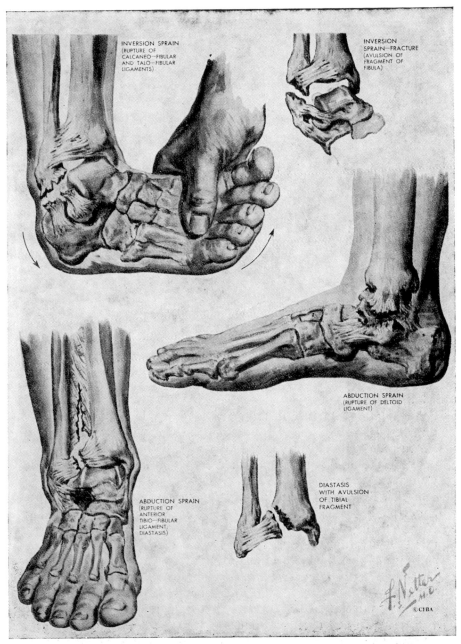

INVERSION SPRAIN
(RUPTURE OF
CALCANEO—FIBULAR
AND TALO—FIBULAR
LIGAMENTS)

INVERSION
SPRAIN—FRACTURE
(AVULSION OF
FRAGMENT OF
FIBULA)

ABDUCTION SPRAIN
(RUPTURE OF DELTOID
LIGAMENT)

ABDUCTION SPRAIN
(RUPTURE OF
ANTERIOR
TIBIO—FIBULAR
LIGAMENT;
DIASTASIS)

DIASTASIS
WITH AVULSION
OF TIBIAL
FRAGMENT

Fig. 9-1. *(Continued).* Major sprains and sprain fractures of the ankle and foot. (© Copyright 1969, CIBA Pharmaceutical Company, Division of CIBA-GEIGY Corporation. Reprinted with permission from CLINICAL SYMPOSIA illustrated by Frank H. Netter, M.D. All rights reserved.)

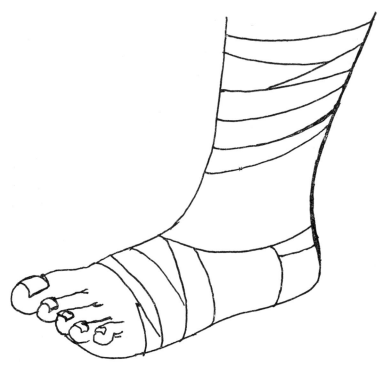

Fig. 9-2.   Figure-eight pressure bandage for injuries to the ankle.

tions the athlete to localize the pain. Some gentle palpation of these areas may be done to localize the injury. After rendering appropriate measures to control hemorrhage and extravasation of hemorrhagic exudate into the surrounding tissue, he notes all his observations in a permanent training-room record.

Step 2. An elastic bandage is first immersed in ice water and then applied to the ankle and the foot in a figure-eight technique, extending it down to the base of the toes (Fig. 9–2). Following this an ice bag or towel filled with finely cracked ice is applied to the site of the injury and held in place by a second elastic bandage. This should be kept in place for 30 to 60 minutes; then a sponge rubber donut is held in place at the site of the injury by an elastic bandage. The duration of the ice compress is determined by the severity of the injury. In mild sprains, one application may be sufficient. In a moderate sprain, it may be necessary to apply cold compresses for 2- to 3-hour intervals until swelling is controlled. If the sprain is severe, continuous application of cold compresses for 48 hours is necessary; this occasionally requires hospitalization of the athlete. To prevent frostbite, ice and skin should not be in contact with each other.

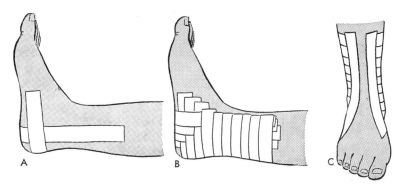

Fig. 9-3. Open front basketweave taping for a sprained ankle.

Another method of compression is the open basketweave strapping, provided the injured ankle is properly prepared (Fig. 9–3). The application of an open basketweave strapping to a sprained ankle is only indicated when the anticipated swelling is minimal or nil. Physicians who are not as adept at taping as trainers may prefer to use elastic bandages for injured joints to allow for swelling. The attending physician will decide whether elastic bandages or open basketweave adhesive strappings are to be used for acute ankle sprains.

Step 3. The athlete is provided with crutches of proper size and instructed in their proper use. He is not to bear weight on the injured foot. He is instructed to elevate the injured leg above the hip during waking hours and during sleep, to place the injured foot and ankle on two pillows, which aids gravity in the drainage of the swollen ankle. He is also to apply a cold compress to the injured ankle.

The athlete is referred to the doctor the same day and instructed to see him before going to bed. The attending physician examines the athlete and decides whether or not an x-ray picture is indicated.

Definitive Treatment (Follow-up Care). The following day the doctor reappraises the ankle. He looks for pain, swelling, tenderness, ecchymosis, joint restriction, and laxity. Even with the most adequate first-aid measures to control hemorrhage, some does occur. However, within 24 to 48 hours, the attending physician will be able to pinpoint and diagnose the pathologic condition and prescribe proper therapy.

Mild Sprains. Mild ankle sprains with minimal swelling, tenderness, ecchymosis, and limitation of motion.

First Day
1. Immerse foot and ankle in ice water (45° F) for at least 20 minutes (a sock should be worn to prevent frostbite). If ice water is not available, an ice bag with finely cracked ice may be secured to the site of injury with an elastic bandage.

2. Apply open basketweave strapping with 1½- to 2-inch adhesive tape or an elastic-bandage dressing to the injured ankle depending on the amount of objective and anticipated swelling.
3. Continue with crutches and no weight bearing on injured leg.
4. Keep leg elevated above hip during waking hours and on two pillows while asleep. The athlete must be instructed to remove an elastic bandage at bedtime if he is wearing one. To not do so would be to invite increased pain and swelling as the result of the pooling of the blood as the circulation slows down during sleep.
5. Take analgesics for pain if necessary as prescribed by the attending physician.

Second Day

MORNING

1. Repeat first day treatment.

AFTERNOON

1. Repeat morning treatment.
2. Encourage athlete to do isometric exercises of muscles of the entire leg as well as active motion of the hip, knee, ankle, and foot.
3. The athlete should be trying protective progressive weight bearing to pain tolerance.
4. Keep leg elevated.
5. Continue with analgesics as occurrence arises (PRN-Pro Re Nata)

If by the beginning of the second day post-injury hemorrhage has stopped and exudate is under control, contrast baths can be started. If not, contrast baths can be started on the third day post-injury. This technique stimulates circulation, aids lymphatic drainage, and facilitates healing. The procedure consists of applying alternating hot and cold applications to the injured areas. The first and last applications are always with hot water (105 to 110° F). The time interval varies with the trainer's or therapist's choice. It runs from 4 to 10 minutes for hot and 1 minute for cold (45 to 55° F). The most frequently used variable is 4 minutes to 1 minute. The entire treatment runs about 20 minutes. As noted before, a sock shall be worn to increase the athlete's tolerance for ice water. Buckets or plastic, rectangular wastebaskets may be used for the contrast bath.

Third Day

MORNING

1. Contrast baths as described before.
2. Repeat second day's afternoon treatment.
3. Soreness can be relieved by adding 2 cups of epsom salts to every gallon of hot water.

AFTERNOON

1. Immerse leg in whirlpool between 105 to 11° F for 15 minutes.
2. Follow with light, gentle massage of foot, ankle, and lower leg for 5 to 10 minutes.
3. Apply a 2-inch elastic bandage using figure-eight and locked heel.
4. Discard crutches if pain is minimal and there is no limp with full weight-bearing.
5. Keep leg elevated when not weight-bearing.

6. Encourage walking and active exercises of the entire leg to aid in milking out the residual exudate.
7. Analgesics and other medication should be stopped.

The athlete can return to his sport in less time depending on his response to treatment.

Sprains with moderate tearing of the ligamentous fibers or severe sprains with definite rupture of one or several ligaments are best treated by flexible, removable casting, or surgery respectively; however, early appropriate first-aid measures to reduce hemorrhage are also necessary before casting or surgery.

Moderate Sprains. Sprains with moderate swelling with or without ecchymosis, local tenderness, and painfully guarded ankle mobility are treated with a removable type of plaster immobilization. Supportive measures such as bed rest, continuous cold compresses for 48 to 72 hours, elevation, elastic bandaging, and analgesics are instituted. A stirrup-type removable plaster splint is applied after hemorrhaging has ceased and preceded by cotton padding material. Commercially prepared stirrups air splints, such as devised by Stover, are also available. The instep and Achilles-tendon area are left uncovered. Isometric exercises for the splinted leg are encouraged. The athlete uses crutches with no weight bearing on the injured leg. Keep leg elevated when not on crutches. The ankle is examined frequently, active and passive ankle motion is done, and contrast baths for the injured ankle are permitted. When there is no longer any appreciable tenderness on palpation of the injured ligament, progressive and protected weight bearing of the injured foot to pain tolerance is permitted. Approximately 1 week post-injury, pain, discomfort, and swelling should have lessened considerably. Physical therapy efforts should now be actively implemented to facilitate the removal of the remaining traumatic exudate and swelling. Modalities such as cryotherapy, hydrotherapy, ultrasound massage, therapeutic and isokinetic exercises by use of cybex and other muscle-strengthening equipment should be used in their proper sequential manner to effect maximum benefits from treatment. This requires the coordinated efforts of the athlete, trainer-therapist, and physician. It may take as much as 2 or 3 weeks of rehabilitation for an athlete to recover sufficiently to return to competition.

Severe Sprains. Severe sprains with rupture of one or more ligaments produce abnormal motion at the ankle joint. These athletes should be hospitalized and the ankle treated with continuous cold compresses, elevation, and analgesic medication. The joint laxity should be confirmed with comparative stress x-ray films. Some authors have shown that arthrographic determination of the ligament rupture prior to surgery is helpful. The ligaments are then repaired surgically, after which a short leg cast is applied. The initial cast is removed in 4 weeks and a walking cast applied. Therapy directed to other parts of the musculoskeletal system should be encouraged throughout the complete care of this athlete.

An athlete treated for an injured ankle is functionally ready for competition if he can perform simulated rope skipping or hopping without undue pain, limp, or supportive strapping.

The healing time, the duration of treatment, and the athlete's response vary with the severity of the sprain, the immediate first-aid measures, and the definitive therapy employed. The use of heat and massage and resumption of full weight bearing too early may start additional hemorrhaging and minimize the effect of early first-aid measures to reduce swelling. If the athlete still has a perceptible limp, he should not be discharged from treatment. The use of a protective wrapping or strapping to support an injured ligament until the athlete can walk and run without a limp is recommended. Returning an athlete to competition before maximal benefits have been gained may result in a chronically painful and disabled ankle. With this type of sprain, the mutual coordination of the physician's and trainer's skills and the cooperation of the athlete in most cases brings about excellent results. The axiom "once a sprain, always a sprain" should not apply here.

Strapping the Ankle. Anatomically and physiologically, the ankle is best suited for the benefits of protective strapping and wrapping. Adhesive-tape strapping aids considerably in the prevention of ankle sprains, and also reduces the severity of sprains that might occur despite the strapping. The tape is applied so that the athlete is capable of complete dorsiflexion and plantar flexion of the ankle joint (hinge motion); it practically eliminates completely inversion, eversion, and rotation of the ankle.

Prophylactically, in an uninjured ankle, 1½-inch adhesive tape is applied with the foot at a right angle and the heel in slight eversion; a heel lock is added to stabilize the heel and the talus. This strapping prevents the heel from rolling under and takes the strain off the lateral ligaments. The ankle strap makes the ankle mortise snug by bringing the tibia and fibula together at the ankle joint. This allows full hinge motion of the joint and at the same time provides effective protection against external rotation, which causes a sprain of the anterior tibiofibular ligament, the most commonly injured ligament of the ankle.

Adhesive strapping of the ankle is also used in the treatment of sprains and the prevention of re-injury. In sprains, the ankle must be strapped in position so that the strain is taken off the injured ligament. A small wedge placed on the appropriate side of the heel of the shoe continues to protect the ligament off the field.

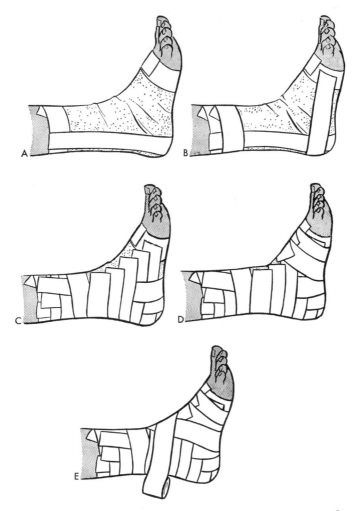

Fig. 9-4.   Closed basketweave taping for support. *A,* Pre-taping underwrap to help prevent blisters. Anchors are applied, as well as the first stirrup. *B,* Second anchor, first horseshoe. *C,* Horseshoes and stirrups completed. *D,* Two anchors are applied around the arch. *E,* Apply figure-eights lightly over the ankle to hold open the ends of the horseshoes.

Many excellent methods of taping are available to give protection to the ankle. Moreover, since many trainers devise their own variations of taping methods, we will illustrate only one classic form of taping the ankle.

The Gibney (basketweave) adhesive-tape strapping gives effective support and may be applied closed or open. The closed basketweave (Fig. 9–4) is an excellent support and when properly applied, practically eliminates rotary and side-to-side motion of the ankle while permitting full plantar and dorsiflexion of the foot.

Closed Basketweave (Right Ankle).
1. Use skin protectant.
2. Use pre-taping underwrap.
3. Anchor meets in the front.
4. Stirrup is applied from the medial side of ankle, close to edge of Achilles tendon.
5. Horseshoe applied as far down on the side of foot as possible.
6. Second anchor applied.
7. Second stirrup, second horseshoe, fourth anchor.
8. Third stirrup, third horseshoe, fifth anchor.
9. Fourth and fifth horseshoe, sixth anchor.
10. Second, third anchor around arch.
11. Start figure-eight from inside of foot.
12. Figure-eight under arch and back over ankle front.
13. Figure-eight completed and an anchor applied around other anchors on top of tape.

After the ankle and foot are sprayed with a skin protectant, blisters and other skin irritations can be prevented by use of an underwrap.

The closed Gibney basketweave is best indicated for practice, games, and the prevention of re-injury in moderate, severe, and complicated ankle sprains. It is especially useful when the anterior tibiofibular ligament has been sprained, which may lead to a permanently weakened and widened mortise.

The open basketweave may be used therapeutically for an acute ankle sprain. This type of strapping not only helps to reduce the swelling, but allows some swelling to occur. In addition, the ankle is supported, which reduces the pain felt by the athlete. If the ankle presents a moderate amount of swelling or a moderate amount is anticipated, do not use any type of adhesive strapping, since this may cause circulatory impairment with ensuing pain and discomfort. Apply an elastic bandage and refer the athlete immediately to the doctor, who is in the best position to prescribe what type of strapping or wrappnig is indicated.

When there is a question as to whether or not a collateral ligament of the ankle has ruptured, x-ray pictures of the ankle should be taken, with the hindfoot held in forced inversion or eversion, depending on which side of the ankle the ligament rupture is suspected. The degree or lack of talar tilt helps determine the diagnosis. Using local procaine or sedating the athlete before manipulating the ankle reduces the pain and anxiety usually associated with this stress testing.

Ankle Wrapping. There are as many different methods of preventive ankle wrapping with elastic and nonelastic bandages as there are adhesive strapping techniques. Elastic wraps are better used to treat ankle sprains than for prophylaxis. Although adhesive taping is superior in the prevention of ankle injuries, fabric wraps have materially reduced the incidence of ankle injuries because the same anatomic and physiologic fundamentals are followed in their application. Wraps may be used successfully for prevention of injury for athletes without prior ankle injuries and for those who are sensitive to tape. They are applied smoothly over the athletic sock around the foot and ankle with two figure-eight turns incorporating a heel lock. This also prevents blisters and skin irritation. The wrap is secured either with a few small pieces of adhesive tape or a few turns of adhesive tape in a figure-eight. Obviously, ankle wrapping is easily applied by the athlete, inexpensive, and easily laundered.

If the athlete has an ankle that has been injured, adhesive tape is the strapping of choice. For all games and contests, adhesive taping, even though more expensive, is recommended.

Knee Injuries

The knee joint is the largest articulation in the body and one of the strongest for the normal activities of daily living and working. Yet, it is the joint most vulnerable to athletic trauma because of its construction, function and location. Nature has endowed the knee with a system of intricately designed and ingeniously arranged ligaments which, in harmony with powerful muscles, maintain the stability of the knee at any point of motion. However, the knee is structurally deficient to withstand the tremendous forces to which it is subjected in athletics. The femur, tibia, and patella articulate in such a manner as to allow two basic types of motion—flexion-extension and rotation. The anatomic make-up that allows these motions in what is basically a hinge joint also makes the knee more subject to injuries in athletics. This is because the slightly concave surfaces of the tibial condyles and their loosely-held menisci give an insufficient repository for the convex, dissimilar-sized femoral condyles against the direct, lateral, and rotary forces to the knee (Fig. 9–5). The patella moves up and down between the femoral condyles and lifts the tendon of the quadriceps muscle away from the axis of motions of the knee joint.

The quadriceps muscles are the main extensors of the knee; this extensor apparatus is mainly responsible for man's ability to stand, walk, and run. Unfortunately, because of its delicate mechanism and late evolutionary appearance, it is unstable and easily deranged by any injury severe enough to restrict activity. A loss of muscle volume, tone, and control may follow restriction of activity, resulting in quadriceps

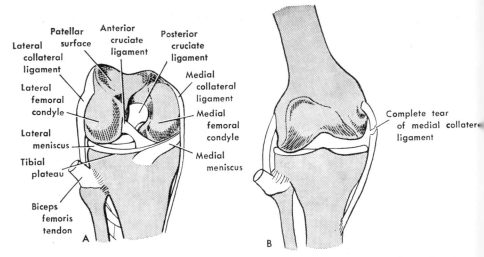

Fig. 9-5. Anterior views of the right knee joint. *A*, Normal joint, knee flexed. *B*, Knee in slight valgus with tear of the medial collateral ligament. Note the two menisci positioned on the plateau surface of the tibia.

weakness and inadequate joint protection. The forces required of the quadriceps mechanism during activity are large. In stair-climbing, a force three to five times that of body weight is necessary to maintain knee equilibrium. Similar forces are needed in kicking a football. The knee is most stable in extension. The bulk of knee injuries involve the medial structures because most traumatic forces are directed from the lateral to the medial aspect with the knee in a bent position.

As noted before, there is a rotary component to knee function—the tibia rotates medially in flexion, and in extension, it rotates laterally in the so called "screw home" mechanism. Associated and controlled motions of the menisci place them in position to distribute the load on the joint. With the many synchronous movements of the component parts that occur in the moving knee as well as its anatomic deficiencies, it is understandable why this joint is so easily injured in its exposed position. It is difficult to protect the knee from sudden blows and from the rotary forces of turning and twisting quickly when the foot is fixed to the ground while running at high speeds. The knee must also be stable in extremes of motion. The collateral and cruciate ligaments cannot accomplish this stabilization alone—there must be a harmonious working relationship of all muscles and ligaments to enable the knee to function efficiently.

The detailed anatomy and physiology of the knee is beyond the scope of this book and the reader is encouraged to read works by Kaplan, Clancy, Kennedy, Slocum, Larson, James, Nicholas, Noyes,

Palmer, Smillie, O'Donoghue, Helfet, Frankel, Nardin, Hughston, MacIntosh, Marshall, Rockwood, Green, and others to enhance his understanding.

First-Aid Measures (First 24 Hours). *Step 1.* The trainer questions the athlete about where, how, and when the accident occurred. Was the knee ever hurt before? Was the knee struck by another player or by the ground? Did it happen while running and then twisting the knee to avoid another player or to "cut back" into a play situation? Did it happen during a tackle, block, or pile-up? Was the knee struck from the medial or the lateral side, or from front or behind? Was the knee injured when it was straight, bent, or turned medially? Was the foot fixed to the ground? Did the knee "give way?" Did the athlete feel two bones slipping over one another in the joint? Was he unable to straighten the knee because it felt locked? Was the inability to stand or bear weight associated with a tearing sensation or "giving way" of the knee accompanied by excruciating pain (suggestive of a ligament tear) or a snapping, painful pop (suggestive of an isolated damaged meniscus)?

The trainer carefully inspects the bony and visible soft-tissue landmarks, looking for deformity, swelling, and ecchymosis. He questions the athlete in order to localize the pain. Some gentle palpation of these areas may be done to detect tenderness and swelling. The trainer tests range of motion of the knee, but does not test for ligamentous instability.

Step 2. An elastic bandage first immersed in cold water is applied in a figure-eight fashion about the knee. Then an ice bag or towel filled with crushed ice is applied to the knee and secured to the knee with another elastic bandage; this is kept in place for 1 or 2 hours. After the cold compress application, a felt padding shaped to the anterior contours of the knee is secured to the knee to compress the exposed joint capsule, thus preventing the collection of blood, lymph, and synovial fluid in the intra- and extracapsular tissues. The athlete may go home with this wrap, but the trainer must check that it is applied snugly but not tightly.

As with ankle sprains, the duration of the ice compress is determined by the severity of the injury. In mild contusions and sprains of the joint, one application may be sufficient. In a moderate contusion or sprain, it may be necessary to apply cold compresses in 2- to 3-hour intervals until swelling is controlled. If the injury is severe, the athlete should be hospitalized and swelling checked with cold compresses continuously for 48 hours and with analgesic and anti-inflammatory medication if necessary.

An alternate method is to immerse the injured knee in ice water for 30 minutes. After removal, thoroughly dry the skin and wrap the knee in underwrap for a distance of 4 inches above and below the joint. Then apply a 6-inch square of soft sponge rubber with space for the patella cut out; secure to the knee with an elastic bandage. Weight-bearing is forbidden until the athlete is seen by the physician.

Step 3. The athlete is supplied with appropriately sized crutches and cautioned not to walk on the injured leg. He is instructed to keep the leg elevated above the hip during waking hours. During sleep, place the injured leg on two pillows. This aids gravity in draining the swollen knee.

The athlete is referred to the doctor and instructed to see him immediately. The attending physician examines the athlete and decides whether or not an x-ray study is indicated.

Definitive Treatment (Follow-Up Care). The earlier a physician systematically examines an acutely injured knee, the sooner a diagnosis can be established and definitive treatment started. The presence or absence of joint laxity can be determined more reliably when the physician examines the injured knee immediately after the injury. The examination must be done carefully and under ideal conditions that allow privacy. All clothing, taping, and wrapping is removed. The uninjured knee is used for comparison.

Inspection. The doctor looks for the presence or absence of a limp. He observes the position of the knee with the athlete in erect and supine positions. He notes whether or not deformities are present. He notes the location and degree of swelling, determining whether it is in the joint, bursa, or soft tissue surrounding the knee, and whether it is synovial effusion or hemorrhage. Rapid swelling in a knee joint suggests hemorrhage. He must decide whether the intra-articular effusion, which causes increased articular pressure and distention with or without pain, should be aspirated; this procedure is not without risk of serious infection.

Palpation. The doctor palpates the bony and soft-tissue landmarks. Tenderness and swelling along the course or at the tibial or femoral attachments of the collateral ligaments indicate ligament injury. Tenderness over the medial-joint space with inability to extend the knee completely suggests an associated damaged meniscus. Ballottement of the patella indicates effusion into the knee joint.

Range of Motion. The physician tests the range of motion of the knee joint, being fully aware that intra-articular effusion limits motion at the extremes of flexion and extension. Most athletes maintain an injured knee in slight flexion because the capacity of the joint is greatest in this position. Spastic hamstring muscles may also keep the knee flexed. Inability to extend the knee completely does not always signify a torn cartilage, but a torn cartilage should be suspected if the condition persists after considerable treatment, provided the history and other findings corroborate such a diagnosis. The appropriate rotary motions of the femur and tibia must be observed during the range-of-motion tests, which include the Helfet, Lochman, MacIntosh lateral pivot shift, Slocum tests and others. Eliciting a click in the knee during the McMurray test suggests a cartilage injury.

Ligament Stability. We are primarily concerned with the collateral and cruciate ligaments and capsular structures. The medial collateral ligament is the knee ligament most commonly sprained, usually from a blow to the lateral side of the knee when the foot is fixed to the ground. This same type of blow may also lead to a torn anterior cruciate and medial meniscus, resulting in the "unhappy triad of O'Donoghue." Hyperextension and hyperflexion forces can cause multiple ligamentous injury.

The lateral aspect of the knee is less frequently involved than the medial side, and the lateral collateral ligament is infrequently injured. However, a tremendous force to the medial aspect of the knee may cause a tear of the lateral collateral ligament, along with injuries to the biceps femoris tendon, peroneal nerve, and popliteus tendon. Posterior cruciate ligament tears are most commonly injured in severe hyperflexion and hyperextension injuries, and also in conjunction with injuries of the anterior cruciate and collateral ligaments. It has also

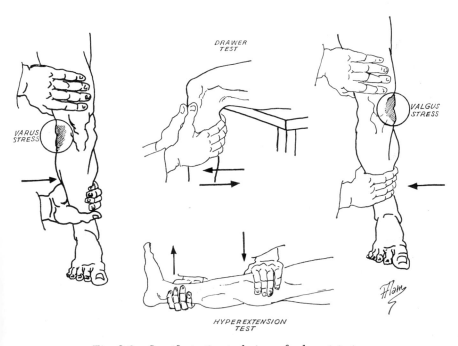

Fig. 9-6. Specific testing techniques for knee injuries.

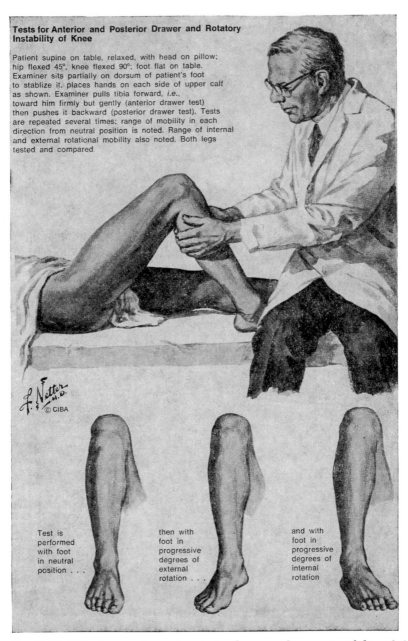

Tests for Anterior and Posterior Drawer and Rotatory Instability of Knee

Patient supine on table, relaxed, with head on pillow; hip flexed 45°, knee flexed 90°; foot flat on table. Examiner sits partially on dorsum of patient's foot to stablize it, places hands on each side of upper calf as shown. Examiner pulls tibia forward, *i.e.*, toward him firmly but gently (anterior drawer test) then pushes it backward (posterior drawer test). Tests are repeated several times; range of mobility in each direction from neutral position is noted. Range of internal and external rotational mobility also noted. Both legs tested and compared

Test is performed with foot in neutral position . . .

then with foot in progressive degrees of external rotation . . .

and with foot in progressive degrees of internal rotation

Fig. 9-7.   Tests for anterior and posterior drawer and rotary instability of the knee.

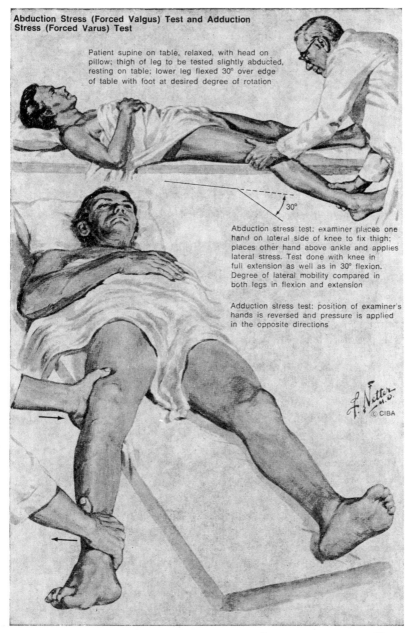

Abduction Stress (Forced Valgus) Test and Adduction Stress (Forced Varus) Test

Patient supine on table, relaxed, with head on pillow; thigh of leg to be tested slightly abducted, resting on table; lower leg flexed 30° over edge of table with foot at desired degree of rotation

30°

Abduction stress test: examiner places one hand on lateral side of knee to fix thigh; places other hand above ankle and applies lateral stress. Test done with knee in full extension as well as in 30° flexion. Degree of lateral mobility compared in both legs in flexion and extension

Adduction stress test: position of examiner's hands is reversed and pressure is applied in the opposite directions

Fig. 9-7. *(Continued)*. Abduction stress (forced valgus) test and adduction stress (forced varus) test. (© Copyright 1977, CIBA Pharmaceutical Company, Division of CIBA-GEIGY Corporation. Reprinted with permission from CLINICAL SYMPOSIA illustrated by Frank H. Netter, M.D. All rights reserved.)

been shown that the posterior capsule is one of the main stabilizers of the knee and is frequently injured with ligaments of the knee.

The physician should examine the injured knee within 30 minutes after the accident, before pain, swelling, muscle spasm, and the athlete's anxiety make the examination difficult. If this is not feasible, the trainer performs a cursory examination and follows with the appropriate first-aid and supportive measures to relieve pain and swelling. When the physician finally does get to examine the athlete, repeated examinations should be done, including stress testing of the knee under x-ray control if a ligament tear or rupture is suspected. The use of local anesthetic and sedation before stress testing reduces the pain and anxiety usually associated with this procedure. Stress testing of both knees is done to check out any physiologic laxity of the ligaments of the uninjured knee. Knee-joint stability is tested while the knee is held in terminal extension, in 30 or 90° of flexion, and the lower leg positioned in neutral, or internal or external rotation. Valgus (abduction) or varus (adduction) forces are then directed to the flexed or extended knee. Push and pull forces are directed to the upper tibia in the positions of the lower leg as noted. The nature and extent of the instability is noted. The extent of the joint laxity ranges from < 0.5 cm, which is 1 + (minimal); < 0.5 cm to 1 cm is 2 + (moderate); and > 1 cm, which is 3 + (marked). Figures 9-6 and 9-7 by Netter are illustrative of these tests.

Marshall's table (Table 9-1) is a useful and easy-to-read schematic of ligamentous prime stabilizers and lines of defense against forces causing knee-joint disruption. However, Marshall states that in spite of the disagreements on this concept in the knee literature, it still serves as a useful and practical guideline for physicians testing a knee for stability. It helps in the understanding of the laxity of the knee joint and its pathologic correlation with the suspected ligaments and capsular tissue causing this joint instability. The reader is encouraged to read authors such as Hughston, Hoppenfeld, Netter, Larson, and others who have made great contributions to knee testing.

After taking his own history and physical examinations, and reviewing the x-ray findings and the information noted by the trainer, the physician should be able to pinpoint the pathologic condition and prescribe the proper treatment in 24 to 48 hours after the injury.

Arthrogram and Arthroscopy. Until recently, a detailed history, physical examination, and conventional x-ray films were all that was available to the attending physician to assist him in arriving at a diagnosis and rendering appropriate care. Now we have arthrography and arthroscopy, which aid the physician in pinpointing the pathologic condition.

With an arthrogram, a special radio-opaque dye is injected into the

Table 9-1.   *"Lines of Defense"* *

tress	Knee Position	Relative Importance†
Valgus (medial side)	Extension	1. Superficial MCL, 2. ACL, post. cap. 3. Deep MCL 4. PCL
	Flexion	1. Superficial MCL 2. ACL 3. PCL
Varus (lateral side)	Extension	1. ACL, LCL, poplit. 2. PCL
	Flexion	1. LCL
Hyperextension		1. ACL 2. Post. cap. 3. PCL
Anterior tibia (anterior drawer)		1. ACL 2. MCL
Posterior tibia (posterior drawer)		1. PCL
Rotation of tibia, external	Flexion	1. MCL 2. ACL, LCL, poplit. 3. Post. med. cap.
	Extension	1. ACL, MCL
Rotation of tibia, internal	Flexion	1. ACL, PCL 2. LCL 3. Poplit., IT, band
	Extension	1. ACL 2. LCL, poplit., IT band 3. PCL

*When the knee is stressed, ligaments have a relative importance in preventing instability.

†ACL: anterior cruciate ligament. IT band: iliotibial band. LCL: lateral collateral ligament. MCL: medial collateral ligament. PCL: posterior cruciate ligament. Poplit.: popliteus. Post. cap.: posterior capsule. Post med. cap.: posterior medial capsule.

Marshall, J.L., and Rubin, R.M.: Knee ligament injuries—a diagnostic and therapeutic approach. *In* Injuries in sports: recent developments. Orthop. Clin. North Am., 8:641–668, 1977.

knee joint under local anesthesia. A series of x-ray pictures are taken in multiple projections to follow the flow of the dye in the joint. Although the arthrogram provides fairly accurate information about whether or not the meniscus is torn, it is not that accurate about ligament tears unless there is a complete rupture of the capsule and ligament. Popliteal cysts are also visualized in arthrograms of the knee. Arthrograms are useful with musculotendinous cuff and capsular tears of the shoulder.

Although arthroscopy has been around quite a while (1920s), the advancement of fiber optics and the smaller-size arthroscopy tube have led to its popular use among orthopedic surgeons. It has resulted in a significant reduction in major surgery of the knee with its attendant postoperative morbidity, prolonged hospitalization, increased expenses, and loss of income for the professional and recreational athlete and the working man.

The arthroscope is inserted into the knee joint through a less than 1-inch surgical incision with the patient under local anesthesia. Its major benefit is its ability to diagnose meniscal, ligament, and capsular tears, floating loose bodies, and chondromalacia of the patella. It also helps to identify malalignment subluxation. With this added information, unnecessary surgery is avoided, leading to other forms of therapy, such as conventional casts, fabric immobilizer splint with velco fasteners, and rehabilitation for partial ligament tears of the knee.

If arthroscopy reveals a slight tear of the meniscus, it can be repaired through the arthroscope, leaving most of the meniscus intact. Complete meniscectomy, when indicated, via the arthroscope tube has been reported by Cavanough of Colorado. Intra-articular shaving through the arthroscope of the cartilaginous surface of the patella in chondromalacia is also performed. Floating loose bodies and debris are easily washed out through the arthroscope. Retinacular releases can also be done through the arthroscope.

If the arthroscope confirms significant tears of the ligament, these are best repaired by a conventional surgical approach and repair with its attendant, increased postoperative hospitalization and longer rehabilitation program. Although most arthroscopy procedures are done in a hospital setting with a 1- or 2-day stay, outpatient arthroscopy is now being done by Pevey and others under local anesthesia. However, it is reported that, with outpatient arthroscopy using general anesthesia, arthroscopy accuracy is above 90%.

According to Tongue and Larson, arthrography and arthroscopy used together have a 98% accuracy for meniscal lesions and an 82% accuracy for medial collateral ligament disorders.

Contusion. Contusion of the knee with minimal synovial effusion, pain, swelling, tenderness, limp, and limitation of motion, usually following a direct blow to the front of the knee.

First 48 Hours
1. Repeat ice and compression treatment if swelling has not been checked.
2. Apply a knee immobilizer to keep knee straight and discourage bending.
3. Quadriceps setting exercises to pain tolerance are started immediately. The athlete tenses his quadriceps muscles as hard as he can for 5 seconds, relaxes the muscles momentarily, and then repeats the exercises for as many times as he can in a 5- to 10-minute period. For total leg strength, the athlete should do 300 quadriceps contractions daily in the intervals best suited for himself.

4. In conjunction with quadriceps setting exercises, the athlete should also do straight-leg raising exercises following such series of quadriceps sets. The knee must be held in full extension throughout the straight-leg raise.
5. Hip abduction exercises while side-lying on the uninjured side with the injured knee held in full extension to maintain the strength of the hip abductors of the injured leg.
6. The muscles of the lower leg on the injured side are included in the total leg program of resistance exercises using a towel or belt or on isokinetic equipment designed for dorsiflexion, inversion or eversion, and plantar flexion, both with knees flexed or extended.
7. Keep leg elevated above hip during waking hours and on two pillows while asleep.
8. Continue with crutches and avoid weight-bearing on injured leg if limp is present.
9. Analgesics for pain and anti-inflammatory medication is prescribed when necessary by the attending physician.

After 48 Hours
1. Discontinue knee immobilizer.
2. Use moist hot packs for 20 to 30 minutes or immerse injured leg in a whirlpool between 105 to 110° F for 15 minutes; still others have their athletes immerse their full bodies in the whirlpool between 105 to 110° F for 15 minutes. Some trainers use the contrast baths routine.
3. Next the athlete places himself in a supine position on the treatment table and elevates his injured leg for about 10 minutes to allow swelling to drain from the injured knee.
4. This is followed by 5 to 10 minutes of massage to disperse the remainder of the intra-articular swelling.
5. Then perform range-of-motion exercises for the knee to pain tolerance.
6. Progressive resistance exercises for the quadriceps, hamstrings, hip and lower leg muscles using isokinetic equipment if available to achieve total leg strength beginning with short arc knee movements. If such equipment is not available, ankle weights or aluminum sandals and a metal handle with removable collars can be used starting at 5 pounds and going up to 10 and 20 pounds and then switch over to an isotonic knee-strengthening machine to full range, first starting with short arc movements.
7. Swimming can also be used for knee-exercise therapy.
8. Dry the knee and apply a dry elastic bandage.
9. The athlete continues his exercise program at home.

Fortunately, most effusions are small and resorb in a few days if immediate measures of cold application, compression bandaging, and restriction of knee motion to check swelling are instituted. Although an elastic wrap for the knees for practice or games gives safe psychologic support, it is not wise or necessary to apply preventative adhesive tape strappings for this condition. The athlete may discard his crutches and bear weight as soon as there is no limp and he is able to extend his knee easily against a resistance of 10 to 15 pounds. Normalcy is usually achieved in about 1 week.

Aspiration of the knee is indicated only when there is a large accumulation of intra-articular fluid and capsular distention. Significant accumulations of blood in the effusion should be aspirated to relieve pain and prevent adhesions. The technique of aspiration must be done with strict asepsis, preferably in a hospital or doctor's office.

Sprains. The knee is more vulnerable to ligament sprains than any other kind of injury. Injury to the medial collateral ligament is the most frequent knee injury of any type (Tables 9-2 and 9-3). A mild sprain results in either ligamentous stretching or mild tearing or both without any impairment of ligament strength. A moderate sprain results in the ligament being partially torn. A severe sprain follows complete rupture

Table 9-2. Ligaments Involved in Knee Sprains Among Harvard College Athletes Over a 30-Year Period.

Medial collateral ligament	405
Lateral collateral ligament	98
Crucial ligament	31
Medial collateral ligament and medial meniscus	59
Medial collateral ligament and lateral meniscus	14
Medial collateral ligament and lateral collateral ligament	8
Medial collateral ligament and crucial ligament	11
Lateral collateral ligament and lateral meniscus	6
Tibiofibular ligament, superior	6
Patellar ligament	3
Unspecified	45
TOTAL	686

Table 9-3. Knee Injuries in Harvard College Athletes Over a 30-Year Period.

Ligament sprains	668
Joint contusions	305
Muscle contusions	95
Dislocations (partial)	32
Muscle strains	29
Lacerations and abrasions	26
Superficial contusions	20
Infrapatellar bursitis	21
Infected abrasions or furuncles	15
Hyperextension	7
Meniscus	81
Osgood-Schlatter disease	2
Congenital anomaly	1
Miscellaneous	1
TOTAL	1,303

of one or more ligaments, which may result in some degree of separation or even dislocation and the knee's giving way. The pathologic and clinical findings vary with the nature and extent of the external force to which the knee is subjected. Clinically, mild and moderate sprains are differentiated by the amount of pain, swelling, ecchymosis, tenderness, limp, limitation of motion and joint laxity. In the severe type, joint laxity also is observed. All three conditions are treated differently. An injured athlete walking off the playing field unaided may still have a serious knee injury requiring surgery.

Immediate Treatment (on the field)

1. Examine the athlete carefully to determine the nature and extent of the injury and how to remove the athlete from the playing field.
2. Treatment in athletic training room:
   a. Have athlete take a shower.
   b. Apply a 4-inch elastic bandage previously immersed in cold water. Elevate the injured leg. Apply an ice bag or cold pack to minimize swelling and secure to injured knee with another elastic bandage. This is kept in place for at least 1 hour.
   c. Remove cold compresses, dry skin thoroughly, and wrap injured knee with a fresh, dry elastic bandage.
   d. Apply a knee immobilizer.
   e. The athlete is provided with proper sized crutches with instructions in crutch-walking and cautioned to avoid weight-bearing on the injured leg. The athlete is instructed to keep the injured leg elevated above the hip during waking hours. During sleep, the athlete is instructed to remove the elastic bandage and knee immobilizer and place the injured leg on two pillows. Leg elevation aids gravity in draining the swollen knee. The duration of the cold compresses for overnight treatment is determined by the severity of the injury.
   f. As soon as possible, the athlete is referred to the attending physician who examines the athlete and determines the nature, extent, and treatment of the injury.

Mild Sprains. Mild sprain of the medial collateral ligament with minimal pain, swelling, tenderness, limp, and limitation of motion.

First Day

MORNING

1. Repeat ice and compression treatment if swelling has not been checked.
2. Continue with elastic bandage and knee immobilizer.
3. Continue with crutches and avoid weight-bearing on injured leg.
4. Keep leg elevated above hip during waking hours and on two pillows while asleep.
5. Analgesics for pain and anti-inflammatory medication as prescribed by the attending physician.

First Day

AFTERNOON

1. Repeat morning treatment.

Second Day

MORNING

1. Repeat first day's treatment.
2. Encourage athlete to do quadriceps setting exercises—about 300 during day at intervals most suitable for the athlete. Straight-leg raising exercises follow quadriceps' sets.
3. Hip abduction exercises in a side-lying position on the uninjured side with injured knee held in full extension.
4. Active range-of-motion exercises for the hip, foot, and ankle; guarded exercises for the injured knee.
5. Continue exercise program at home.

Second Day

AFTERNOON

1. Repeat second day's morning treatment.

Third Day

MORNING

If swelling is still present, repeat second day's treatment. If swelling has subsided, exudate is under control, and pain and discomfort are lessened, the following can be used:

1. Immerse injured leg in whirlpool bath between 105 to 110° F for 15 to 20 minutes. Some trainers use a contrast-bath routine.
2. Remove from whirlpool bath, dry and follow with gentle massage of the upper foreleg, knee, and thigh for 5 to 10 minutes.
3. Begin with resistance short-arc extension and gradually progress to repetitions and range-of-motion exercises.
4. Place elastic bandage about knee.
5. Apply knee immobilizer.
6. Keep injured leg elevated when not ambulating.
7. Continue with crutches until limp, pain, and swelling are no longer present and progress onto weight-bearing activities, while periodically testing with protective weight-bearing to grade degree of recovery.
8. Encourage walking as long as it does not increase exudate. Walking and exercise of the leg help milk out traumatic exudate.
9. Continue exercise program at home.

Third Day

AFTERNOON

1. Same as morning treatment.
2. Discontinue knee immobilizer.

Fourth Day

Pain and discomfort should have lessened considerably by now and should not impede intensified efforts to facilitate removal of the traumatic exudates and reduction of swelling and rehabilitation of the quadriceps, other leg muscles, and joints for total-leg strength.

1. Remove elastic-bandage support and immerse leg in a whirlpool bath for 20 to 30 minutes.
2. Remove leg from whirlpool, dry, and follow with gentle massage of the upper foreleg, knee, and thigh for 15 minutes.
3. Progressive resistance quadriceps exercise routine is best accom-

plished with isokinetic and isotonic exercise equipment if available. Otherwise, it is done in the following manner:

a. Use an aluminum exercise sandal weighing about 2½ pounds, metal handle with removable collars, and iron discs weighing 2½, 5, 10 and 12½ pounds. (Ankle weights may be used in place of exercise sandals.)

b. The strength of the uninjured leg must be used as a guide in the rehabilitation of the injured leg. The athlete sits at the edge of the examination table and a weighted sandal is applied to the foot of the uninjured leg. He is asked to straighten his knee 10 times. Then iron discs in 2½- or 5-pound increments are added to the sandal. The greatest amount of weight he is able to lift while straightening the uninjured knee is the maximal strength that the injured leg must achieve. This testing can be done while the injured leg is recovering from the immediate symptoms and signs of the injury.

c. The injured leg is now tested by applying the weighted sandal to the foot; in a similar manner, the maximal weight that can be lifted 10 times is noted.

d. The athlete must exercise his injured leg daily by extending it 10 times with 50% of the maximal weight established in "c"; 10 times with 75% of the maximal weight established in "c"; and 10 times with the full weight established in "c."

e. The athlete should be encouraged to increase the maximal weight established in "c" whenever he can; he follows the same pattern of exercise, making appropriate increases in 50 and 75% of the new maximal weight.

f. When the treated leg is able to extend the same weight as the uninjured leg 10 times, the maximal benefits of treatment have been gained and normal strength achieved. Extending the knee 10 times with 50 pounds attached to the exercise sandal is not an unusual feat for college and professional football players.

4. Keep leg elevated when not weight-bearing.

5. Discontinue crutches and bear weight as soon as there is no limp and the athlete is able to extend his knee easily against a resistance of 10 to 15 pounds.

6. Encourage walking and active exercises of leg to help milk out traumatic exudate.

7. Analgesics and other prescribed oral medication should be discontinued when there is no longer any pain.

Fifth Day

1. Same as fourth day's treatment.

This type of injury may take 5 to 10 days of treatment. Whirlpool treatment may be alternated with moist hot packs followed by a light, fingertip massage twice daily for the duration of the treatment. An elastic-bandage support for the knee should be continued until all the swelling has been resorbed and full range of knee motion and maximal strength of the musculature that activates the knee have been achieved.

Moderate Sprains. With a moderate sprain of the medial collateral ligament with pain, ecchymosis, swelling, limp, and painfully guarded motion, treatment depends on whether or not there is slight joint laxity. With no joint laxity, the athlete is placed in a knee immobilizer and on crutches for 3 weeks. In addition to cold compresses, elevation, analgesic and anti-inflammatory medication, elastic bandages, and restrictions on weight-bearing, a knee with marked effusion or distention should be aspirated under strict aseptic precautions. The aspiration is repeated if necessary. By the third or fourth day, with pain, tenderness, and swelling lessened, continuous hot moist packs are applied to the knee and the athlete is started on isometric exercises. No weight-bearing is permitted on the injured leg. The knee is rehabilitated with whirlpool, massage, and progressive resistance exercises in the same manner as described for the mild sprain. It takes a minimum of 3 weeks of intensive rehabilitation efforts to reach a competitive edge. Knee braces with single- or double-sided hinged splints made of plastic or metal material forming a bridge over the knee are useful to prevent reinjury.

If a knee is moderately sprained and also shows some minimal or slight laxity along with effusion, this joint laxity may be associated with subclinical tears of the anterior cruciate or medial collateral ligament and associated meniscus tears. Because a further workup, such as an arthrogram, examination of the knee under general anesthesia, and an arthroscopy may be necessary to ascertain the knee joint pathologic condition, hospitalization is indicated. If the workup indicates surgery is unnecessary, one of us (M.N.) waits until pain, discomfort, tenderness, and swelling have lessened considerably and applies a plaster cylinder cast on the third or fourth day with a knee held between 20 to 30° in flexion. Some physicians use removable, variable-position knee immobilizers or commercially prepared plaster splints. The athlete is discharged from the hospital on the same day following cast application. The athlete continues with crutches and does not bear weight on the injured leg. Isometric exercises are reinforced along with other rehabilitation efforts. The cast is removed 3 to 4 weeks post injury. If a variable-position knee immobilizer is used instead of a cast, physical therapy and rehabilitative measures can be started much earlier. The knee is rehabilitated with whirlpool baths, massages, progressive-resistance exercises, and other exercise modalities (see "Rehabilitation" at the end of this section).

Severe Sprains. Severe sprains of one or more of the collateral or cruciate ligaments are responsible for abnormal laxity at the knee joint. These athletes are best treated in a hospital with continuous cold compresses, elevation, anti-inflammatory and analgesic medication, and other supportive measures. After a diagnosis has established the extent of the damage, surgical repair of the injured structures should be done soon thereafter. A padded, long-leg plaster cast is applied with the knee flexed between 20 to 30°; the cast remains on for 6 to 8 weeks. During the wearing of the cast, therapy to other parts of the musculoskeletal system must be encouraged to render complete care to the athlete. Whenever plaster-cast immobilization is used, no weight-bearing is permitted because synovial reaction is usually present. As this reaction subsides, weight-bearing is started.

Meniscus Tears. The semilunar cartilages (menisci) move backward during flexion, pressing the posterior halves between the posterior surface of the articulating femoral and tibial condyles. The menisci move forward in extension, and the anterior halves are snugly held between the opposing femoral and tibial condyles. The medial meniscus, in addition to its tibial attachments, also is attached at its periphery with the deep layers of the medial collateral ligament. A traumatic force directed to the lateral aspect of the knee that is strong enough to separate the medial aspects of the femoral and tibial condyles also places the medial collateral ligament and capsule under strain. If the force is great enough, it may also damage the medial meniscus because of its attachments and position. The medial meniscus is most frequently injured when a partially flexed knee is struck by a sudden blow on its lateral aspect as the femur rotates medially on a tibia that has been secured by the foot fixed to the ground. The same injury may also occur without any external force when the knee is quickly turned inwardly with the foot fixed to the ground while running or cutting at high speeds.

Tear of the medial meniscus under the circumstances described above is characterized by the knee giving way, pain, swelling, tenderness, limitation of motion, and a true history of locking. In questionable cases of cartilage or ligament tears, the recent use of arthrography and arthroscopy in experienced hands has proven to be a valuable diagnostic procedure in determining the integrity of these structures.

Treatment varies with the age of the athlete, his response to treatment, the number of recurrences, and his desire to continue in athletics. Junior high, high school, and college athletes who suffer torn semilunar cartilages for the first time and are confirmed to be undisplaced by arthroscopy are treated operatively or conservatively depending on the size of the tear. Conservative care includes hospitalization, leg traction, plaster cylinder, crutches, and no weight-bearing for 1 month. During the cast immobilization, quadriceps setting exercises are strongly emphasized, as well as isometric exercises of the other leg muscles. After the cast is removed, local moist heat, massage, and progressive resistance exercises for the quadriceps and hamstring muscles are started. The player can return to the game only after a full range of knee motion and maximal thigh muscle strength have been achieved. Recurrence of meniscus injury is usually an indication for surgical removal of the meniscus if the athlete intends to continue in the sport that caused the injury. Bucket handle and some other less complicated meniscal tears can be surgically removed by operative, arthroscopy. Athletes who have suffered several recurrent meniscal injuries in a sport have not required surgery because they finally discontinued the sport, concentrating instead on one that did not subject their knees to such trauma.

The rehabilitation of the injured knee that has been operated on and/or casted requires a considerable amount of coordination of the skills of the attending physician, trainer, and physical therapist. The athlete and the coach also play an important role. The athlete must show patience, determination, and motivation to achieve maximum benefits from treatment. He must not try to hurry along his return to competition before recovery has been reached. Most young athletes are too impatient to allow nature to heal in its own time. They may actually retard full recovery if they pressure the medical personnel to allow them to get back to competition before its time.

In addition to the personal equation and whirlpool baths, there is some isokinetic equipment that can be used to help recovery along, such as Cybex II, Nordic Ski track, treadmills, and bicycles. Swimming is another useful modality in the rehabilitation of the injured knee. However, this equipment must be used properly and sequentially in the athlete's recovery. The trainer-therapist's ingenuity and skill allows the rehabilitating athlete to benefit from this equipment. In addition to equipment, active exercises must be used to keep muscles distal and proximal to the traumatized joint active throughout the rehabilitation process. Flexibility/stretch exercises also play a role in the injured athlete's total rehabilitation.

Strapping the Knee. The application of an elastic bandage with or without a sponge rubber or felt pad or strapping with adhesive tape, aids considerably in supporting the sprained knee. This support enables the athlete to move the knee with less pain. The bandaging or taping is applied in a figure-eight manner, so that the loops cross directly over the injured ligament, which has been placed in a relaxed position. This gives a feeling of support, strength, and security to the knee. Slocum limits adhesive taping to convalescent treatment in knee sprains, but questions its value for the prevention of injuries. Thorndike disagrees and recommends a Duke-Simpson tape strapping to prevent reinjury of the knee ligaments. In some parts of the country this tape job is still being used. This topic is just as controversial among trainers—many do not tape knees for preventive purposes for practice or games. We do not subscribe to the practice of routinely taping a knee post-injury to

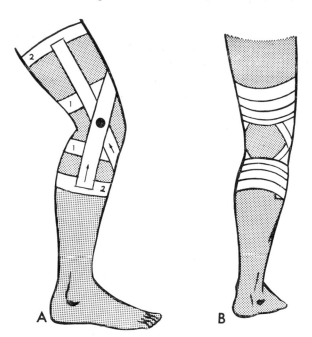

Fig. 9-8. General method for taping the knee. The skin of the knee area approximately 7 inches above and below the midline of the patella is prepared by shaving and cleaning and the application of an even coat of skin protectant. The athlete sits or stands and maintains his knee in slight flexion while the adhesive tape is applied. He can maintain flexion by placing his heel on a spool of 1½-inch tape. *A,* Anchor strips "1" and "2" are applied. All vertical strips of tape must cross over each other at the exact center of the knee joint (black dot). As each pair of vertical strips is applied, secure with anchors above and below. *B,* If there are both internal and external sprains, the tape should be applied on both sides of the knee, and the anchors should go around the leg. The completed job consists of eight vertical strips with four anchors above and four anchors below.

prevent a reinjury. If, in the judgment of the medical staff, a protective knee strapping is indicated, however, the tape job indicated in Figure 9-8 can be used, despite its psychologic implications. Many trainers use their own versions of this basic knee strapping technique.

Unfortunately, some physicians permit trainers to ply their knee-strapping techniques and skills on players with "floating cartilages," or chronically unstable and weak knees in the mistaken belief that this will help the knee to withstand the rigors of a sport. This should not be permitted; rather, the player should be disqualified from the sport that is wrecking his knees and transferred to one that does not expose the knee to such trauma. It is doubtful whether any braces, devices, or strapping or wrapping methods can protect the knee against the violent forces of some body-contact sports.

Maximal development of power and strength of the musculature that moves and stabilizes the knee is an absolute prerequisite for sport participation. Formulation of new safety rules and better enforcement of existing rules to prevent knee injuries are necessary to reduce the incidence of injured knees in contact sports such as football, soccer, and ice hockey. Artificial turf is being used with the expectation of reducing the incidence and severity of knee injuries. As yet there is insufficient evidence to warrant any definite conclusions.

Artificial Turf. In the summertime and early fall, artificial turf's characteristic of retaining heat makes playing difficult and causes a skin burn of the elbows and knees on contact. It is great for upkeep and maintenance, but its medical benefits are far from conclusive, and the "jury" is still out concerning its applicability on the high school level. Its suitability for use in the pros is another matter.

Chondromalacia. Since the first edition of this book and the onset of the fitness mania, chondromalacia now ranks as one of the most common sports disorders. It is most frequently seen in adolescents and young adults. It is only occasionally seen in oldsters. In chondromalacia, the gliding patellofemoral joint motion that we take for granted becomes painful and disabled because of the tremendous amount of biomechanical strains and stresses placed on this joint in running and jumping sports such as basketball, jogging, running, tennis, and volleyball. The undersurface of the patella is somewhat protected from the bony condyles of the femur by the interposition of the fat pad. When the knee flexes repetitively, as it does in athletic activity, however, the patella loses the protection of the fat pad. Therefore, as the knee cap descends distally, the articular surface of the patella makes increasingly more bony contact with the distal end of the femur as the patella moves in the groove between the femoral condyles. At the same time, the patellar tendon is placed under greater tension causing a compressive force directly on the patella within the patellofemoral articulation.

Other anatomic and biomechanical factors affecting the tracking mechanism of the patella between the femoral condyles add to the pathophysiologic changes of the patellofemoral articulation, which lead to increased biomechanical pressure on the articular surface of the patella. I (M.N.) refer to imbalance of the musculature on the lateral and medial sides of the patella as well as the lateral and medial retinacular ligaments and iliotibial band. These muscles and ligaments play a role in keeping the tracking of the patella on the cartilage-covered groove between the femoral condyles during the constant flexion and extension of the knee during athletic activity. There are other anatomic conditions that lend themselves to pathophysiologic movements that aid in the development of chondromalacia causing pain and disability of varying degrees in the athlete. The malicious malalignment syndrome starting at the hips with an increased femoral neck anteversion, increased Q angle, hypermobile patella, increased external tibial torsion, and pronated flat feet are all causes leading to chondromalacia. Essentially, the causes of chondromalacia are traumatic—malalignment of the patella and resultant maltracking between the femoral condyles —and idiopathic. Pathologically, there is an early softening, then roughening, and subsequent fibrillation of the articular (undersurface) of the patella. These pathologic changes cause a disruption of the normal gliding motion of the patellofemoral articulation. Pain and discomfort may be only minimal. As the athlete continues participating on the involved knee, increasing degeneration sooner or later causes the athlete to become sidelined. This is a difficult condition to treat unless it is recognized and treated in its earliest stages. At this early level, medical help can be instituted to curb its progression.

The diagnosis is not usually difficult to establish. It is important that the athlete describe to his doctor the disability, the site, as well as the time of occurrence of the pain. The pain may be described as peripatellar or even retropatellar. The most frequent site of pain is along the medial border of the patella. In some runners, the pain may lessen during a run only to worsen near the end of the run. Going up and more frequently, going down stairs causes pain. Stiffness of the knee with prolonged sitting or the knee "giving out" may cause the athlete to seek out his doctor's help. Joint-line tenderness is frequently present but not associated with meniscal tears.

The clinical examination leaves no doubt as to the diagnosis. Tenderness of one or both patella facets may be elicited. Flexion and extension of the knee usually produces crepitus that can be felt by the examiner's hand. If the degeneration is marked, the crepitus is even audible to the athlete. Passive motion of the patella laterally may produce anxiety or an apprehension sign. Compression testing of the patella manually against the femoral condyle with the knee extended or pushing the proximal pole of the patella distally as the athlete is asked to contract the quadriceps muscle with the knee extended produces pain with a chondromalacic condition. Extending the knee from 30° of flexion against resistance is used to elicit patellar pain. If pain is produced with the aforementioned tests, chondromalacia is probably present. Other signs confirming chondromalacia would be atrophy of the thigh and even the calf, and perhaps effusion.

Conventional x-ray views of the involved knee may show no bony or periosteal pathologic condition. However, tangential (sunrise views) may reveal an increased femoral sulcus angle with an inadequately developed lateral femoral condyle and perhaps a "jockey cap" appearance of the patella. If there is some accompanying arthritic spurring, it may be picked up on the anterior, posterior, lateral, or tunnel views.

The management and care of chondromalacia patella is best handled in a conservative manner using rest, physical therapy, which includes a combination of cryotherapy and moist heat, isotonic and progressive-resistance isometric exercise routine, and in some cases, infrapatellar restraining braces and straps. Occasionally, because of the intense pain and discomfort exhibited by the athlete, it may be necessary to temporarily immobilize the involved knee of the athlete with a plaster cylinder cast or a commercial knee immobilizer, along with the use of crutches and partial weight-bearing until the knee becomes manageable, for the remainder of the conservative therapy. Pain can be reduced by rest and early cryotherapy for 3 or more days, followed by moist heat. The knee can then be built up with an isotonic and progressive-resistance isometric exercise program as formulated by De-Haven, et al. His 82% recovery rate in athletes from contact as well as recreational sports who sustained this condition speaks well for his program. Brody, in his monograph on running injuries, is equally emphatic on a conservative program for runners with chondromalacia. He further adds that an orthotic may correct excessive rotation and pronation, thereby correcting the tracking problem. If the temporary orthotic is helpful, it can be replaced by a well-tolerated shoe orthotic, obviating the need for wraps, horseshoe braces, infrapatellar straps, and derotation braces about the knee. Surgery for chondromalacia is rarely recommended or performed.

Jumper's Knee

Although this pathologic entity was described by Sinding-Larson and Johansson for adolescents and by Smillie for adults as patellar or quadriceps tendonitis, it was Blazina who popularized it as the "jumper's knee," aided by the publicity extended to a big-time basketball player who suffered this clinical disorder. Clinically, it is a tendonitis of the quadriceps tendon insertion at the superior pole of the patella and/or the inferior pole of the patella. It is brought on by repetitive-jumping athletic activities with sudden decelerating forces, active or violent, active extension of the knee such as is seen in rebounding or in trying to stop quickly in basketball. These activities cause maximal stresses and strains of the knee leading to microruptures of the quadriceps tendon at superior and inferior attachment sites to the patella. Basketball and volleyball are classic athletic activities that bring on these abnormal stresses. It is also seen in high jumping, long-jumping, platform diving, triple jumping, cross-country running, figure skating, tennis, and other recreational and competitive athletic activities.

Clinically, the history brings out the abnormal forces to which the quadriceps-tendon attachment sites are subjected during an athletic activity. At first, an aching pain is felt that disappears with varying amounts of rest. As the disorder progresses, the athlete may experience a sense of fullness about the tendon-attachment sites, which will be described as swelling. With further progress, the athlete may even describe a feeling of "giving way" momentarily, which is quite different than true locking or catching.

The athlete is best examined in supine position with the entire leg exposed. In most cases, a tenderness can be elicited at the inferior pole of the quadriceps attachment. Effusion of the knee is usually absent. Although signs of ligamentous or meniscal damage are not present, it is not uncommon to find other patellar disorders, such as patellar subluxability, patellar chondromalacia, genu recurvatum, genu valgum, and others.

Although x-ray films of the knee in multiple view, including intercondylar and skyline views of the patella, may initially be negative or perhaps show a radiolucency at the involved patella pole, a number of radiographic abnormalities have been described, such as a periosteal reaction of the patella, elongation of the involved pole, fatigue fractures of the inferior pole or other radiographic abnormalities.

Treatment of this condition depends on the stage of the disorder when the athlete seeks medical help. If pain or discomfort is experienced only after the activity has ceased, we are usually dealing with a mild form. Ice compression is applied immediately to the knee, and it is followed by elastic bandaging and more ice compression the same evening. A felt horseshoe conforming to the patella and secured by the elastic bandage can be helpful. The best treatment is rest from the sport and the athlete is advised to stop playing until the acute symptomatology disappears. Ice compression, elastic bandaging, and rest are continued until symptoms disappear.

In mild cases, the athlete is put on a hip-flexion and abduction exercise program. As the acute pain lessens, the athlete is put on an isometric exercise program for his quadriceps to increase his tolerance to pain. No knee-bending exercises are permitted. Moist hot packs to the knee are helpful prior to competition when the athlete is ready to return to his activity. A scout x-ray film of the knee should be taken. The young athlete with only a mild case finds it difficult abstaining from his sport even though participating will aggravate it. So the microruptures worsen, and finally, mucoid degeneration sets in.

Clinically, the athlete experiences pain and disability during and after cessation of the activity. Even though the athlete is advised against continuing in the sport, he usually elects to continue. Despite the use of medication, ice compression, rest, wet heat, exercises, and a patella-restraining brace, the athlete may experience no relief. At this point, the attending physician may elect to inject a corticosteroid at the site of the pathologic condition. If he does, the athlete must be advised that injection of this material has led to weakened tendons and in some cases, to tendon ruptures. Multiple injections should not be done. The physician must monitor the gastrointestinal status and periodic blood counts if certain medications are prescribed that require such surveillance.

If none of the recommended treatments help and the athlete persists in playing the sport, there is a surgical option available. Removal of the inferior pole of the patella or surgical removal of the degenerated quadriceps and patella-tendon site with supplemental reefing can be done.

Shoulder Injuries

The shoulder is a complicated structure of multiple bones, joints, muscles, ligaments, nerves and vascular structures whose main function is to move the arm on the trunk. Because the shoulder has relatively little inherent bony stability, it is suitably designed for producing large ranges of motion of the arm, which are so essential in athletics. In fact, it is the most mobile joint in the body. This mobility is achieved through the harmonious working of strong ligaments and powerful muscles. These muscles also provide bulk, and together with the ligaments ensure a firm anchoring of the component parts.

The shoulder is best known for its functions in ball throwing in such sports as baseball, football, and basketball. However, the shoulder also plays an important role in throwing a left hook, stroking a tennis ball, swimming, driving a golf ball, throwing a shotput, flinging a javelin, hurling a discus, and thrusting a foil. In addition, the shoulder may be used to protect a boxer's chin or head from a punch, perform a rugged block or tackle, or form a line of resistance to a forward moving opponent. The offensive and defensive use of the shoulder complex varies with the size of the object that has to be moved bodily or propelled by a piece of equipment, as well as the demands of the competition. This usage is most effectively realized with proportionate assistance from foot, leg, hip, trunk, and contralateral upper extremity movements in a coordinated and integrated manner.

The bony components of the shoulder include the clavicle, the head of the humerus, the sternum, the scapula, and that portion of the thorax over which the scapula moves. These bones and accompanying ligaments form four separate yet interdependent joints. These joints are listed in the order of frequency of injury:

1. Acromioclavicular.
2. Glenohumeral.
3. Sternoclavicular.*
4. Scapulothoracic.†

* Infrequent.
† Rare.

The muscles of the shoulder contribute to the size of this region, making it quite prominent and more easily injured in contact sports because of its exposed position and usage. The shoulder is also prone to injuries because of the tremendous leverage forces to which it is subjected. Slocum, Bateman, Brewer, Neer, Cox, Rowe, DePalma, Allan, and Stewart, have described and analyzed the mechanism of throwing as well as the stresses and strains to which the structures of the shoulder are subjected as a result of it. The unnatural motions of throwing a baseball, including the tremendous forces braking the momentum of the follow-through, make pitchers more prone to shoulder, arm, and elbow injuries, especially those pitchers who depend on curve and screw balls. The reader is encouraged to read these informative articles to understand the anatomy, physiology, and the mechanisms of injury that lead to these clinical conditions, which at times are difficult to diagnose.

In this book, traumatic conditions of the acromioclavicular and glenohumeral joints are considered, since these occur more frequently and the cause of the injury is quite apparent. The glenohumeral joint, with its heavy overlying musculature, and the acromioclavicular joint, lacking such anatomic protection, sustain contusions varying with the nature and extent of trauma. They are rarely of a serious or disabling nature. Additional protection is also provided with protecitve equipment. In addition, shoulder and arm conditions that are seen frequently in baseball players are discussed.

First-Aid Measures (First 24 Hours). *Step 1.* The trainer questions the athlete as to how, when, and where the injury occurred. Was the shoulder ever hurt before? Did the injury result from a blow, fall, or twist? Did it happen during a tackle, block, pile-up, or throwing motion of the arm? If he fell, did he land on his hand, elbow, arm or shoulder? If he fell on his hand, was his body weight moving forward, causing his elbow to bend? If he fell on his elbow, was the arm flexed and internally rotated or extended and externally rotated? If he fell on his arm, what was its position on impact? If the arm was struck a blow, what was its position from the trunk? If the athlete heard a clicking noise, had a sensation of something "catching," or felt bones slipping over one another in the shoulder, at what point and in what position was the arm from the trunk? If he fell on his shoulder, what aspect of it took the brunt of the force? Is he able to move his arm or does he have to support the arm and shoulder because of the pain? Answers to these questions help in understanding the mechanism of the injury and the probable clinical conditions resulting from it.

The trainer carefully inspects the bony and visible soft-tissue landmarks, looking for deformities, deltoid flattening, position of the arm to the trunk, swelling and ecchymosis. He questions the athlete to locate the site of pain. Some gentle palpation of these areas may be done to elicit tenderness and swelling. The trainer then tests the range of motion of the arm on the trunk, immediately stopping if the pain is great with any attempted motion.

Step 2. If the history of trauma suggests acromioclavicular joint injury, the trainer must take steps to check swelling and immobilize the injured shoulder with an elastic compression bandage and ice therapy before referring the athlete to the attending physician. This is done in the following manner:

1. The shoulder and arm are immobilized with a sling.
2. The lower arm (forearm) is placed diagonally across the chest and the entire upper extremity is tied high in a sling to elevate the scapula.
3. An ice compress is applied to the injured area to check swelling.

If the trainer suspects a separation or dislocation of this joint, he must immediately contact the team physician for further instructions. In any event, the injured athlete is referred to the doctor and instructed to see him immediately. The physician decides whether an x-ray study is indicated. If the history suggests a glenohumeral-joint dislocation, the athlete's arm is placed in a sling and the attending physician is immediately contacted. This is an emergency that needs immediate care by a physician, who will tell the trainer to send the athlete either to his office or to the hospital emergency room, where a closed reduction is done. If this is unsuccessful, the athlete can be admitted to the hospital and the reduction performed under general anesthesia. In the interim, the trainer applies ice therapy to the shoulder and the shoulder is protected from further injury.

Definitive Treatment (Follow-Up Care). The mechanism of injury and subsequent pathologic condition of the acromioclavicular or glenohumeral joints are usually quite apparent, unlike clinical conditions resulting from the act of throwing, which usually require more extensive investigation to make a diagnosis. The attending physician takes his own detailed history and makes a careful examination under ideal conditions in privacy, with clothing, taping, and wrappings removed. The uninjured shoulder is used for comparison. The doctor should have no difficulty in arriving at an accurate diagnosis and starting proper treatment.

Acromioclavicular Joint. This is the most frequently injured joint in the shoulder complex. Contusions, sprains, separations, and dislocations of this joint result most frequently from a sideway fall onto the lateral aspect of the shoulder (lateral edge of the acromion—more commonly referred to as the "point of the shoulder"). This injury may also occur from a direct blow to the acromion during a hard block, by a shoulder striking another shoulder during body contact, or by a direct downward force on the shoulder. A player who is "piled on" from behind while rising from a prone position may suffer an acromioclavicular injury.

The degree of injury varies with the nature and extent of the traumatic force. The term "shoulder separation" is commonly used when the trauma is great enough to produce a separation or dislocation at this joint, with an accompanying deformity. A separation may be severe enough to warrant a closed reduction and immobilization with slings, elastic bandages, adhesive dressings, strappings, or bracing; this may be difficult to achieve, because of the small size, large range of motion and anatomic relationship of the acromioclavicular joint to the chest and shoulder girdle. The attending physician must use that method by which he can best restore the joint to its normal position and keep it there until the torn ligaments have fully healed.

CONTUSION AND MILD SPRAIN (first degree sprain). Contusion and mild sprain of the acromioclavicular joint following minor trauma is usually associated with pain, local tenderness, swelling and limitation of arm movement. This condition is best treated with ice therapy to the injured joint and the use of a sling for 24 to 48 hours. The upper limb is tied high in a sling and ice therapy applied to the injured joint. The immobilization is removed after 48 hours, and if pain and swelling have been controlled, physical therapy consisting of ice therapy, and range-of-motion exercises of the shoulder are done, at first passively and then actively, to pain tolerance. If early return to athletics is warranted, additional protection to this joint can be provided with a sponge rubber pad placed over the acromioclavicular joint and adhesive strapping. A novel protective device by D'Andrea to reduce direct trauma to the injured acromioclavicular joint can be fashioned with an inflated appropriately sized bicycle inner tube taped on the under surface of the shoulder pad which keeps the shoulder pad off the acromioclavicular joint. The valve stem is covered with foam rubber and positioned beneath the shoulder pad and not externally exposed.

SEPARATION (second degree sprain). Second degree sprain (separation) of the acromioclavicular joint with incomplete tears of the acromioclavicular joint capsule and ligament can be recognized when the outer end of the clavicle (at least ½ inch the depth) is prominent and shows a joint laxity with the inferior surface of the clavicle at or just below the superior surface of the acromion accompanied by pain, local tenderness, and restriction of arm movements. The joint separation (increased space between the clavicle and the acromion) can be demonstrated by x-ray examination done while the athlete holds 10 to 15 pound weights in each hand to produce downward traction.

The attending physician can perform a reduction with the trainer acting as an assistant. A properly fitting Kenny Howard brace is ap-

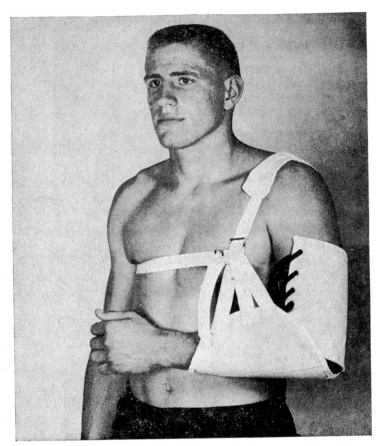

Fig. 9-9.   Kenny Howard brace. (Courtesy of Kenny Howard.)

plied (Fig. 9-9). This maintains the reduction by depressing the clavicle and elevating the acromion to insure a properly reduced acromioclavicular joint. Analgesic and anti-inflammatory medications are prescribed when necessary. The athlete is instructed to keep an ice bag on his injured shoulder for the next 48 to 72 hours. One of us (B.T.) uses only a sling as prescribed by his attending physician.

The following day the athlete is examined by the doctor, who checks the pulses, nerve function, and the status of the immobilization. He also starts the athlete on isometric exercises of the shoulder-girdle muscles on the injured side as well as the muscles of the immobilized limb. This immobilization remains for 3 to 4 weeks. X-ray pictures are again taken on the second week and after the immobilization has been removed.

Following removal of the immobilization, physical therapy consisting of Hydrocollator heat, massage, and exercises facilitates recovery. This can be hastened if done twice a day. A program for rehabilitation is described on page 205, following the discussion of glenohumeral dislocation.

DISLOCATION (third degree sprain). In dislocation of acromioclavicular joint, a deformity is noted, with the distal end of the clavicle elevated above the acromion and the presence of a marked separation of these bones equal to the depth of the lateral end of the clavicle or more. Dislocation results from ruptures of the acromioclavicular joint capsule and ligaments and the coracoclavicular ligaments. X-ray films show widening between not only the acromion and distal end of the clavicle, but also the coracoclavicular distance. Pain, tenderness, deformities at the acromioclavicular joint and restricted arm movement make the diagnosis easy. Physicians vary in their approach to this problem; some prefer surgery, others recommend more conservative measures, such as the Kenny Howard brace.

If conservative measures fail and the adult athlete wants a cosmetically more attractive shoulder, surgery is indicated, even though the recent trend is not to operate on this condition. The surgeon can select from many operative procedures if this is his judgment. A primary repair of the ruptured capsule and ligaments without any bone work is an acceptable method. The literature suggests that excision of the distal end of the clavicle is an excellent procedure provided no more than 1 to 1½ cm of the bone is resected and the trapezius, deltoid, periosteum, and capsule are sutured to their origins to contain the bone end of the clavicle in its proper place. The distal end of the clavicle must be bevelled. Some surgeons, after excising the distal end of the clavicle, use a Dacron Velour graft ligament reconstruction. Early mobilization and, as a rule, no special taping or pads are necessary postoperatively. The same type of physical therapy is given as for separation of the acromioclavicular joint. After sufficient physical therapy including an intensive program of resistance exercises has produced a normal range of motion, muscle strength-athletic activities may be resumed. Postoperative care lasting up to 3 to 4 weeks or more must be anticipated.

Glenohumeral Joint. This is the most mobile joint in the body because of its loose, relaxed ligaments and the lax articular capsule that binds the large round head of the humerus into the shallow oval cavity of the glenoid fossa and its attached labrum. The arm is moved about at the shoulder joint by the deltoid, pectoral, biceps, triceps, and latissimus dorsi muscles in a coordinated manner with the rotator cuff muscles, which also contribute strength and stability to this joint by firming the position of the head of the humerus into the glenoid fossa. Anteriorly, the deltoid protects the shoulder joint well against direct trauma, but the subscapularis muscle is now regarded as a prime protector against a dislocation. Inferiorly, the capsule is vulnerable; superiorly, it is protected by the acromion.

CONTUSIONS. These are common occurrences in athletics and usually cause pain, tenderness, and restriction of shoulder motion. A careful history of the injury and the basic examining procedures of observation, palpation, and joint-function tests make the diagnosis obvious. If a fracture or dislocation is suspected, a roentgenogram should be taken. Treatment is with ice therapy and limitation of shoulder motion for 24 to 48 hours. Wearing a sling for a day or two helps, followed by local moist hot packs, light massage, and active exercises to pain tolerance.

SPRAINS. The ligaments of this joint are seldom sprained because they are so loose and allow a great range of motion.

DISLOCATION. This joint dislocates more frequently in athletics than all other major articulations considered together. Pain, deltoid flattening and inability to move the arm are characteristic of dislocation. The large head of the humerus slips out from the shallow respository of the glenoid fossa and its attached labrum, contusing, stretching, and tearing through supporting soft tissue in its path, most frequently as a result of indirect trauma. The humeral head is moved out of its normal articulating position by forces that cause the humerus to act as a lever or by forces that are transmitted through the shaft of the humerus. As the shoulder is placed in abduction and external rotation (overhead throw), the subscapularis muscle moves upwardly exposing the unprotected anterior capsule through which the humeral head dislocates anteriorly. This causes a flattening of the side of the shoulder because the humeral head is normally positioned under the deltoid muscle. This dislocation is confirmed by palpation. Moseley adds that most anterior dislocations follow an anterior-inferior direction because the tendon of the long head of the triceps affords strong support to the inferior capsule when the arm is in full abduction. In addition, the greater portion of the head of the humerus projects anteriorly to the biceps tendon, which further predisposes to an anterior-inferior dislocation. The head of the humerus is most commonly in a subcoracoid position following dislocation; this can be confirmed by inspection or palpation. Subclavicular and subglenoid dislocations have been noted, but these are rare. With the anatomy so distorted, shoulder motion is practically nil and any active or passive attempt to move it causes severe pain. Usually, with an anterior dislocated shoulder, the athlete is unable to place the hand of the arm of the injured shoulder onto the uninjured shoulder. Some of the more common histories associated with anterior dislocations are the following:

1. Fall on outstretched hand as body lunges forward, causing the elbow to flex and exerting maximal stress on shoulder capsule.

2. Fall backward on the point of elbow with the arm in backward extension.

3. Movement of the arm into a position of abduction, horizontal extension, and external rotation.

4. A blow on an abducted and externally rotated arm during a poorly executed tackle, when the momentum of the runner forces the tackler's abducted arm backward into horizontal extension, levering the head out of the joint.

5. Direct blows to the posterior aspect of the shoulder can cause anterior dislocation.

No athlete is immune to this clinical condition. I (M. N.) have reduced shoulder dislocations in boxers that occurred following the delivery of a blow, in tennis players as a result of a serve, and in basketball players who have crashed into a wall. Although posterior dislocations of the glenohumeral joint are rare, they do occur as a result of direct blows or a fall anteriorly on the shoulder as well as forced internal rotation of the adducted arm.

The doctor's examination includes determining the status of the axillary nerve, since this is frequently injured in shoulder dislocations. The ulnar nerve can also be injured but rarely the radial. Hypoesthesia of the lateral aspect of the shoulder or a weakness of shoulder abduction by the deltoid strongly suggests an injury to this nerve. However, the presence of nerve injury does not alter the immediate treatment. The x-ray pictures must be taken of the shoulder to confirm the diagnosis as well as the possibility of associated fractures.

The best treatment is immediate closed reduction of the dislocation on the field of play if the athlete is seen within minutes of the injury. The athlete is placed supine on the ground or floor. The doctor kneels on one knee and then exerts straight traction on the dislocated arm by grasping and pulling the athlete's hand and wrist while the trainer exerts counter-traction. An audible thud in the region of the shoulder as well as a normal rounding out of the flattened deltoid signals a successful return of the humeral head to the glenoid.

If straight arm traction is unsuccessful after a few minutes, take the athlete off the field. Appropriate pre-reduction analgesic and/or muscle relaxant are given; then use the Kocher method of reduction. In this method, with the elbow held in flexion and the arm adducted and externally rotated, traction is exerted on the arm as it is carried into forward flexion and then internally rotated. (Caution: fractures of the humerus have occurred with this method.)

If the injury is not seen within minutes of the trauma, it is usually necessary to use general anesthesia to relax the powerful shoulder muscles of the athlete, which resist reduction, especially when muscle

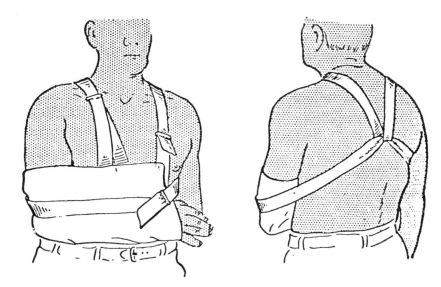

Fig. 9-10. The wrap-around shoulder sling eliminates pull on the neck and secures the arm in internal rotation and adduction. (Reproduced by permission from Rowe, C.R., and Marble, H.C.: Shoulder girdle injuries. *In* Cave, E.F. (ed.): Fractures and Other Injuries. Copyright © 1958 by Year Book Medical Publishers, Inc., Chicago.)

spasm, pain, and anxiety are also present. The reduction must be as gentle as possible to prevent further soft-tissue damage.

After a traumatic dislocation of the shoulder has been reduced, immobilization in adduction and internal rotation in a wrap-around sling for 3 weeks have been shown to reduce the high incidence in recurrent dislocation up to 40 years of age as much as 10 to 15%. Post-reduction x-ray films must be taken. The neurovascular structures are checked periodically.

There are significant differences of opinion concerning postreduction management and treatment for high school, collegiate, and professional athletes. However, there is agreement that high school and collegiate athletes must have full recovery of normal strength in all the muscles of the shoulder before they resume play. For high school and intercollegiate athletes, one shoulder dislocation per season is sufficient to ban the athlete from further competition that season. These primary reduced shoulder dislocations are immobilized for no less than 3 weeks, followed by a period of physical therapy including progressive resistances exercises.

Under 20 years of age, the recurrence rate is 94%; at 20 to 40 years of age, there is a 74% recurrence rate; and over 40 years of age the recurrence rate is 14%. In a football player, a recurrent dislocation should be repaired and football disallowed until this is done. In the 40-years old and over group, 2 weeks of immobilization are sufficient. Protective harnesses for reduced dislocations are available but are ineffective and not recommended.

The professional athlete is in a class by himself, often being permitted to return to active competition in 7 to 10 days with a restrictive harness limiting abduction, extension, and external rotation; the harness is worn for about 4 weeks while a rehabilitative program of progressive resistive exercises is simultaneously carried out. This traditional program of limited immobilization has led to increased incidence of redislocations. If the dislocation recurs, a surgical repair is performed followed by the usual rehabilitation.

Whenever a shoulder is to be immobilized with either a sling or Velpeau type of dressing for a period of time exceeding a week, a program of rehabilitation of the muscles must begin at the onset of the immobilization to prevent muscle atrophy. Isometric exercises of the shoulder and arm should begin as soon as pain permits. If the forearm muscles are also included in the immobilization, the muscles of this part must also be exercised.

Following removal of the immobilization, Codman exercises are encouraged. These are both isotonic and stretching exercises that are aided by the force of gravity. Some muscles need more strengthening than others; this is determined by testing. The following inexpensive equipment is useful for exercising: rubber ball, finger exercisers, bouncing putty, finger ladders, shoulder wheels, metal handle with removable collars, and iron discs weighing 2½, 5, 10, 12½ to 50 pounds. Klein recommends a reconditioning program of seven specific progressive-resistance exercises that produce significant functional gains in chronic shoulder injury, dislocations, and instability. Isometric exercises following termination of the regular exercise program are done to maintain the strength of the shoulder-girdle muscles.

Shoulder Lesions in Baseball. Baseball players are plagued by the same clinical conditions of the shoulder, arm, and elbow as anyone else in the general population. However, the constant wear and tear and great strain placed on these parts are responsible for the more frequent occurrence of injury in professional baseball players and especially pitchers. Professional and Little League baseball pitchers can each claim a distinctive yet different lesion in the shoulder that may result from pitching. The shoulder is most frequently the cause not only of sore and tight (stiff) shoulders, but also of sore and tight (stiff) arms. Some of the more common ailments are strains of frequently used muscles or their tendinous insertions, subacromial or subdeltoid bursitis, bicipital tenosynovitis, osteoarthritis of the shoulder joint, loose bodies in the shoulder joint, exostosis at posterior-inferior rim of the

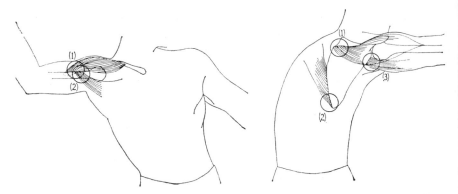

Fig. 9-11. (Left) The preparatory phase of pitching, which represents traction and tension arcs. (1) Anterior insertion of deltoid; (2) insertion of pectoralis major. Periosteal tears that occur in this area frequently respond quickly to trigger point injection. (Right) Follow-through phase. (1) Posterior origin of the deltoid; (2) insertion of the rhomboid major; (3) long head of the triceps at its origin from the infraglenoid tuberosity. If a pitcher has not warmed up sufficiently and puts abnormal effort into the follow-through, stretching and tearing may result. (Slocum, D.B.: Mechanics of some common injuries to the shoulder in sports. Amer. J. Surg., 98:395, 1959.)

glenoid, luxation of the biceps tendon from the bicipital groove, supraspinatus tendon fraying, nonspecific inflammation and others. Elbow conditions are considered elsewhere (page 214).

Since a variety of clinical conditions may be responsible for a disabled shoulder and arm, an effort must be made to locate the source of trouble. It is important to take a detailed history. In addition to the usual examination techniques of inspection, palpation, range of motion, and muscle testing, it is absolutely necessary to observe, study, and analyze the player's throwing motion from stance to follow-through. Slocum has divided the act of throwing into four steps or phases:

1. Initial stance.
2. Wind-up preparatory phase.
3. Initial forward action of arm.
4. Follow-through.

In order for a physician to pinpoint the pathologic condition responsible for the ballplayer's ailing arm, he must have a thorough understanding of the mechanism of throwing. He will then be able to observe, study, and analyze the player's throwing or pitching pattern, thereby enabling him to arrive at an accurate diagnosis. He does this by correlating the appearance of the symptoms with the anatomy and the phase of the throwing mechanism in which these appear. Routine and special x-ray views including the West-Point view and including arthrography, as well as arthroscopy help considerably in visualizing any bony, periosteal, or soft tissue pathologic condition.

The protracted "sore arm" that is the bane of pitchers may be due to a variety of causes. As noted before, the pathology may be in the shoulder, arm or elbow. Only the most frequent clinical conditions of the shoulder responsible for the sore arm are discussed here.

PERIOSTEAL-TENDINOUS AND MUSCLE TEARS. During the preparatory phase of the wind-up, the anterior deltoid and pectoralis major muscles are stretched as the arm is drawn back and into abduction and external rotation. The insertions of these muscles may be injured by tension. During the follow-through phase, the scapular insertions of the posterior deltoid, rhomboid major and long head of the triceps are fully stretched. These muscles can be easily injured as a result of an overload.

These lesions cause local pain and discomfort. They are easily localized by palpation as well as by studying the throwing pattern. An injection of local anesthetic combined with a steroid at the trigger point, is both diagnostic and therapeutic. The injected area is treated by cryotherapy for 24 hours. Ultrasound may be helpful and is instituted the day after an injection. The pitcher uses a 5-pound steel ball, the exact size of a conventional baseball, in a series of exercises carefully designed to strengthen and rehabilitate sore arms. The exercises simulate the various motions, including wind-up and follow-through in the act of throwing. It is also recommended the pitcher rest for 1 to 2 weeks following the injury depending on the extent of the injury. This applies equally to swimmers, tennis players, and others who sustain similar injuries.

EXOSTOSIS ON POSTERIOR-INFERIOR RIM OF GLENOID. As a result of the tremendous throwing and braking forces to which the capsule and its coverings at the shoulder joint are subjected in the follow-through phase of pitching, pathologic changes occur in the posterior capsule and adjacent triceps tendon. Bony deposits may form at the posterior-inferior rim of the glenoid following excessive strain and overuse. This condition is a distinctive lesion of professional baseball pitchers. These deposits cause local pain and discomfort posteriorly in the shoulder. Tenderness can commonly be elicited in the posterior axillary fold, yet pain may be felt anteriorly in the deltoid because of pain referred by way of the circumflex nerve when it has been irritated. Pitching causes increased pain and discomfort. After a couple of innings of hard pitching, the pitcher may find it difficult to continue.

Routine A-P or P-A x-ray views of the shoulder may not reveal the lesion; it may be necessary to x-ray the shoulder while positioned in external rotation with the x-ray tube tilted 5° cephalad. The best and quickest way to manage these lesions is by injections and physical therapy. The point of maximal tenderness is injected with a 1- or 2-ml combination preparation of local anesthesia and corticosteroid. If the athlete gets relief, he may continue to perform. The injection may be repeated if pain recurs after a suitable interval.

If no relief is experienced after three injections plus physical therapy, it may be necessary to have the pitcher change his pitching style from overhead to a side arm or ¾ style, provided he is young enough to make such a change. Operative treatment for this condition has a poor prognosis for returning the athlete as a successful pitcher.

BICIPITAL TENOSYNOVITIS. Suspect this condition when the athlete complains of local pain and discomfort over the front of the shoulder in the region of the tendon of the long head of the biceps, when there is marked tenderness with palpation over this tendon in the bicipital groove, or tenderness on rolling the tendon under the examiner's fingers. The diagnosis is firmly established when testing of the biceps muscle against resistance produces pain in the region of the bicipital tendon (Yerguson's Maneuver).

If the pitcher is not a professional, the arm should be placed in a sling and painful movements avoided. Daily physical therapy, consisting of moist heat and ultrasound, is indicated and a nonsteroidal anti-inflammatory such as aspirin. If the condition does not subside in 1 week, then an injection of a corticosteroid and local anesthetic should be considered at the site of maximal tenderness under strict aseptic precautions. Resumption of pitching duties, of course, depends on the athlete's response to treatment and is usually allowed in a graded manner.

In the professional pitcher, this lesion is best treated early with an injection of a corticoid combined with a local anesthetic, the injected area is treated by cryotherapy for 24 hours. Following this ultrasound may be used. In this manner, the pitcher is relieved of his pain and kept active but probably misses his regular rotation. However, repeated injections of corticosteroid into a tendon are not without the risk of inducing subsequent tendon rupture.

The doctor must be alert to the fact that, if this clinical condition goes unrecognized, it may lead to a rupture of the long head of the biceps with characteristic deformity of the biceps. This complication is best treated surgically upon early recognition.

FOCUS OF INFLAMMATION. Infrequently, a ballplayer will have a sore and disabled arm or shoulder that is difficult to diagnose. Because many team physicians are orthopedically and surgically oriented, the diagnosis remains an enigma after their examinations. A complete medical check-up by a physician oriented in internal medicine is then indicated. Various medical conditions such as arthritis, gallbladder disease, kidney infections, cardiac conditions, and others may be the cause of his pitching difficulties. Rarely, a dental problem may be responsible for the ballplayer's wretchedness and poor performance.

LITTLE LEAGUER'S SHOULDER.   This is a fracture of the proximal epiphyseal cartilage of the humerus in Little League pitchers. It is usually accompanied by sharp pain in the shoulder region and a marked reduction in pitching efficiency. Localized tenderness, painful shoulder motions that become intensified with testing of the various shoulder muscles against resistance, and radiographic widening of the translucent line of the epiphyseal cartilage in a Little League pitcher usually establish the diagnosis.

Treatment of these athletes is the use of a sling for several days and discontinuance of all participation until symptoms are resolved. The prognosis is excellent. According to Torg, this translucency may take 8 to 12 months to reossify.

Anterior Instability and Transient Recurrent Subluxation of the Shoulder. Periodically, a physician is consulted by an athlete who has a disabling shoulder condition that causes recurrent episodes of pain and disability. Because the condition has not improved, the athlete has decided to see his doctor. The patient's history and complaints strongly suggest glenohumeral joint instability. Vigorous, and sometimes violent, repetitions of overhead athletic activities of the shoulder and arm, as are used in racquet, throwing, and swimming sports, can lead to this disabling entity. Blazina and Satzman highlighted this syndrome in a 1969 report, which caused practicing orthopedists to give more attention to this clinical entity. They added that following an injury, the entire upper extremity may be limp, feel numb, or tingle. Rowe and Zarins stated that following a transient subluxation, the athlete may complain of a sudden sharp, stabbing, paralyzing pain. The arm may "go dead," which prevents the athlete from using the arm above shoulder level. Rowe and Zarins named this the "dead arm syndrome."

According to Protzman, many West Point cadets, whose training includes hand-walking by grasping the rungs of overhead ladders as well as large amounts of pull-ups, have sustained anterior shoulder instability disorders and subluxations. Rockwood adds that even a minor fall or such minor activities as swinging a badminton or tennis racquet can lead to transient subluxation.

This clinical disorder may also appear in nonathletes, especially in those who do heavy overhead work.

The physician must pay particular attention to the patient's history because at times that may be the only guide available for selecting proper therapy. The patient usually describes a sensation of looseness and instability in the shoulder. Patients may say, "My shoulder comes out," "My shoulder is about to come out," "My shoulder slipped (or is slipping) out," or "My shoulder voluntarily slipped back in." Others may say, "My shoulder hung up and then went back into place." It is important for the doctor to ascertain what the shoulder position had been

8

when the symptoms commenced. The majority of these disorders occur as a result of abduction, extension, or external rotation of the shoulder. Here, the head of the humerus transiently subluxes over the anterior rim of the glenoid, causing anterior shoulder pain. The pain lessens when the humeral head relocates itself. Pain is also felt posteriorly because of the checkrein function of the shoulder's posterior structures, which prevents further subluxing of the humeral head. Knowledge of prior trauma or operations is important since it can help the physician make an appropriate judgment for treatment.

A careful examination is done with the patient standing, sitting, or lying in a supine position. Testing for anatomic contours, muscle strength, and range of motion is best done with the patient standing. More precise testing of the shoulder is done with the patient in a sitting or supine position and the elbow of the involved upper extremity on either the examiner's hip or a pillow. Tenderness and instability can be elicited. Anterior pain is almost always present with anterior-inferior instability.

A clicking, snapping, or clunking noise may be heard during range of motion of the shoulder. These noises may be related to movement of the head of the humerus as it subluxes over the rim of the glenoid or returns to its normal position.

External rotation and abduction of the shoulder produce in the patient a positive sign of apprehension, indicative of anterior shoulder instability and subluxation. If an athlete starts guarding or resisting external rotation when the shoulder is in 90 degrees or less of abduction, then a subluxing shoulder must be suspected. A comparative examination of the noninjured shoulder and arm must also be done.

The physical examination should be followed by an x-ray examination that includes anteroposterior views of the shoulder in internal and external rotation, lateral axillary views and a West Point view. The West Point view described in Chapter 9, is a tangential view of the anteroinferior rim of the glenoid. Although an acute anterior subluxation of the shoulder may not show any demonstrable bony disorder, chronic anterior subluxations may reveal an avulsion fracture of the anteroinferior rim of the glenoid, irregularity of the glenoid rim, calcific deposits anterior to the rim of the glenoid, and defects of the humeral head.

Treatment of the patient depends on the type and degree of subluxation. Rockwood classifies subluxations as types I and II, caused by trauma, and types III and IV, voluntary and involuntary atraumatic, respectively.

Type I is treated first with a muscle-strengthening exercise program directed to the three parts of the deltoid and to internal rotator muscles. If this treatment fails and the shoulder continues to subluxate, operative treatment is indicated. The surgeon performs the shoulder reconstruction operation with which he is most familiar. For a type II subluxation, if the athlete has a history of one or multiple dislocations interspersed with intermittent subluxing episodes, a standard shoulder reconstruction operation is indicated. Anterior redundant capsular pouches must be eliminated surgically.

Type III and type IV may have genetic, muscular, neurologic, and neuropsychiatric bases. The cause of the patient's disability must be accurately established. A rehabilitation program is always beneficial. Surgery should not be performed if there is a neuropsychiatric component. It may be helpful to send such patients to a psychiatrist for consultation and therapy.

Types III and IV can seem interchangeable at times. Determining the type of atraumatic subluxator (voluntary or involuntary) prior to treatment is important. Rockwood emphatically states that whenever surgery is indicated, the anteroinferior redundant pouch must be eliminated.

Impingement Syndrome. Neer's pioneering research on the shoulder led to our present understanding of painful disorders of the shoulder seen in athletes, such as the impingement syndrome. He demonstrated that the shoulder's functional arc of elevation is forward, not lateral as was commonly believed. He also showed by cadaver dissection how the overhead motion of the shoulder could produce the impingement syndrome. Impingement occurs when the greater tuberosity impinges the soft tissue against the anterior edge of the acromion and the coracoacromial ligament. Cadaver dissections of older persons showed marked degenerative changes and osteophyte formation on the undersurface of the anterior acromion. In other cadaver specimens, thickening and even osteophyte formation was noted in the coracoacromial ligament.

Rathbun and McNab's microvascular research on the subclavian artery provided additional etiologic evidence of the impingement syndrome. Injection of a micro-opaque substance into the subclavian artery, which carries the blood supply to the rotator cuff, revealed an avascular pattern in the supraspinatus tendon and intracapsular portion of the biceps tendon when the arm is held dependent at the side of the body. Accordingly, these tendons are more vulnerable to degenerative changes. Since these relatively avascular tendons course together over the humeral head, McNab suggested that this avascular pattern is conducive to development of the impingement syndrome.

This syndrome gained wider clinical recognition and acceptance from Hawkins and Kennedy's cross-Canadian letter survey, conducted on 2496 Canadian swimmers of major swimming clubs following the 1976 Olympic Games. Fifteen percent of the swimmers that specialized in freestyle and butterfly strokes were discovered to have shoulder disability of the impingement type. Johnson, in a more recent report, found that between one half and two thirds of the world-class swimmers surveyed have had significant shoulder problems. Johnson adds backstroke swimmers to the category of freestyle and butterfly swimmers.

Kennedy's cadaver dissections of the shoulder confirmed Neer's findings. Impingement was also shown to occur at the acromioclavicular joint, subacromial bursa, infraspinatus, and long head of the biceps. Johnson states that a rigorous training program that involves as much as 16,000 strokes per week or 660,000 strokes per season produces overuse syndromes as a result of the subdeltoid bursa's inability to keep pace with the lubrication demands of the shoulder. Accordingly, inflammation results. When examining athletes with shoulder complaints, physicians must be aware of the close anatomic relationships of the important shoulder structures that exist within a small area, and they must consider that one or several of these structures may be the cause of pain and disability. This clinical disorder is also seen in such competitive and recreational athletes as tennis and racquetball players, baseball pitchers, quarterbacks in football, and other athletes who participate in predominantly overhead sports.

The impingement syndrome occurs in all age groups, from teenage swimmers to geriatric tennis players. Repeated loading of the shoulder as the arm is brought vigorously into a forward flexed position above the horizontal plane causes repeated impingements and progressive wear and tear of the bony and soft tissue structures. In addition to the bony and soft tissue changes that take place, rotator cuff tears do occur in later stages.

Neer and others divide the progressive development of this syndrome into the following three stages.

STAGE I—EDEMA AND HEMORRHAGE. The first stage results from overuse-overhead activities in such sports as baseball, tennis, and swimming and typically affects athletes under age 25. Pain is usually minimal and occurs with activity, although it is sometimes described as resembling a toothache and occurring primarily at night. Tenderness may be elicited at the anterior acromion and greater tuberosity, the biceps and supraspinatus tendon may be tender and may cause bicipital groove pain, and crepitus may be present. A test for impingement syndrome is done in the following manner: The arm is flexed forcibly against the anteroinferior surface of the acromion; if 10 ml of a local anesthesia injected into the patient's subacromial impingement area causes relief of pain, the diagnosis is confirmed. Stage I is reversible.

Conservative care consisting of rest, oral anti-inflammatory medications, and physical therapy is recommended for treating this stage of the condition. When the pain lessens, additional measures are instituted, such as stretching of the muscle and capsule, muscle strengthening, and corrective measures to eliminate faulty athletic movements and to produce proper biomechanical moves. The athlete must warm-up properly to ensure loosening and flexibility of the joints, muscles, and tendons and activation of the lubrication mechanism. Training programs must include flexibility and strengthening exercises to help prevent shoulder problems. Subluxing shoulders, frozen shoulders, and acromioclavicular arthritis must be ruled out.

STAGE II—FIBROSIS AND TENDINITIS. As impingement continues without relief, the disorder becomes chronic and more difficult to treat. Additional inflammatory scarring occurs in the subacromial bursa, supraspinatus tendon, and biceps tendon. Tenderness is frequently elicited over the biceps and supraspinatus tendons as well as other areas of the shoulder. The shoulder joint becomes progressively stiffer (crepitus may be present). Although this condition is seen more frequently in the 25- to 40-year-old age group, it is also seen among 50- and 60-year-olds. Clinical testing must be precise to ascertain which structures are causing pain and disablement.

In this stage, it is important to either confirm or rule out the presence of coracoacromial ligament involvement. This can be done in the following manner. The humerus is forcibly flexed to 90 degrees and then forcibly rotated internally, which causes the greater tuberosity to impact the supraspinatus tendon against the anterior surface of the coracoacromial ligament. The previously described impingement injection test is then performed. One of the characteristic signs of this stage is the athlete's reluctance to bring his arm down vigorously from an abducted, overhead position, such as that used in serving a tennis ball, or in executing an overhand stroke in racquetball, or in performing a swim stroke. Soon the patient avoids all athletic activity because of the anticipated pain and weakness. The patient has now reached a stage of irreversibility, in which either surgery or complete avoidance of the offending activity is indicated.

The type of surgery indicated depends on what pathologic process is responsible for the patient's condition. A chronic subacromial bursa may have to be removed, or a coracoacromial ligament may have to be resected. In any event, the patient must be told to expect a lengthy rehabilitation program to recover a normal range of motion and strength. A return to competitive athletics at the same level of proficiency should not be anticipated, but a return to recreational athletics can be.

STAGE III—BONE SPURS AND TENDINITIS. The third stage is character-ized by continuing shoulder problems, running a gamut of minimal to severe pain, weakness, and limitation of motion of the shoulder-arm complex in patients over age forty. Chronicity can be punctuated by recurrent attacks of tendinitis that may be severe enough to awaken the patient from sleep. Progressive degeneration of the tendon leads to par-tial or complete rupture of the rotator cuff and the biceps tendon. A complete cuff rupture is evidenced by tenderness over the greater tu-berosity, atrophy of the infraspinatus and supraspinatus muscles, and weakness of abduction and external rotation. Crepitus and the impinge-ment sign aid in diagnosis. Bony excrescences of the coracoacromial ligament and of the acromion's anterior and undersurface help the phy-sician to localize the pathologic process responsible for this stage of the disorder. If conservative care fails and surgery becomes necessary, an-terior acromioplasty and/or repair of the rotator cuff tear may be indi-cated. Cervical radiculitis and neoplasm must first be ruled out.

In all three stages, a thorough history must be taken, followed by a meticulous examination. An x-ray examination and impingement in-jection test should be conducted. Rest, oral anti-inflammatory medica-tion, and physical therapy must be utilized in all three stages. Ice applied after activities is usually beneficial. Limited use of corticoste-roid injections into the subacromial bursa may be helpful. Ultrasound and TENS have also been effective in chronic, refractory cases. Arthro-grams are best reserved for Stage III.

Such preventive measures as muscle stretching and strengthening must be practiced by athletes prior to competition, as part of a training and conditioning program. If in Stages II and III an operation is planned, the athlete must be advised that rehabilitation is important for his total recovery. He also must be advised that following surgery he might not be able to reach his former competitive level. If the ath-lete follows the reconditioning program conscientiously, however, he should be able to reach a satisfactory recreational capability.

Elbow Injuries

The elbow is an interesting anatomic arrangement of three joints formed by the articulating surfaces of the distal humerus (capitellum and trochlea), proximal radius and ulna and adjoining muscles, liga-ments, synovium, nerves, and vascular structures. Its primary function is to move the forearm to and from the arm as well as to rotate it. The hand, by virtue of its connection to the forearm, moves with it. The forearm can also act as an extension of the arm. Flexion and extension (hinge) movements of the elbow occur at the capitellum-radial head and the trochlea-ulna articulations. These motions are done with a reasonable degree of inherent mechanical stability because of the accurate adaptation of the trochlea to the semilunar notch of the ulna. The biceps and brachialis muscles that run anterior to the joint produce flexion of this joint. The triceps muscle, which runs posterior to the joint, produces extension of this joint. These are strong muscles

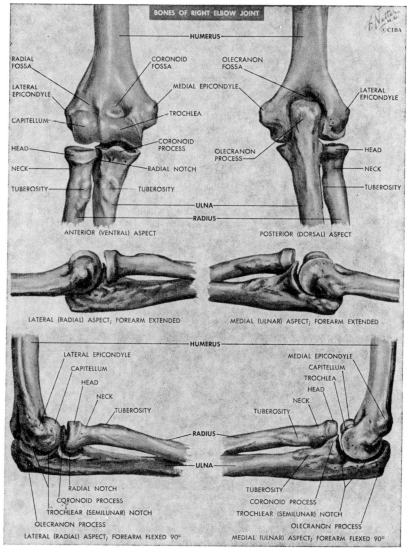

Fig. 9-12. Bones of the right elbow joint. (© Copyright 1969, CIBA Pharmaceutical Company, Division of CIBA-GEIGY Corporation. Reprinted with permission from CLINICAL SYMPOSIA illustrated by Frank H. Netter, M.D. All rights reserved.)

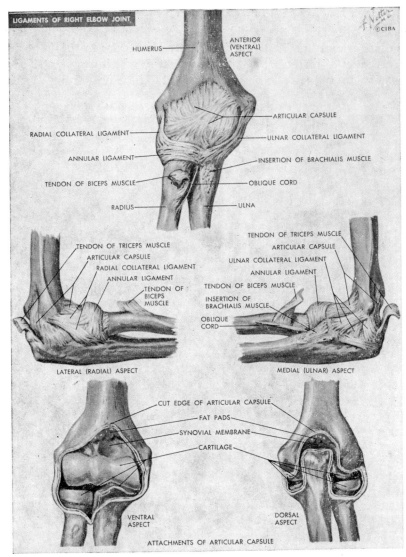

Fig. 9-13. Ligaments of the right elbow joint. (© Copyright 1969, CIBA Pharmaceutical Company, Division of CIBA-GEIGY Corporation. Reprinted with permission from CLINICAL SYMPOSIA illustrated by Frank H. Netter, M.D. All rights reserved.)

that also aid the ulnar and radial collateral ligaments in stabilizing the joint. The distal humerus just proximal to the condyles, anteriorly and posteriorly, has been adaptively thinned to accommodate the coronoid and olecranon processes of the ulna. Because of the bony weakening, this part of the humerus is not infrequently fractured when the curved beak of the olecranon recesses into the olecranon fossa when the elbow is fully extended.

The proximal radius and ulna are bound together by a strong annular ligament. These articulate with each other as well as with the capitellum and trochlea, respectively, to produce pronation and supination of the forearm. These movements are produced by muscles that originate from bony processes of the distal humerus, the medial and lateral epicondyles. At the medial epicondyle, flexor and pronator muscles originate. The pronator teres muscle produces forearm pronation; the flexor muscles produce wrist and finger flexion. The origin and the muscles of this epicondyle may suffer a painful disabling condition seen in baseball pitchers. At the lateral epicondyle arise the supinator and extensor muscles. The supinator muscle produces forearm supination; the extensor muscles produce wrist and finger extension. The disabling "tennis elbow" involves the origin of muscles at this epicondyle.

In athletics, the shoulder and elbow work in concert to produce one or a combination of the fundamental movements of flexion, extension, pronation, or supination of the forearm. This movement is seen in sports in which throwing is dominant, such as a baseball, javelin, and in boxing with the proper execution of a left jab, when the forearm and hand are flung forward at the elbow. The elbow not only is contused and sprained in a manner similar to other joints, but is also subjected to powerful repetitive hyperextension movements and rotary forces of the forearm, such as occur in baseball pitching, javelin throwing, golf, tennis, jai alai and others, which can result in pathologic changes in the joint and structures about it.

Any trauma to the elbow that causes swelling may be serious, especially if swelling occurs in the antecubital fossa, which is tightly bounded by the bicipital aponeurosis. The lack of "give" in this space may cause an unyielding tightness and pressure on the nearby blood vessels, leading to arterial impairment. Although the median, radial and ulnar nerves course about the elbow, only trauma to the ulnar nerve has practical implications in athletic injuries. This nerve is superficially placed in the ulnar notch (commonly known as "Funny Bone") and is not infrequently contused, causing a sharp momentary pain, tingling or numbness to radiate down the inner side of the forearm to the ring and small finger.

The elbow joint is frequently threatened with a marked loss of function because of development of myositis ossificans and adhesive capsulitis following muscle contusions, fractures, and dislocations of the bones of this joint. The reader is encouraged to read the anatomy, physiology, and kinesiology of the elbow.

First-Aid Measures (First 24 Hours). *Step 1.* As with other injuries to joints, the trainer takes a complete history, placing special emphasis on the mechanism of the injury. Did the injury result from a blow, fall, or twist? What was the position of the part at the time of the injury? Did it happen during a tackle, pile-up, arm lock, hitting the boards or gym floor, throwing motion, or during a tennis match? Is he able to move his elbow or does he have to carry this injured upper extremity by holding the wrist of the injured limb? Did he feel an electric-like momentary pain, tingling or a numbness radiating from the inner side of the elbow to the ring and pinky fingers? The trainer makes a careful examination of all surfaces of the injured elbow, inspecting the soft tissue and bony landmarks looking for deformities, swelling, and ecchymosis. He looks for the points of the olecranon and both epicondyles and palpates them, looking for a triangular outline formed by these bony prominences when the elbow is held flexed at 90°. Unnatural depressions and prominences must be noted. He palpates the radial pulse. He gently tests for range of motion and immediately stops if the pain is too great. He tests for finger approximation, spread, and extension.

Step 2. If the trainer feels reasonably certain that there are no fractures or dislocations, he renders first-aid care similar to that for other injured joints, the emphasis being directed to checking hemorrhage and extravasation of fluid into tissues by applying cold water or ice packs and compression bandaging. The injured athlete is referred to the doctor and instructed to see him before going to bed.

If the trainer suspects a fracture or dislocation, the athlete's arm is placed in a sling and the physician is immediately contacted. This is an emergency, and the physician will instruct the trainer about splinting and referring the athlete to his office or the hospital emergency room. Closed reduction is performed either with appropriate medication or with general anesthesia after the athlete has been admitted. A cold compress is applied to the elbow during the interim. Delay in appropriate treatment can lead to disastrous complications such as Volkmann's contracture.

Definitive Treatment (Follow-Up Care). *Contusion.* Because the back of the elbow is superficial and exposed and has practically no protective muscle padding, it is frequently contused from blows to it or falls in football, wrestling, basketball, tumbling, and ice hockey. Since the point of the elbow and its overlying soft tissues are prominent, reaction to trauma is rapid and readily observable. Subsequently, serious prolonged disability in contused elbows is infrequent because early and effective first-aid measures to check hemorrhage and extravasation of fluid into the joint can be started. The use of ice compresses, sponge rubber padding, and elastic compression bandaging for 24 to 48 hours materially reduces swelling. This is followed by ice,

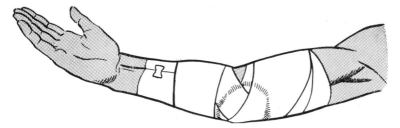

Fig. 9-14. Bandaging a contused elbow. Cover the tender spot of the elbow with a felt or sponge rubber "donut," and wrap with an elastic bandage. Note that the antecubital space away from the injury is left unwrapped.

massage and guarded active exercises. A sponge rubber pad should be worn in competition to prevent re-injury (Fig. 9-14).

If the superficially placed olecranon bursa has become distended, the same type of treatment is rendered. However, some team physicians may prefer to aspirate the bursal sac, which must be done under strict aseptic precautions. Although this may reduce the recovery time, it does carry a risk of infection.

If chronic or recurring bursal effusions appear or the bursa becomes thickened, a search must be made for the chronic or repetitive source of trauma, which will be removed. It may even be necessary in such cases to remove the bursa surgically if the pathologic condition continues.

Sprain. Elbow sprains rank low in the incidence of joint injuries. Although twisting of the elbow in any direction can produce a sprain of this joint, sprains occur in athletics most commonly when the back of a fully extended elbow is struck a blow while the athlete's hand and shoulder are held in a fixed position, as in a football pile-up. This injury occurs also in a basketball game when a player's arm is forced into hyperextension when caught between two players. The elbow may also be sprained when a player strikes a gym wall, floor, or earth with his outstretched hand and braced elbow to keep his body from colliding with the immovable mass. Acute onset of pain, tenderness, swelling, and marked restriction of elbow function should make one suspect a sprain of the elbow joint.

In our experience, sprains of the elbow are due mainly to hyperextension injuries and involve the anterior capsule. Some authors disagree, stating that the pathologic condition is predominantly a tear of one or both origins of the flexor and extensor muscles at the medial and lateral epicondyles of the humerus. This can easily be determined by careful palpation to localize the greatest point of tenderness, followed by testing of various muscles against resistance. Contraction of an injured muscle group causes pain at its point of origin. If there is significant pain, an x-ray study will determine whether an avulsed chip of bone from the epicondyle is present. A nondisplayed fracture of the radial head can mimic this condition and may not appear on x-ray films for up to 2 weeks.

The immediate treatment is the application of cold compresses, elastic bandage compression and support of an arm in a sling until seen by the doctor. The doctor applies a bivalved padded plaster cast for the upper extremity with the elbow held in 90°; this is worn for 7 to 10 days, depending on the severity of the injury. Joint aspiration has little to offer in the treatment of this condition. Following cast removal, whirlpool and massage of the area are started. Active exercise is done during the whirlpool therapy. Progressive-resistance exercise is started as the range of elbow motion increases. Following each treatment, the elbow is wrapped with an elastic bandage. A program of isometric and isotonic exercises of the upper extremity is performed at home by the athlete hourly for 5 minutes. The use of a sponge rubber or tennis ball for the hand aids in the restoration of muscle strength. Avoid forceful flexion or extension of an injured elbow to increase range of motion.

The athlete may return to participation after a full range of painless motion and muscle strength have been regained. A protective tape strapping is applied that allows flexion beyond 90°, but limits extension to 20° less than the zero starting (neutral) position. This is worn for 1 to 2 weeks following return to competition (Fig. 9-15).

Javelin Thrower's Elbow. Although the configuration of bones that articulate to form the elbow joint are suitably structured for flexion and

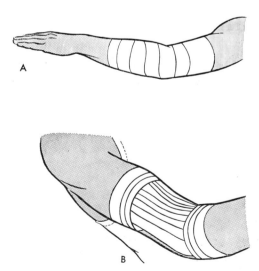

Fig. 9-15. *A*, Compression bandage applied for effusion of the elbow joint. *B*, Method of taping for injuries of the elbow.

extension (hinge motion), the humerus-ulna (trochlea-olecranon) articulation is not anatomically suited for some of the lateral and medial movements of the ulna of the elbow that occur in the javelin throw. The ulna abducts when the radius crosses it in pronation; the ulna adducts when the radius returns in supination to its parallel position with the ulna. The movements of the ulna at the trochlea are not generally well known and may be the reason for many obscure cases of elbow pain.

However, these proximal ulnar movements are considered the mechanism of injury in the "javelin thrower's elbow." There is a coordinated movement of powerful forearm pronation and elbow extension as the javelin is hurled on its way. As the olecranon moves medially during forearm pronation, it exerts tremendous pressure on the medial side of the joint, placing the ulnar collateral ligament under great strain. Although gradual in onset, pain may be acute after a violent throw. It disappears with rest and reappears with effort. On physical examination there may be nothing to see except perhaps some tenderness and slight swelling or fullness along the medial aspect of the elbow. There is usually a full range of painless motion. Muscle testing is usually normal as are x-ray studies. However, the history is a give-away. The best treatment is prevention, that is, the use of correct throwing techniques. The reader is encouraged to read J. E. Miller on the Javelin Thrower's Elbow.

Another, rarer type of javelin thrower's elbow follows a hyperextension injury to the tip of the olecranon, including a fracture. This is more difficult to treat because of recurrence and may eventually necessitate surgical removal of the olecranon tip.

Elbow Injuries in Baseball Players. Certainly a majority of our readers are familiar with the scene of a baseball pitcher on a mound, rearing back, and firing a baseball towards the batter at a velocity in excess of 100 miles an hour. He may have to pitch inning after inning with such power because a "no hitter" is within his grasp. Or he may have to bear down exceptionally hard because of a game situation. The power of each pitch is generated in the large area of the shoulder and arm and is transmitted through the narrower elbow with an increased limb velocity to effect maximal transmission of energy through the forearm and hand.

With an understanding of the anatomy and physiology of the shoulder and upper extremity and the biomechanics of the complicated act of pitching, which may average between 100 to 140 pitches in a regulation nine innings of a baseball game, the reader should be able to appreciate why the elbows of pitchers are so frequently injured. The repetitive throwing stresses the medial reinforcing soft tissue restraints for the same reason that the capitellum is compressed. Therefore, attenuation of the medial ligament system from valgus strains occurs, which leads to pain, instability, and loss of function. Such was the case of Tommy John, a veteran left-handed hurler of the Angels team. His pitching arm was salvaged by Dr. Frank Jobe, who replaced a withered and torn medial collateral ligament with a palmaris longus tendon from his right forearm. The forearm is repeatedly subjected to the powerful extension force of the contracted triceps muscle at its insertion in the olecranon. This causes it to be flung forward at the elbow prior to the release of the ball and the follow-through. The elbow in particular is subjected to a great deal of stress in pitching; this stress, according to Elleman, causes compression of the radial head and may be partly responsible for osteochondrosis of the radial head. In addition, rotary forces of the forearm and flexion and extension of the wrist are powered by muscles that arise from the medial and lateral epicondyles of the humerus. The muscles that predominate depend on whether the hand is supinated with a snap or flexed sharply at the wrist to accomplish a desired curve, hop, sinker, or slide of the ball. These pitchers are more prone to elbow injuries than those who depend on a fast straight ball. Muscle ruptures, medial collateral ligament sprains, and ruptures in the elbow have also been described.

Pitchers who throw breaking stuff—curves, sliders, sinkers, and screw balls—cause the upper extremity and its joints to move unnaturally, thus placing great strain on the arm, elbow, and shoulder. This causes degenerative changes of the hyaline cartilage at the tip, margins, and articular surfaces of the olecranon, medial surface of the coronoid process of the ulna, and the adjacent surfaces of the condyles of the humerus. Such changes result in synovial thickening, hypertrophic arthritic changes, spurs, osteochondritis, and loose bodies. Although most frequently seen in veteran professional pitchers, degenerative changes are also noted in adult pitchers who regularly take their stint on the mound and in other players. Olecranon fractures have been described in baseball players as well. All of these conditions can cause pain, swelling, restricted and painful elbow motion.

Loose bodies caused by cartilage and/or bone are most frequently located in the olecranon fossa, at the tip of the coronoid process, and about the radial head. They may mechanically obstruct extension in the elbow to varying degrees. Loose bodies have also been noted in the ligamentous tissue and tendinous attachment in the region of the medial epicondyle of the humerus beneath the ulnar nerve. They may produce a paresthesia of the ulnar distribution of the hand by irritating the ulnar nerve in its vicinity. It is not unusual to find loose bodies in the olecranon fossa of pitchers in their late teens who have been pitching regularly for a number of years. This is the end result of a chronic Little Leaguer's elbow or aseptic necrosis involving the capitellum, radial head, or both. Yet some authors state that the incidence of aseptic necrosis of the radial head or capitellum or both is rare or low.

Treatment of elbow injuries when joint changes are suspected requires the taking of comparative x-ray pictures of the injured and uninjured elbows. The injured elbow should receive physical therapy consisting of local heat and massage. Physical therapy to the elbow in a whirlpool bath is also beneficial. Injections of a combined corticosteroid and local anesthesia should be tried for points of tenderness. Intra-articular injections may also be given when indicated, and certainly should be tried before surgery is contemplated. However, the benefits must be weighed against the risk of joint destruction, which may follow intra-articular corticosteroid injections. This has been aptly termed "steroid-induced arthropathy." Surgical removal of an isolated but symptomatic spur, exostosis, or ossicle may have a favorable prognosis. However, when surgical removal of loose bodies is performed because they cause the elbow joint to lock, the prognosis for the resumption of a pitching career is uncertain. Treatment of olecranon fractures is well documented in other texts.

Another type of Little Leaguer's elbow has been described for some young pitchers who develop pain, tenderness, and swelling in the medial epicondylar area following maximal pitching effort in Little and Pony League baseball. These clinical findings stem from an avulsion fracture of the epiphysis of the medial epicondyle, which occurs as a result of an extremely vigorous contraction of the flexor-pronator muscles. This produces forearm pronation and wrist and finger flexion to propel the ball on its way to the batter. The epiphysis and attached muscles are displaced downward, away from their normal anatomic site in various degrees of displacement. Inadequate preliminary warm-up, inexperience, and a poorly coordinated pitch may contribute to the incience of this injury.

In elbow injuries of children in which a fracture or dislocation is suspected but not obvious clinically, comparative x-ray pictures are taken of both the injured and uninjured elbow. Special care must be exercised by the attending physician in the interpretation of adolescent elbow radiographs because of age-related normal variants of the ossification patterns of epiphyses in children. A definite separation and wide displacement of the epiphysis of the medial epicondyle is best treated with open operation and internal fixation followed by application of a padded long arm cast with the elbow positioned at a right angle. If the epicondylar fragment with its attached muscles can be replaced and reattached satisfactorily by a heavy suture material, this should be done. If the reduction cannot be maintained by a suture material, it should be fixed with a Kirschner wire, which is incorporated into a padded cast with the elbow held at a right angle. This cast is worn for about 1 month. If the postoperative course has progressed satisfactorily clinically and radiographically, the arm is placed in a sling with resumption of graded activity for approximately 2 more weeks. Active elbow motion is encouraged. Passive elbow motion should be avoided. In some cases the player is also advised to take up another sport.

A slight separation of the epiphysis can be adequately treated by resting the arm in a posterior padded splint for 3 weeks. Preliminary cold packs and elastic compression bandaging are started and continued for 48 hours to check the swelling. The elastic compression bandage is removed after all swelling has ceased, but the arm is maintained in the splint with the elbow positioned at a right angle. Graded activity of the muscles and elbow joint is started when all acute pain, tenderness, and painful motion have disappeared. These active exercises and joint motions are continued progressively until full return of joint mobility and muscle power have been obtained. These athletes are also directed to take up another sport.

Pitchers subject muscles about the elbow to a tremendous strain which causes them to develop a painful localized condition of "tendinomyositis." The flexor-pronator group of muscles that arise from the medial epicondyle are most commonly injured. However, injuries of muscles that arise from the lateral epicondyle have also been described.

It is not unusual for a young pitcher to develop an acute episode of tendinomyositis, which may cause these muscles to go into spasm from fatigue or other reasons after a number of innings of pitching. The player is unable to extend the elbow completely because this tightened muscle spans the elbow joint. With early adequate ice therapy, light massage, and rest, this spasm may disappear in 24 to 48 hours.

If the pain, spasm and restricted and painful elbow motion persist, additional treatment with a synchronized sound-stimulator unit can be used to relieve pain and spasm and restore motion. If pain is significantly disturbing to the adult athlete, analgesics and muscle relaxants may be used beneficially provided that sound clinical judgment determines their need.

The use of anesthetic injections locally with or without the combined use of a corticosteroid is an important therapeutic tool in the management and treatment of such clinical conditions. Injections should be reserved for chronic, protracted, and recurrent cases that do not respond to rest and physical therapy. When I (M. N.) decide to inject a painful, tender tendinomyositis, I employ a long-acting corticosteroid. I inject 1 to 1.5 ml accurately into the tender site under aseptic conditions, but not into the joint, using a disposable syringe with a 22-gauge, 1½-inch needle. A maximum of three injections are given, spaced about 7 to 10 days apart. Each injection is followed by cryotherapy for 24 hours. If relief is forthcoming, it usually occurs by the third injection. If not, do not inject again.

Rest is also important in the treatment of these injuries. The amount of rest depends on the extent of the injury and its progress with treatment. Slings, padded-molded-posterior plaster splints and padded long-arm casts are used. In all of these, the elbow is held at a right angle. At first I use a sling to provide rest, but if the elbow does not improve within a week, I switch over to a padded long-arm cast with the elbow and wrist immobilized and the fingers free. I believe in resting an elbow in a cast before I entertain the use of injections. There is no one best way to treat these conditions; only the doctor's experience, skill, and success determine how he manages and treats these difficult and at times chronic injuries.

Hand, Wrist, and Finger Injuries

There are more than 20 joints in the wrist, hand, and fingers, which are formed by 28 bones bound together by a complicated system of ligaments, strengthened at points by insertions of tendons. These small and closely fitted joints are moved by 33 muscles, most of which originate at the elbow and forearm and insert as long slender tendons near the joints they move. These muscles offer no protective padding to direct injury of these parts. These moving parts have snugly fitted surfaces with little tolerance for any derangement and anything altering the shape of the joint surfaces or the consistency of the soft parts limits motion.

Because these parts are complex, exposed, and vulnerable to injury, and considering their importance to an athlete in athletics and his social and economic well being, practical prophylactic measures must be taken to prevent injuries and reduce the severity of those that do occur. The incidence of injuries is materially reduced if a protective wrapping is used, similar to the bandages used by boxers for their hands and wrists. Such a wrapping adds extra padding to the thinly-

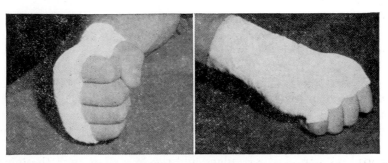

Fig. 9-16. Protective wrapping for the hand and wrist of boxers. (Novich, M.M.: Prevention and treatment of athletic injuries. Merck Report, *65*:15, 1956.)

muscled metacarpals and strength to the ligaments. As a result, the likelihood of contusions, fractures, sprains and dislocations is reduced. In the event of fractures or dislocations, serious displacement of bone ends usually does not occur. Consequently, with the anxiety of injuring the hands reduced, the athlete uses them more efficiently for both offense and defense. This is especially true for football linemen as well as boxers (Fig. 9-16). The use of commercial forearm and hand pads prevents a multitude of minor contusions, abrasions, and bruising of the forearm, wrists, and hands.

First-Aid Measures (First 24 Hours). *Step 1.* As with other injuries, the trainer takes a complete history, placing special emphasis on the mechanism of the injury. Was the hand stepped on? Was it contused or squeezed? Was the part pulled, bent, or twisted? What was the position of the part at the time of injury? The trainer also makes a careful examination of the injured part or parts, looking for swelling and deformities. He gently palpates these areas for tenderness and swelling. He gently tests for range of motion, immediately stopping if the pain is great with any attempted motion.

Step 2. If the trainer feels reasonably certain that there are no fractures or dislocations, he renders first-aid care similar to that for other injured joints, the emphasis being directed to checking the hemorrhage and extravasation of traumatic exudates into tissues by ice water or ice packs and compression bandaging where feasible. This is extremely important in preventing stiffness and fibrosis of joints, which occur rapidly if the movable parts remain bathed in serofibrinous exudate. If the pain, tenderness, swelling, and joint restriction are greater than dull or annoying, he refers the athlete to the team physician with instructions to see him before going to bed. If the trainer suspects a fracture or dislocation, he immediately puts in a call to the attending physician for further instructions. The physician will decide whether an x-ray picture is indicated. The trainer notes all his observations in a permanent training-room record.

Definitive Treatment (Follow-Up Care). *Contusions.* Contusions are common everyday occurrences in most sports, many of which are trivial and ignored. Fewer would result if wraps and flexible pads were used more commonly. Such protection is especially necessary for those athletes who must use the hands aggressively in both offensive and defensive play in body contact sports. If the injury is serious enough to produce pain, swelling, tenderness, and marked restriction of wrist, hand, or finger motion, the athlete should consult the trainer or doctor. The trainer immerses the injured part in ice water or applies ice packs for 30 minutes. After thorough drying, the injured part is splinted and wrapped with an elastic bandage and put in a sling, with the injured part positioned higher than the elbow. If the wrist, hand or several of the fingers have been moderately contused, splinting of these parts for 24 to 48 hours with an appropriately sized padded plaster splint secured with an elastic bandage is recommended. The hand and forearm are placed in a sling with the hand positioned higher than the elbow, which helps to relieve painful motion and limit swelling. During sleep the hand and forearm should be placed on a sloping bed of pillows.

The use of whirlpool or moist hot packs, massage and exercises for these injured joints 48 hours following injury is suggested. Pain, tenderness, and swelling have lessened by this time, and these modalities aid in the absorption of traumatic exudates. Early physical therapy and especially joint mobilization reduce the likelihood of fibrosis, adhesions and stiffness in the wrist, hands and fingers. Squeezing a rubber sponge in lukewarm water is an efficient and inexpensive method to aid maximal restoration of wrist, hand and finger function.

Sprains. Sprains of the fingers and thumbs commonly occur in athletics when fingers are bent or twisted beyond their normal range of motion or are jammed by an external force. They are usually accompanied by pain, swelling, and restricted, painful motion commensurate with the injury, which may require x-ray films to rule out fractures. An important component in finger sprains is partial or complete rupture of the collateral ligament or capsule of these small joints leading to instability and/or capsulitis, which may persist for months and lead to permanent limitation of motion. These must be protected and treated by a physician familiar with these injuries. Stress testing of the collateral ligament will confirm the diagnosis. Therapy is started to limit the swelling by immersing the hand in ice water. After thorough drying either adhesive tape or a metal finger splint, such as aluminum with foam rubber padding, is applied, depending on the extent of the injury. If adhesive tape is used, the finger (or fingers) is immobilized in 20° to 30° flexion by taping it to the neighboring finger. The mobile, uninjured finger allows use of the injured finger, but at the same time protects it. If a thumb has been jammed or sprained at the metacarpalphalangeal joint, it is splinted to the hand and wrist by a figure-eight adhesive tape or bandage application. It is best not to splint fingers in extension if more than one joint is involved. Splinting is discontinued after local tenderness and painful motion have subsided, and is followed by whirlpool, massage and active exercises. Protective strapping of the finger or thumb should be continued when the athlete returns to competition to prevent re-injury.

PROTECTIVE SPLINTING FOR FINGER SPRAINS. For mild to moderate sprains of finger joints, the injured finger can be splinted to its neighboring finger with three pieces of ½-inch adhesive tape, which is kept on for several days. Athletes may continue to compete with this dress-

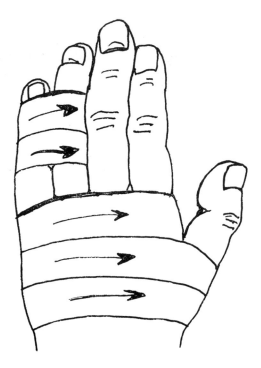

Fig. 9-17. Splinting for moderate sprain of the finger. The injured finger is taped to the neighboring finger. Taping of the hand is optional.

ing with some guarding of the finger. The splint is kept on until all local tenderness and painful motion have disappeared (Fig. 9–17).

For severe sprains, more rigid fixation is necessary, and metal splints such as aluminum with foam rubber padding are popular provided no fractures were present. The metal splint is bent slightly to allow positioning of the finger in 20° to 30° flexion. The finger is secured to the splint with several strips of ½-inch adhesive tape and kept on for 7 to 10 days. No participation is allowed during this phase of treatment.

SPRAINED (JAMMED) THUMB. Most physicians fail to diagnose the area of the thumb that is painful. Is it a dorsal or volar sprain? Does it hurt in abduction or adduction? Fractures, dislocations, and especially collateral-ligament injuries of the thumb are frequent and should not be overlooked. Stress x-ray films are useful for diagnosing ligament injuries.

PROTECTIVE STRAPPING FOR A SPRAINED (JAMMED) THUMB. An underwrap or skin protectant is first applied to the thumb and wrist. The idea is to tape the thumb to prevent painful motion. A 1-inch adhesive tape strapping is applied as a figure-eight spica of the thumb and wrist— these parts are held in a position of function (Fig. 9-18). This dressing

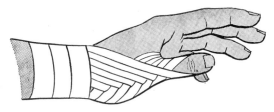

Fig. 9-18. Strapping for a sprained thumb.

prevents extremes of abduction and extension of the thumb. Such protection is continued until tenderness has been eliminated and normal, pain-free motion has returned. Fractures and dislocations of these parts are frequent and should not be overlooked.

Tendon Injury. Although "baseball fingers" are most commonly seen in baseball players, especially catchers, this injury occurs not infrequently in other sports. The most common mechanism of injury is when the tip of any finger is struck a direct blow, causing a forced flexion of the distal phalanx of the finger while the tendon is actively contracted. This produces an avulsion or disinsertion of the extensor tendon with or without an attached fragment of bone from its insertion in the base of the terminal phalanx. A deformity of the distal phalanx at the distal interphalangeal joint results, described as a "drop finger." The same injury may also result when the extensor tendon has been contused sufficiently. The athlete complains of local pain, tenderness, and inability to actively extend the terminal phalanx.

Fresh ruptures can be treated adequately by the application of a volar or dorsal metal splint with the distal interphalangeal joint in slight hyperextension. X-ray films are taken before and after the application of the immobilization, which is maintained for 6 to 8 weeks. For successful reattachment of the tendon, treatment must be started within 7 to 10 days. Surgical procedures do not produce sufficient relief from the deformity and disability to warrant their frequent use. In reliable athletes, the position of slight hyperextension is maintained with an intramedullary pin across the (D.I.P.) joint.

CUT OR LACERATED FINGER OR TORN FINGERNAIL. For emergency care, medicated cream is put on the cut. A finger cap made commercially or made with 1½- to 2-inch adhesive tape 5 to 6 inches in length is placed on the cut. In order to make a finger cap, the tape is twisted around the distal phalanx of the finger with ½-inch tape on and off finger. The open end is molded and trimmed in the shape of the finger.

Wrist Sprains. The wrist is frequently sprained when it is accidentally put through a range of motion greater than that which is normal. This may occur from a multitude of events, resulting in stretched or sprained radial or ulnar collateral, volar, dorsocarpal, and distal radioulnar ligaments. The intensity of the pain, tenderness, swelling, and joint restriction varies with the severity of trauma. Those cases that are mild respond quickly with early application of cold compresses or ice water for about ½ hour, followed by splinting with elastic bandages or adhesive tape. A padded, molded, removable metal or plastic splint may also be used. The wrist is placed in a functional position of extension (dorsiflexion) of 15°. The splint is secured to the wrist with an elastic bandage with fingers left free to move. Heat, massage, and exercises to the wrist begin the day following the injury. A protective strapping of three overlapping strips of 1½-inch tape is placed about the wrist daily following treatment, and also to prevent re-injury when the athlete returns to competition. The attending physician examines the wrist daily to determine its progress and when the athlete may resume play.

If the wrist does not respond to such treatment or if there is point tenderness, x-ray films should be taken to determine the presence of any bony or periosteal pathology. The application of a padded plaster cast with the wrist extended (dorsiflexed) 15° (position of function) for 10 to 14 days or longer gives a moderately or severely sprained wrist the complete immobilization so necessary to achieve maximal restoration. The fingers are left free to move. A word of caution: the wrist that remains "sprained" should make the doctor suspect a fracture of the carpal navicular, and requires follow-up x-ray examinations of the wrist from multiple views. Early diagnosis can be aided by bone scan in difficult cases.

After removal of the cast, whirlpool, massage, and exercises are necessary to aid in the absorption of traumatic exudates. Early joint mobility reduces the likelihood of fibrosis, adhesions and stiffness in the wrist. Exercises facilitate restoration of normal muscle strength. Athletic participation may be resumed when the wrist is neither tender nor painful upon effort and has a normal range of motion and muscle strength. Protective strapping and appropriate padding of the wrist and forearm are indicated to prevent reinjury.

MUSCLE INJURY

The second largest category of athletic injuries involves the muscles and tendons and infrequently the fascial covering of some muscles. Muscle injuries predominate in this category and result from strains and contusions. Frequently, muscles may become disabled by going into painful spasm or cramp for a variety of reasons.

A muscle strain can occur at any point from its origin to insertion: tendon, musculotendinous junction, or muscle belly. Sometimes they are referred to as a pulled muscle or tendon depending on the site. Fascial tears with muscle herniation are almost clinically indistinguishable from muscle tears. The severity of the injury ranges from a tear of a few or many fibers as a result of overstretching to a complete rupture of the muscle or tendon.

For the purposes of our discussion, it is sufficient to know that these injuries result when the tensile strength of the muscle or tendon fibers is exceeded by the forces to which these tissues are subjected. Strains can result after a vigorous contraction against resistance, as is frequently seen in back injuries of weight lifters following a lifting incident. In tendons, excessive force can cause overstretching and even rupture of a tendon at or near a point of maximal length, as is seen in a skier who falls forward without release of his bindings and can severely stretch or even rupture his Achilles tendon. This is also seen in football and basketball players. Conditions predisposing to both muscle and tendon injuries are insufficient conditioning, myostatic contractures, limited joint function, incoordination between opposing muscle groups, fatigue, improper warm-up, lack of skill, and pre-existing degenerative changes in the muscle and tendon.

These injuries are usually sudden, painful, and immediately disabling. However, pain and disability may develop later. The nature and extent of disability depends on the location and the number of muscle and tendon fibers, and blood vessels ruptured at the site of the injury. Tenderness, swelling and ecchymosis are the most frequent signs of these injuries. The athlete may hear a sharp snap or tear emanating from the injured tissue at the time of the injury. Testing the strength of a single muscle group against resistance aids in localizing the injury.

Muscle strains occur at many anatomic sites. Some strains are characteristic of specific sports; others may occur in several types of athletic activity. No athlete is immune from strains, regardless of his sport. The preponderance of injuries are minor muscle strains that heal in 1 to 7 days, depending on the extent of the injury. Only the more frequent muscle strains and pulled tendons are discussed here.

Muscle Strains and Pulled Tendons

In muscle strains, the torn muscle fibers and their blood vessels hemorrhage, resulting in swelling, ecchymosis, and restricted function. In order to prevent the formation of excessive restrictive fibrous scarring when these torn muscles heal, hemorrhage and swelling must be immediately checked with cold applications for no less than 30 minutes and preferably longer, compression bandaging, and elevation where possible. These techniques should be continued at home. Slings, splints, crutches and other supportive measures should be used to rest or limit activity of the injured part when indicated. Analgesic and anti-inflammatory medication should also be used.

Following these first-aid measures, healing of the injured muscle by the formation of a strong mobile scar is hastened with heat, massage, and gentle exercises if swelling has stopped. Activity is graded until the scar in the muscle is more mature. After the injured muscle has developed maximal flexibility and strength, the athlete is then fit to return to his sport. A protective strapping may be used to prevent reinjury. Premature return to sports can result in reinjury and a chronic problem.

Trapezius Muscle. This is a superficial, large, trapezoidal muscle located on the back of the neck, shoulders, and upper back; it is easily palpated. It has widespread origins from the occiput, ligamentum nuchae, and spinous processes of C7 to D12 and insertions into the

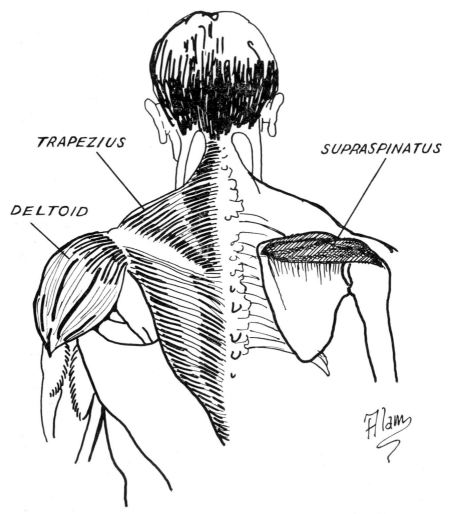

Fig. 9-19.   Muscles of the upper back and shoulder that are involved in athletic injuries.

clavicle, acromion, and spine of the scapula (Fig. 9-19). Because of its location, the trapezius is intimately associated with movements of the head, neck, shoulder girdle, and arm. Strains of the trapezius occur most frequently in football, wrestling, and gymnastics. In football, the trapezius muscle may become strained as a result of being suddenly stretched while in a contracted state in a variety of situations. In wrestling, it may result from attempting to break a securely held head-hold. The trapezius may also be strained as a result of a gymnast not flexing his head and neck properly in a forward roll. Tears of this muscle most frequently occur at the angle of the neck and at the clavicular attachments. In boxing, the trapezius may be severely strained when a powerful punch is thrown and misses its target. In this case, the whole muscle may be torn off the spine of the scapula, with severe bleeding.

Pain, tenderness, and swelling at the site of the injury usually depend on the extent of the trauma. Frequently, this muscle goes into spasm following injury, causing a kink in the neck, a stiff neck, and even an inability to move the injured shoulder and the upper extremity on the same side. Testing neck movements as well as the different portions of the trapezius muscle against resistance aids in localizing the injury.

Severe strain with marked bleeding requires the immediate application of cold compresses, compression dressings and rest in a sling to stop the hemorrhage. This treatment may be combined with an adhesive strapping (Fig. 9-20) and a sling applied between treatments if the shoulder sags on the injured side. Analgesic and anti-inflammatory medication may be given. If swelling is anticipated, cold compresses are continued. If not, cold compresses are replaced by heat application and followed by massage and exercise. The exercise program is graded progressively until normal strength and flexibility are obtained. The

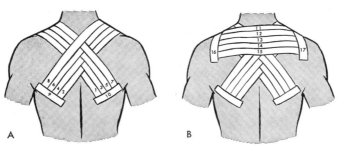

A   B

Fig. 9-20. Method of strapping for trapezius strain. *A*, The diagonal strips help to immobilize the upper back and are applied from the bottom of the shoulder blades to the top of the opposite shoulder. *B*, The horizontal strips help to anchor the diagonal strips and provide further immobilization.

sling and adhesive strappings are discarded when the shoulder can be supported normally without discomfort.

Rotator Cuff Muscles. The subscapularis, teres minor, infraspinatus and supraspinatus muscles are collectively called the "rotator cuff" and envelop the humeral head at their insertions into the humerus. In addition to activating rotation and abduction movements of the shoulder, these muscles also impart strength and stability to the relatively unstable shoulder joint. This effect is accomplished by making the joint snug when these muscles are contracted. These muscles are most frequently strained near their bony insertions into the humerus as a result of a violent contraction of any or all the muscular components during weightlifting or when an athlete falls on an arm or outstretched hand. Football players and baseball pitchers may incur this injury as a result of throwing a football or baseball. Although any of the rotator cuff muscles may tear, the supraspinatus muscle is most frequently injured.

Supraspinatus Muscle. In addition to the acute pain and tenderness usually localized to the part of the cuff that is injured, active motion of the shoulder is restricted. Testing abduction of the shoulder against resistance causes increased pain and the arm falls limp to the side.

The immediate first aid is to apply cold compresses to the injured muscle. Rest and support of the injured muscle can be accomplished by an adhesive strapping (Fig. 9-21) and a sling. The following day cold packs, massage, and gentle exercises are started and then the adhesive strapping and sling are replaced. The supportive strapping and sling can be reapplied daily when rest and restricted activity of the injured muscle and upper extremity are necessary. This regimen is continued until acute symptoms subside. Then heat, massage, and a graded exercise program are started. We use the pendulum exercise holding a 1-pound weight (Fig. 9-22) because it is easy to understand and do, and it provides an objective measure of improvement. Following a pendulum exercise routine, active assistive exercises using a towel and

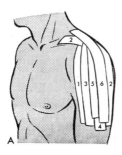 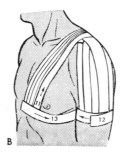

Fig. 9-21. Method of strapping for strain of the supraspinatus muscles. *A,* Tape is applied upward toward the shoulder under firm tension. *B,* Tape is applied from the chest toward the middle of the back. Arm anchor (12) should be applied so that it does not restrict the circulation of the arm.

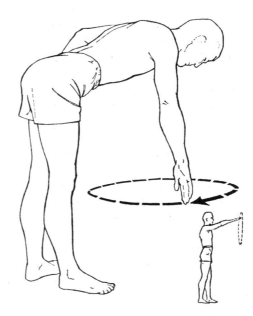

Fig. 9-22. Pendulum exer-
cise routine.

broomstick are recommended. Isometrics and strengthening exercises
are later instituted for total rehabilitation of the shoulder. Disability
varies from a few days to a few weeks, depending on the sport. An
x-ray study of the shoulder is indicated if any bony or periosteal
pathology is suspected. Surgical repair is necessary if a complete disruption of the rotator cuff is present.

Deltoid Muscle. This large, triangular, and superficially placed
muscle fits over the shoulder joint (except for the axillary region) like
the cap of a sleeve. It has a widespread origin from the clavicle, acromion, and scapular spine and inserts into the deltoid tuberosity of the
humerus. Because this muscle consists of anterior, middle, and posterior parts, it can raise the arm at the shoulder in forward, sideward,
and backward directions respectively. The anterior part is most frequently strained, especially in foobtall, when an arm tackle fails to
bring the runner down but the force of the speeding runner succeeds
in stretching the deltoid muscle without levering the head of the humerus out of the shoulder joint. The middle and posterior deltoid may
be strained in any sport following movements of the arm against resistance in the lateral and posterior directions respectively.

Pain, tenderness, swelling, and localization of the pain by the athlete
as well as testing active motion of the arm against resistance help to
make the diagnosis. The first aid is the same regardless of which part
of the deltoid is injured. Cold applications and adhesive strapping support similar to that used for supraspinatus strains may be used with a

sling if immobilization is necessary for 24 hours or longer. The exercise program is similar to that described for supraspinatus strain.

Intercostal Muscles. Each side of the rib cage is enclosed by a thin, two-layered sheath of 11 adjacent internal and external intercostal muscles that occupy the entire length of the intercostal spaces. Their primary function is to aid in respiration. These muscles lift the ribs during inspiration and may contract during voluntary expiratory efforts. Violent and repeated coughing can cause strain in these muscles.

This muscle injury may be so excruciatingly painful that the athlete restricts his breathing and takes shallow breaths to ease the pain brought on by regular respiratory excursion. At times, an actual tearing can be felt and the athlete may be rendered immobile, afraid to move his trunk or arm because of the pain. Point tenderness is usually present and perhaps even some swelling.

The best treatment is immediate application of an adhesive strapping of the injured part, extending from just beyond the midline in front or from just beyond midline in the back to support the chest and limit the chest excursion (Fig. 9-23). This gives the injured muscle a chance to heal. Cold compresses may be applied to the injured site of the chest muscle for 30 minutes or more; these may be continued at home. The tape should not be removed for 3 to 7 days. The strapping should be reinforced if it starts to pull away at the edges, and may be removed when acute symptoms have subsided. Following removal, moist hot packs, massage, and breathing exercises can be started. The use of a rib cage protector may prove beneficial following removal of the tape. Pulmonary problems such as pneumonia may complicate these injuries.

If a rib fracture is suspected, an x-ray picture should be taken of the rib cage. If the x-ray pictures do not show a fracture, a follow-up x-ray

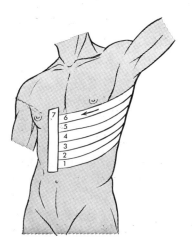

Fig. 9-23. Method of taping for rib strain. The tapes begin and end beyond the midline on the unaffected side to immobilize the injured ribs. An anchor strip, like no. 7, is also placed on the back.

study should be done in 10 days if the pain in the chest continues. It is not unusual for follow-up x-ray pictures to reveal a rib fracture that was not present on the original study.

Tennis Elbow. This condition is most frequently seen in tennis players, but is not confined to them. There is no unanimity among authors as to its pathology; it has been variously described as a radiohumeral bursitis, radiohumeral synovitis, epicondylitis and epicondylalgia. This ambiguous pathologic condition may account for a group of clinical conditions that occur about the lateral aspect of the elbow, having a similar onset, symptoms, and signs. In more experienced players, the pain can be felt on the medial side as well. Such conditions have been noted in golfers, fishermen, handball, racquetball, paddleball, badminton, and squash players, pitchers, and others. There is, however, agreement that these ailments stem from the repeated demands of these sports on the elbow, by which it is subjected to sudden, changing, forcible and, at times, unnatural motions. The experts agree that beginner's backhand frequently causes lateral epicondylitis, whereas the advanced player's extremely hard serve can cause medial epicondylitis. Players who use the two-handed backhand develop fewer elbow problems from tennis.

We treat the "tennis elbow" as a localized condition of tendinomyositis of the supinator-extensor group of muscles that arise from the lateral epicondyle of the humerus. We believe this condition occurs in tennis players not only from repeated forceful pronation and supination of the forearm with an extended elbow but also represents the sum of microtraumatic injuries (strains) resulting from the complicated biomechanics of gripping a tennis racket, carrying out the stroke, and striking the tennis ball. Not only is it important to put the ball over the net, but it must also be hit to a particular portion of the court, frequently with enough speed and spin to make it difficult, and at best, impossible to return. The racket must properly fit the player's hand in order to strike the ball properly. The proper grip size of a tennis racket will help prevent twisting or knocking the racket out of the hand by the impact of the ball. The best grip is accomplished by a synergistic contraction of the forearm muscles, with the wrist held locked in slight extension and ulnar deviation; this places an additional load on the extensor group of forearm muscles and increases the exposure to trauma. The limb velocity of the stroke, the rotary movements of the forearm during a stroke motion, and the speed of the approaching ball determine the strains and shocks to which the forearm muscles are subjected, both in their bodies and at their condylar origins. The wrist and elbow joints also share in this trauma, but fortunately are only rarely injured.

Development of the "tennis elbow" is one of the hazards of playing tennis regularly. Faulty stroke mechanics hasten the development of tennis elbow. A spin serve accomplished by wrist flexion and ulnar or radial deviation causes additional tension and strains of the extensor muscle group. The forehand and especially backhand strokes, when converted into forearm pronation and supination respectively during the follow-through to produce spin on the ball, are also conducive to this tennis condition. In the forehand stroke, the elbow ends slightly bent, and in the backhand, the elbow ends extended. Chop or slice strokes, especially backhand slices, place even greater stress on the forearm muscles. In a well-executed stroke, there is only a minimum of movement at the elbow and wrist. The wrist should be fixed in slight extension and in slight ulnar deviation at impact.

Clinically, the athlete complains most commonly of pain on or about the lateral epicondyle and in the body of the extensor muscle. The pain may be dull or sharp. Tenderness is usually present about the conjoined tendon of the muscle, and tender areas may also be noted in other muscles about the elbow. The pain in increased by activity and lessened by rest and restricted activity. Pain and weakness radiating down the forearm are commonly experienced when lifting objects with the forearm in pronation and the elbow fully or partially extended. Pain is usually absent when lifting in supination. Testing a dorsiflexed wrist against resistance usually causes pain at the condylar origin of the muscle or in the body itself. Gripping with the forearm pronated causes pain, as when turning a door knob by pronating the hand and opening the door against resistance (door-knob test).

The conservative treatment that was recommended for the tendino-myositis of the muscle arising from the medial epicondyle for baseball pitchers is also indicated for tennis elbow. A counterforce forearm brace is frequently helpful.

Fortunately, prophylactic measures can be taken to prevent these injuries and avoid recurrences. The player must pay proper attention to the selection of a proper racquet and handle size, racquet flexibility and weight, and string tension. The arm and forearm muscles must be exercised to obtain maximal flexibility and strength. In the arm, the brachialis, brachioradialis, and triceps muscles participate more significantly than the biceps. In the forearm, the supinator-extensor muscles and especially the extensor carpi radialis work harder than the pronator-flexor muscles. All of these exercises to develop flexibility and strength are equally useful in handball, paddleball, racquetball, and squash. Proper stroke mechanics are essential. Play should cease when fatigue, improper warm-up, illness, or tension states increase the risk of injury. Warm-up with stretching and flexibility exercises prior to practice or competition reduces the incidence and extent of sprains and strains of the musculoskeletal system.

Low Back. The lumbar paraspinal muscles are located in the lumbar area of the back. They comprise the large muscle mass located between the spinous and transverse processes of the vertebrae, which even extend beyond the transverse process to cover partly the posterior portion of the thorax. These paraspinal muscles are concerned with extension, lateral bending and rotation of the trunk. They are frequently strained in weight lifting, as well as other sports, usually from a lifting incident in which a powerful contraction of these muscles is made against resistance. Movement of the back may or may not accompany this muscular effort. Pain and disability may be felt immediately upon straining, sometimes accompanied by snapping, popping or tearing sounds emanating from the back. However, in many instances the symptoms and abnormal physical findings present themselves the following day or even later. Usually, the pain is localized to one side of the back, and tenderness is felt at the site of the injury. Swelling is not uncommon in most low back strains. The appearance of painful muscle spasm splints the back, adding to the athlete's discomfort and requiring the use of muscle relaxants. Frequently, low back strains are complicated by intervertebral joint sprains.

When a low back has been strained sufficiently to produce pain and disability, I (M. N.) apply adhesive tape strapping to the low back (Fig. 9-24) if I see the athlete soon after the injury. Bed rest for 48 to 72 hours or longer is mandatory, depending on the severity of the injury. Bed rest is best accomplished in a hospital with a board under a firm mattress. However, this may be impractical, so conscientious bed rest on a firm mattress at home and bathroom privileges only are acceptable. Analgesics and muscle relaxants must be prescribed. After the acute symptomatology has lessened, the tape is removed and heat, massage and gentle back exercises may be started. Electrical stimula-

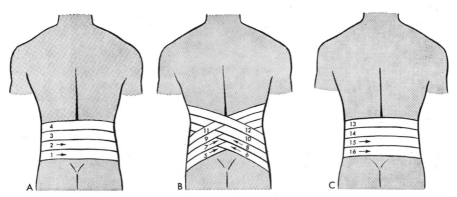

Fig. 9-24.   Taping for low back strain. This method consists of three layers of tape, each shown separately.

tion of muscles combined with ultrasound may be used if pain or muscle spasm does not lessen with hand massage. This apparatus works well with trigger points and painful muscle spasm in the low back. When the athlete has regained a full range of back mobility and muscle strength, he is ready to return to the game.

Groin. The adductor group of muscles located on the medial aspect of the thigh and the iliopsoas muscles account for the bulk of groin strains that occur in athletics. The following muscles comprise the adductor group: adductor magnus, adductor longus, gracilis, adductor brevis, and pectineus. Because of their origin from either the pubic or ischial rami and their insertion into the femoral shaft, their principal action is to adduct the thigh and hip; however, these muscles perform additional movements, depending on the degree of hip flexion. For example, the adductor magnus muscle is able to inwardly rotate the hip. This is used in such actions as "stemming" in skiing and gripping the sides of a horse while riding.

The iliopsoas muscle is comprised of the psoas major and the iliacus muscles. These muscles have separate origins but a common insertion. The psoas muscle arises from the anterior surfaces of the transverse processes, the sides of the vertebral bodies and the corresponding intervertebral discs from T12 to L5. This muscle runs distally in the posterior wall of the abdomen to the iliac fossa, where it joins the iliacus muscle that arises here. Together they insert into the lesser trochanter of the femur, acting as flexors and internal rotators of the hip joint. Acting alone, the psoas major can flex and laterally bend the lumbar spine.

Although pulled groin muscles occur most frequently in running sports, they do occur in other sports. These muscles are strained either as a result of stretching a contracted muscle or an over-contraction mechanism. In horse riders who become unbalanced, these muscles become strained in the process of overcontracting to maintain equilibrium. Gymnasts who land heavily on parallel bars in a straddle position often strain the adductors.

The weather plays a decided influence in the incidence of these injuries. In rainy weather, hyperabduction and hyperextension movements of the hip because of slippery footing result in groin pulls. When an athlete is insufficiently warmed-up in cold weather, a quick change in direction, such as a lineman pulling out, results in similar hip movements and groin injuries. Characteristically, this injury is seen early in football practice and in early basketball season. Fatigue, poor posture, uneven muscle strength, poor flexibility, and overstretching are the primary causes leading to such strains.

Most athletes find this injury disturbing because of its location and interference with mobility. The presenting complaint may be pain or

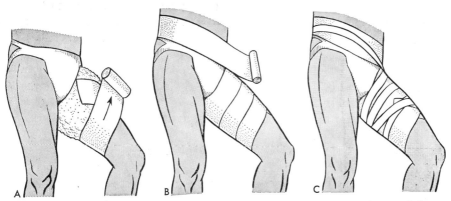

Fig. 9-25.   Bandaging strained muscles in the groin area. *A*, Standing with leg flexed and turned outward, cover the groin area with a padding made from a combine roll. Apply a 6-inch elastic bandage with pressure. *B*, Continue with elastic bandage, wrapping it once around the waist. *C*, Apply adhesive tape.

tightness in the groin. Usually the injury can be localized by palpating the point of maximal tenderness. With the athlete in a supine position, testing the hip against resistance primarily in flexion and adduction helps localize the injured muscle because of increased pain and weakness. The hip is also tested in abduction and extension to determine the status of the muscles concerned with those movements. A complete tear of the origin of one of the adductor muscles can produce a painful lump in the groin which should not be confused with an inguinal hernia.

Treatment is started to check hematoma by use of ice therapy and the application of a single hip spica compression bandage with the hip in 10 to 15° flexion (Fig. 9-25). Bed rest and limitation of activity until all bleeding has ceased is mandatory. The use of moist hot packs or whirlpool may be started on the second or third day provided this does not start the bleeding again. When the symptoms subside, the athlete may be allowed to resume activities gradually.

The activity of the athlete is determined by his response to treatment. His progress should be evaluated daily. The supportive groin bandaging enables the athlete to move about and even run without pain. It prevents further tearing of the injured groin muscles, and should be continued until the athlete has achieved the maximal benefits from treatment.

If an avulsion fracture of the lesser trochanteric or any other sites of muscle attachments to bone in the groin region are suspected, x-ray studies should be made.

Quadriceps. This muscle has already been adequately described (see p. 173). Because of its function and location it is easily strained

9

in sprinters and hurdlers. However, this injury is not confined to track and field athletes, but may be experienced in all sports when a violent contraction or injurious stretch of this muscle occurs during an athletic activity.

Although pain usually depends on the severity of the injury, in general, quadriceps pulls are not as painful as hamstring pulls. The initial step is to control the bleeding with ice therapy and a compression wrap.

For functional testing of the injured quadriceps, and treatment, including the supportive strapping, see "Charley Horse," page 251.

Hamstring. This is a powerful group of three posterior femoral muscles located on the lateral, posterior, and medial aspects of the thigh. They arise from the ischial tuberosity and insert on the lateral and medial aspects of the lower leg. One of these muscles is the biceps femoris, also known as the lateral hamstring. This is made up of two parts: a long head that arises from the ischial tuberosity, which is joined by a short head that stems from the back of the femur. Together the two heads combine and insert into the head of the fibula and lateral condyle of the tibia. The medial hamstring consists of the semitendinosus muscle, which also arises from the ischial tuberosity and inserts on the medial aspect of the tibia near the knee joint. The semimembranosus is the other muscle of the medial hamstring group, which also arises from the ischial tuberosity and inserts into the medial condyle of the tibia. These muscles act as powerful flexors and rotators of the knee; they can also act as hip extensors.

Hamstring pulls are most commonly seen in any of the running sports, especially in track and field competition. Sprinters who uncoil off their starting blocks with maximal effort may pull up lame as a result of a pulled hamstring. This injury may also occur when a runner makes a determined effort to overtake a competitor. Thus, these muscle pulls are appropriately called "sprinter's strain." Swimmers also suffer from hamstring pulls, but not of the intensity experienced by trackmen. Swimmers develop their injuries as a result of a maximal push-off from their starting blocks. Unlike trackmen, football players, and others, swimmers can continue to swim because their main leg effort is powered by the quadriceps and calf muscles. In track, however, the athlete may drop to the ground because of the severity of the pain or may limp to a halt.

The injury occurs anywhere in the muscle, but most frequently it is located at or near the ischial tuberosity. In addition to the pain, swelling and ecchymosis may also appear, depending on the location and extent of the injury. Careful palpation will localize the point of greatest tenderness. The injured muscle usually goes into spasm. Contraction of the hamstring while testing for knee flexion against resistance produces pain and helps localize the site of the injury. A straight leg rais-

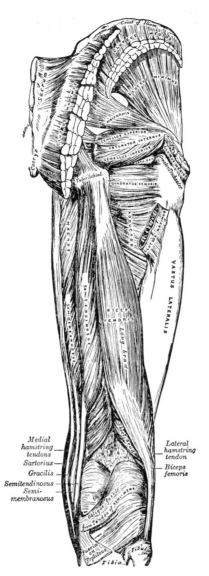

Fig. 9-26. Muscles of the gluteal and posterior femoral regions. (*In* Gray's Anatomy of the Human Body. Courtesy of Lea & Febiger.)

ing test, with the athlete in a supine position with the knee extended, also aids in determining the site and severity of the injury.

If the injury is a minor one, the use of cold compresses, compression dressings and restricted activity for 24 hours may be sufficient. This is followed by moist hot packs, hand massage, and a supportive adhesive strapping for a few days.

tendon is usually obvious clinically by a deformity in the contours of the tendon. A defect or gap between the ruptured ends may be palpated, associated with a Thompson test, which is positive when manual compresson of an injured calf does not result in ankle plantar flexion. Pain, tenderness and swelling frequently accompany this injury. Rupture is best treated in the hospital with either surgical repair or plaster cast immobilization in plantar flexion.

Foot Strain. This condition, as expected, is seen more frequently in running sports. It gives rise to essentially the same signs and symptoms of painful flatfoot. However, flatfoot and other static conditions are frequently absent. The size, shape, contours and static deformities in the feet, if present, usually have no bearing on a young athlete's performance unless the feet have been injured forcibly or gradually.

There is no unanimity concerning the pathology of this condition among physicians conversant with athletic medicine. However, most agree that this is a painful and disabling condition that requires treatment. We believe that this condition results from an overstretching of the plantar structures of the foot due to an overuse syndrome. Although the plantar and spring (plantar calcaneonavicular) ligaments may be injured, the plantar fascia bears the real brunt of this injury. These bands are overstretched either by a severe direct force or by a cumulative effect of repeated strains. Weakening of this plantar structure predisposes to the traumatic injury of these tissues. The plantar fascia is made up of spindle-shaped fibers that break like bamboo when subjected to sufficient stress. An inflammatory reaction results with hemorrhage and swelling. The ends of the torn fascial fibers curl up and become painful and tender nodules on the plantar surface of the foot which are palpable when the foot is dorsiflexed. The plantar fascia may go into spasm and stand out cord-like on the sole of the foot. There are two types of predisposing factors: (1) intrinsic, such as that caused by latent development, overweight or a malfunctional problem; (2) extrinsic and traumatic, such as that caused by improperly fitted shoes or by landing on the tarsus instead of the ball of the foot. Excessive demands made on these feet before they are conditioned to the task invariably bring on the strain syndrome.

Clinically, both feet are usually affected, but the amount of pain and discomfort may vary between feet. There are multiple areas of pain and tenderness located on the plantar surface of the foot. Ecchymosis may occasionally be present. Weight-bearing is painful and causes a limp. Stiffness of the foot may also cause a limp. The calf muscles may shorten secondarily and not infrequently develop cramps, which also occur in the foot. The painful and tender elongated fascial nodules and the spastic plantar fascia have already been described.

First-aid treatment with cold compresses locally for 30 minutes or more is started to check the swelling. If the pain is great and weight-bearing is too painful, crutches should be provided the athlete, who is given instructions not to bear weight on the injured foot. If the pain is severe, bed rest is prescribed until acute pain has subsided. Adhesive tape rest straps for the foot are recommended. The tape starts at the metatarsal phalangeal joints and is taped to the plantar surface of the foot, with the ends crossing each other over dorsum of the foot. The tape extends to the insertion of the plantar fascia into the os calcis. This can be removed daily and reapplied after whirlpool and massage. Manipulation of the foot also contributes to relief. The adhesive strapping is continued until the acute condition subsides. Some physicians and trainers use felt pads secured to the long arch; this is unnecessary once the pain has subsided and the athlete has exercised his weak and strained muscle back to normal strength and flexibility. X-ray films of the foot are taken to rule in or rule out stress fractures or other bony or periosteal disorders.

Common Muscle Contusions

These are minor injuries that are common to all sports; in training room jargon they are known as bruises. Contusions occur in all the muscles described in the section on muscle strains as well as other muscles of the body vulnerable to blows. They heal in 1 to 7 days, depending on the number of muscle fibers and blood vessels injured and the hemorrhage that ensues. Optimal healing can be achieved by minimizing hemorrhage with cold compresses and compression dressings for 24 to 48 hours. Rest and restricted activity of the injured part and elevation where feasible are also indicated. The following day, physical therapy consisting of heat, whirlpool where feasible, hand massage and gentle active exercise are started to facilitate the absorption of the traumatic exudate. Electrical muscle stimulation and ultrasound may be used with contusions of deep muscles. Muscle relaxants may be prescribed if painful muscle spasm is present. Slings, splints, crutches, appropriate protective pads, adhesive tape strapping, or elastic bandage wrappings should be used to immobilize and rest the injured part. Supportive strapping may be used to prevent re-injury.

Shoulder Pointer. This injury results from a direct blow to the top of the shoulder in the area of the acromioclavicular joint and the adjacent deltoid and trapezius muscles. It is seen mainly in football when the shoulder pad does not fit or is worn improperly. This condition may be confused with a minor acromioclavicular joint injury, but it can be distinguished from joint injury in that the pain, tenderness and swelling are noted in the lateral fibers of the deltoid and the middle fibers of the trapezius muscles, and no demonstrable laxity occurs at the acromioclavicular joint.

These injuries respond satisfactorily with ice compresses, shoulder cap adhesive strapping, and the use of a sling for a few days. Complete restoration is aided by moist hot packs, massage, and active exercises of the injured area. Re-injury can be prevented by the use of a properly fitted shoulder pad overlying a foam rubber pad taped to the injured area. The athlete should be ready to return to competition in less than a week.

Hip Pointer. This injury results from a contusion to the iliac crest and the insertions of the anterior and lateral abdominal muscles. It is seen most frequently in football following a blow to this superficial exposed area because of an improperly fitted hip pad. A hip pointer is a more painful and disabling condition to treat than a shoulder pointer because the insertions of the anterior and lateral trunk muscles are further strained with forward, lateral, and rotary trunk movements. Increased intra-abdominal pressure brought on by coughing, sneezing, or laughing also aggravates these injured muscles.

Treatment is directed to comforting the athlete and checking the swelling. The application of an adhesive tape strapping not only restricts the activity of the area, but also aids in compression. Cryotherapy is applied directly to the injured area followed by strapping. Bed rest for one to several days is certainly helpful in restricting and limiting activity. The use of analgesic and anti-inflammatory medication and injections of local anesthesia and corticosteroids are indicated depending on the severity of the injury. Heat and active exercises may be used after the acute symptoms have diminished. Whirlpool baths can also be used. However, following return to competition, the iliac crest must be protected by a sponge rubber pad and regulation hip pads that fit properly.

Low Back. Because of its incapacitating nature, contusion of the low back may cause immediate cessation of play. It is not unusual for an athlete to sink to the ground or stay on his feet with his trunk half-flexed. In both instances, the athlete usually puts his hand on his back to protect it against further injury. This type of injury usually follows a kick or hard blow to the back. In addition to the soft tissue injury, it is necessary to check out any suspected bony injury by x-ray study. Kidney involvement can be evaluated clinically and by urinalysis. Pain, tenderness, and painfully restricted trunk motion are usually present. Hematoma and ecchymosis are present if the blow is hard enough.

Because of the disabling nature of the injury, we believe in immediate bed rest that aids in reducing pain. The pressure of the back on the mattress also aids in preventing swelling. Analgesics and muscle relaxants are prescribed for painful muscle spasm, which is usually present. When pain and spasm have lessened, active exercises may be started in bed and gradually increased until maximal restoration of muscle strength and flexibility have been obtained. As soon as hemorrhage has been controlled, heat and light massage are given to the low back. The use of the whirlpool baths, electrical muscle stimulation, and ultrasound for low-back muscle injuries has been especially useful in achieving optimal results. Conscientious bed rest at home on a firm mattress and bathroom privileges are acceptable, but the athlete must be warned against abusing the privilege of not being under the direct surveillance of the medical and coaching staff while at home. However, his progress will indicate how honest he has been in following orders.

If moderate to severe back pain persists, x-rays may be necessary to rule out fractures, especially of the transverse processes.

Charley Horse. This is a common disabling condition in athletics seen predominantly in contact sports such as football, soccer, basketball, and field hockey; it usually follows a direct blow to the anterior thigh. Depending on the magnitude of the blow, this force either contuses or crushes the entire soft tissue contents of the anterior compartment of the thigh against the femur. This happens frequently in football when the front of an athlete's thigh is struck a blow by another player's head, shoulder, knee, or foot. A loose or improperly fitted thigh pad increases the likelihood of such an injury. Although the brunt of the trauma is borne by the quadriceps muscles, resulting in the rupture of a varying number of muscle fibers and their blood vessels, the subcutaneous tissue with its fraily supported fat cells and blood vessels are concomitantly traumatized as well. This adds to the hemorrhage and ecchymotic discoloration at the site of injury.

Some authors state that a "charley horse" may occur in muscles other than the quadriceps and may also follow a tear or rupture of muscle fibers as result of violent muscular contraction. Although there is no unanimity about the mechanism of injury, there is agreement on the treatment.

The quadriceps muscle, consisting of the rectus femoris, vastus intermedius, vastus lateralis, and vastus medialis, is a large fleshy muscle that covers the front of the thigh and spans the hip; it activates two joints. Because it is a hip flexor as well as a knee extensor, it is an important antigravity muscle vital to maintaining the erect position. This has been discussed earlier in this chapter (p. 173). When the muscle is contused, the severity of the condition is directly proportionate to the number of muscular fibers and blood vessels ruptured and the amount of hemorrhage and traumatic exudate that escapes. The thigh becomes swollen, painful, and diffusely tender. Limping is an expected sign, and running is not attempted.

The hemorrhagic exudate in the thigh may become organized during the process of repair and take on a stone-like consistency when palpated. Active contraction of the quadriceps is quite painful, causing

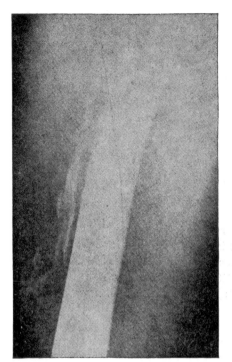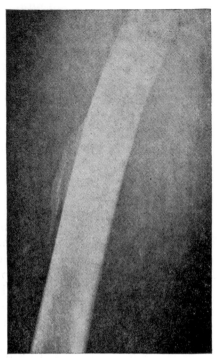

Fig. 9-30. Traumatic myositis ossificans. (Left) During a football block, a 16-year-old boy suffered a direct blow to the right quadriceps muscle 4 weeks before this x-ray picture was taken. In addition to being painful and tender, the right thigh measured 1¼ inches more in circumference than the left thigh. (Right) One year later, this x-ray picture shows progressive ossification of the calcified areas of the quadriceps muscle.

Muscle Spasms and Muscle Cramps

The outstanding physiologic characteristics of muscle function are its ability to contract to stimuli and overcome resistance, its ability to yield to passive stretch, and its ability to relax and give up its tension. These basic properties of muscle function are integrated and coordinated to permit reciprocal contraction-relaxation of opposing muscles and activation of adjacent joints.

When a muscle responds to a stimulus, it reacts by contracting a sufficient number of muscle fibers to move or stabilize a musculotendinous unit to overcome or resist the presenting resistance. Such a reaction is initiated by the muscle's sensory organ or muscle spindle. A discussion of muscle spindle structure and function is beyond the scope of this book. If a greater amount of work is to be done, an increased number of muscle fibers are brought into play. This gradation of muscle contraction is made possible by the recruitment of (i.e., the gradual increase in) a number of activated motor neurons. Motor neurons are nerve cells located in the anterior horn of the spinal cord that innervate the skeletal muscle fiber by a motor nerve. Normal motor performance depends on the right degree of motor neuron activation; the latter depends on the correct balance between excitatory and inhibitory influences impinging upon the motor nerve pool. Trauma, dietary deficiencies, drugs, fatigue, fasciculating illness, myotonic disorders, nerve-root irritation, and psychic stress may interfere with or eliminate this balance and cause muscle spasms or cramps that are quite disabling.

In athletics, painful muscle spasm most frequently results from an acute injury, which need not be severe, or fatigue. The pain resulting from trauma irritates the lower motor neurons, and this leads to reflex protective muscle spasm that splints and limits painful motion of an adjacent joint. The muscle spasm also may become painful, to set up a vicious pain-spasm-pain cycle. Injuries to the neck, shoulder, low back and legs frequently cause painful muscle spasm of the area musculature. Treatment is directed toward correcting the disturbances of the sensory-motor reflex arc. This is done with surface anesthesia, injections, muscle relaxants, moist hot packs, cold packs and electrotherapy. Gentle active motion to pain tolerance accompanies this treatment.

Painful hypertonic muscle contractions that lead to cramps are listed as follows:

1. Fasciculating illness.
2. Myotonic disorders.
3. Metabolic disorders.
4. Psychogenic cramps.

This classification takes into account the diversity of cramps and the varying mechanisms responsible for their appearance. However, this grouping, except for No. 3, does not encompass or explain the appearance of this common athletic occurrence in the healthy athlete.

No athlete is immune to this usually short-lived and disabling condition. The occurrence of cramps in athletics usually results from the following causes.:

1. Loss of salt as a result of excessive sweating.
2. Hyperventilation, causing a carbon dioxide gas loss and respiratory alkalosis.
3. Fatigued state leading to an inability to relax.
4. Circulatory impairment resulting from a tight supportive strap, improperly fitted equipment or shoes.
5. Without any apparent reason.

The following additional circumstances may be associated with the development of cramps:

1. Overstretched and tight muscles anywhere in the musculoskeletal system.

2. Overwork in early season when there is a lack of physical conditioning.
3. A sudden, sharp blow causing intense pain and temporary cramp.
4. Assuming unnatural positions, such as standing at attention for a prolonged period of time.
5. Loss of potassium as a result of urination.
6. Loss or dietary deficiency of other trace elements such as MG, ZN, and CHR.

In the prevention and treatment of cramps, elimination of the cause is the primary consideration. For instance, it is well known that abdominal cramps may occur if a swimmer eats shortly before competing —the implications should be obvious. In cases of excessive sweating with loss of salt, replacement of salt is indicated. Cramps may result from respiratory alkalosis as a result of overexertion in long distance and cross-country running; this can be corrected only by conditioning.

Although cramps are experienced more frequently in the legs, breast strokers can relate many occurrences of cramped cupped hands following trying competition. It is not unusual to see an athlete who is running stop short because of a cramped calf; however, swimmers who maintain their feet in marked plantar flexion while doing a flutter kick instead of using a loose ankle also suffer calf cramps quite similar to those of athletes running on the ground.

Once the cramp has occurred, it can be neutralized by activating the opposing muscle as well as by simply stretching the cramped muscle. This can be also aided by gentle massage.

FRACTURES AND DISLOCATIONS

The third largest group of athletic injuries includes fractures and dislocations. Fortunately, the incidence of these injuries is relatively low, although the athlete who suffers such an injury could not care less about this low incidence. He is concerned only with getting well quickly and back into the game. Diagnosis and treatment offer no great problem in most fractures. Since so many excellent texts cover the diagnosis, treatment and rehabilitation of fractures and dislocations, these topics are discussed only in general terms. However, the reaction of athletes to these types of injuries requires some discussion because they differ considerably from patients usually seen in a medical practice.

An athlete seems not to be aware that treatment and healing varies with the bone that is fractured or the joint that is dislocated. Because of his youthful exuberance, impatience, and excellent potential for restoration, he expects a quick and miraculous recovery, whether he is unable to ambulate because of a fractured ankle or unable to use his shoulder because it is dislocated. In addition to the overt demands and expectations made by the injured athlete on the doctor and the trainer, other pressures, some subtle and some not so subtle, are exerted by the athletic director, the coach and even the parents to accelerate the treatment and heal the athlete in less time than the specialized structures normally need to heal. These lay sources may even offer medical recommendations, usually citing the use of a well-known product or technique. To assist our readers in warding off the questions, suggestions and pressures that are sure to follow fractures and dislocations, some general principles are covered.

The diagnosis and choice of treatment must be based upon the overall clinical evaluation, not upon roentgenograms alone, which are an adjunct to, not a substitute for, clinical evaluation and judgment. Roentgenograms must be taken at the time of the accident in two views, usually anteroposterior and lateral. Additional views are taken if necessary. If the original x-ray pictures are negative for bony or periosteal disorder but pain and disability persist, follow-up x-ray studies are indicated. This is especially true in rib, navicular, and fatigue fractures. It may be necessary to take several sets of follow-up films before a fracture can be definitely included or excluded. Bone scanning is now used in difficult cases.

Most fractured (broken) long bones in young healthy athletes heal with abundant callus in 8 to 12 weeks to permit resumption of athletics. However, a reduced fracture need not be immobilized for so long a period of time if healing is evident clinically and x-ray pictures demonstrate sufficient approximation and callus formation. Young high school and college athletes deposit abundant callus.

The shoulder and elbow joints have a proclivity for forming fibrosis, adhesions and joint restriction following fractures and dislocations. Because of this tendency, guarded joint motion can be started in 10 days to 3 weeks. In elbow dislocations, I (M. N.) use a removable plaster cast or posterior mold and start motion 3 weeks after reduction. Earlier active motion can lead to recurrent dislocations.

Finger fractures and dislocations should be reduced immediately and immobilized on a padded splint in a position of function. However, in most cases, as soon as the pain has subsided, they should be started moving to pain tolerance. Finger fractures require only 2 to 3 weeks of treatment before resumption of play with protective splinting. Reduced finger dislocations should be started on gentle active motion the following day provided the acute pain has subsided. Fibrous ankylosis appears rapidly in these small joints if they are immobilized too long. Fractured toes are started moving actively as soon as the pain has lessened. Again, it is important to obtain painless function rather than a perfect roentgenogram reduction and a stiff digit.

In lower leg fracture, sufficient bone healing may occur in 4 to 6 weeks to permit weight-bearing. In distal fibular fractures, resumption of athletic participation in a non-contact sport may be permitted provided the knee, ankle, and foot have an almost normal range of painless motion and strength. However, there are no hard and fast rules. Each athlete and his fracture must be individually evaluated to determine whether he is fit to return to competition. Chris Evert Lloyd had a stress fracture of the tibia that did not appear on conventional x-ray films. It was detected only in a radioisotope scan test. As a result of this diagnosis, she was advised to change her training regimen until the fracture healed.

A word of caution: attending physicians must have a high index of suspicion of fractures at unusual sites and in particular should look for avulsion fractures. Birnbaum reported an avulsion fracture of the lesser trochanter caused by the contraction of the iliopsoas muscle in the jackknifing motion of serving in tennis that was missed for 14 months despite examinations by four orthopedists and four radiologists. Dependence on x-ray pictures and not on clinical tests, such as a Ludluff's sign, inability to flex the hip while in a sitting position, or the presence of swelling or ecchymosis or both at the base of Scarpa's triangle, leaves reason to believe that the attending physicians did not suspect such a fracture. Unfortunately, by not resting sufficiently, the patient was left with a chronic condition.

In athletics, the major dislocations involve the shoulder, elbow, and ankles. These should be immobilized for no less than 4 weeks to allow satisfactory healing of the torn ligamentous and capsular tissues. The high incidence of recurrences in shoulder dislocations has already been noted (see p. 204).

When an extremity is encased in a plaster cast or dressing, atrophy of the muscles of the immobilized limb is certain to follow even when an athlete makes a vigorous effort to exercise the restricted muscles. The middle fibers of the deltoid and the quadriceps muscle of the thigh atrophy rapidly when the upper and lower extremities, respectively, are immobilized. When the shoulder, arm, or forearm are casted or immobilized with a Velpeau dressing or a sling and swathe, vigorous isometric exercises of the muscles of these parts must be started as soon as the pain subsides. After the period of immobilization, Codman exercises for the injured shoulder provide both isotonic and stretching exercises aided by the force of gravity. This increases the range of motion of the shoulder as well as strengthening of the muscles about the shoulder.

When the lower extremity is immobilized in plaster, the antigravity muscles (quadriceps and calf) atrophy more rapidly in size and strength than the other muscles of the leg. This is the price they pay for escaping so late from their evolutionary bonds. Active isometric exercises of all the muscles of the immobilized limb are started as soon as the pain subsides. However, greater emphasis is directed to the quadriceps than the other muscles. If only the lower leg is encased, the quadriceps is still vigorously exercised as well as the calf and anterior leg muscles. The joints that are not immobilized are also put through a range-of-motion exercise. These maintain the strength, shape, and size of the restricted muscles and minimize the limp after the cast is removed.

Power and strength testing must be done to determine what muscles need further rehabilitation. These tests assist in determining the optimal time an athlete is fit to return to competition. We use inexpensive materials, such as rubber ball finger exercisers, bouncing putty, finger ladders, shoulder wheels, metal sandals, adjustable weights, and stationary bicycles to achieve maximal flexibility and strength of these muscles. If isokinetic/isotonic machines are available, they should be used in conjunction with further therapy.

BURSITIS

This is an inflammation of the bursal sac that causes pain and swelling. The most common sites of bursitis in athletics are the shoulder, knee area, and heel. X-ray study of these sites before starting therapy rules out or confirms the presence of any bony, periosteal, or soft tissue disorder.

Subdeltoid or Subacromial Bursitis. This bursa is composed of an upper subacromial portion, located beneath the upper end of the deltoid muscle and acromion, and a larger subdeltoid part, which is located over the greater tuberosity and rotator cuff and is also covered by the deltoid. This bursa is interposed between the deltoid muscle and the acromion and the humeral head and the rotator cuff; it is frequently inflamed in baseball and basketball players as a result of excessive repetitive throwing motions. Other athletes may relate a history of injury to the shoulder area by a direct blow or a fall on an outstretched hand or point of the shoulder.

In acute cases, the player complains of severe shoulder pain that becomes worse with any shoulder movement, either active or passive. Shoulder motion is moderately restricted, especially abduction and internal rotation. If the bursa is markedly distended, it may cause swelling of the shoulder. The shoulder may feel warm to the touch. Localized tenderness over the greater tuberosity or just beneath the acromion has special significance because of the presence of a bursa at these sites. However, tenderness may be generalized. Passive abduction of the shoulder may cause a sudden increase in pain as the inflamed and distended bursa is put under pressure by the acromion. The athlete usually seeks help early because the condition may be quite disabling. However, diagnosis may be difficult because the shoulder, as noted previously, is a large and complicated anatomic region containing many structures that could be injured or responsible for pain. The physician must take his own detailed history and use examining techniques at his command to arrive at an accurate diagnosis and institute appropriate treatment. Routine and special-view x-ray studies must be utilized.

The trainer is instructed to start the athlete on daily cryotherapy, with modifications prescribed by the physician. Following this, the athlete's arm is placed in a sling, which he should wear until told otherwise by the doctor. I (M. N.) also prescribe an analgesic or anti-inflammatory medication to help reduce the pain and discomfort. As the pain subsides, graduated exercises of the shoulder are started, which are continued even while the arm is still in a sling. The first motions are internal and external rotation, and a few degrees of abduction. These are progressively increased until range-of-motion exercises, such as Codman, ladder climb, and shoulder wheel exercises, can be done to pain tolerance. For those athletes who cannot tolerate cold therapy, Hydrocollator packs, ultrasound and electrical muscle stimulation, and a sling may be used instead, along with the therapeutic exercises. Some physicians inject the site of maximal tenderness with a local anesthetic combined with a corticosteroid. However, I reserve this type of treatment for acute exacerbations of chronic cases that usually show some x-ray evidence of calcification. In chronic cases that do not respond, x-ray therapy may give considerable relief and must be remembered as an effective mode of therapy.

Prepatellar Bursitis. This bursa lies between the skin and the patella. Bursitis at this site results frequently in football and soccer players from direct blows or falls on the knees. To a lesser extent, it is also seen in hurdlers. Prepatellar bursal swelling characterizes this injury, along with redness, warmth, and tenderness. Pain and discomfort may develop along with bursal distention. The swelling is usually localized directly over the front of the patella, but may extend beyond these limits. The knee joint is practically never involved. This condition must be examined, diagnosed and a course of treatment prescribed by a physician.

The immediate treatment in acute injuries is the application of an ice compress followed by a compression bandage, continued until swelling has been checked. Although swelling may continue in spite of such measures, it is consideraby lessened. Pain and discomfort are also diminished.

A sizable effusion extending beyond the confines of the patella usually warrants hospitalization, where repeated aspirations can be performed with strict asepsis. This is followed by a firm pressure bandage and ice compresses. After the swelling has been controlled in high school athletes, I (M.N.) apply a padded cylinder cast to the affected leg to give the knee a chance to heal. This helps prevent recurrence of the swelling, since most high school athletes will not rest the leg if not immobilized.

This type of immobilization is not recommended for trackmen, because they usually have minimal prepatellar swelling. These small prepatellar effusions may be aspirated with a 25-gauge needle and a corticosteroid injected, followed by a firm pressure dressing. Such athletes should be able to return to action within 48 hours.

Retrocalcaneal Bursitis. This bursa is situated between the posterosuperior surface of the calcaneus and the tendo Achilles. It frequently becomes inflamed from friction and pressure caused by ill-fitting shoes. Retrocalcaneal bursitis also stems from kicks to this site and tight heel cords. The athlete complains of pain and discomfort in the back of the heel, which increases with motion and is usually eliminated with no weight-bearing. Some swelling and local tenderness may occur at the bursal site.

This condition must be examined and diagnosed by the physician. In acute cases, complete rest, whirlpool and ultrasound therapy are effective. Raising the bursa above the level of the shoe by the use of a sponge rubber heel inside the shoe eliminates the pressure and friction of the shoe counter on the bursa. A full-length molded insert arch placed inside a regular shoe to distribute the weight over the entire foot sometimes helps. If the condition does not respond to treatment, the bursa may be injected with a combination of local anethetic and corticosteroid once weekly for 3 weeks. This and other foot disorders are on the rise with the present boom in running and jogging.

REFERENCES

Anderson, G., Zeman, S.C., and Rosenfeld, R.T.: The Anderson knee stabler. The Physician and Sportsmedicine, 7:125–127, 1979.
Anonymous: Council on Scientific Affairs: Standard nomenclature of athletic injuries (prepared by the advisory panel on standard nomenclature of athletic injuries). Chicago, American Medical Association, 1976.
———: Knee taping and bracing offer some support. The First Aider, 46:9, 1976.
———: Myositis ossificans: Tribune sports report. Medical Tribune, February, 1976.
———: Stress fractures develop slowly. In Common athletic injuries and their treatment. The First Aider, 49:12–13, 1980.
Balakian, G., et al.: Team doctor tips: field, gym, general. Patient Care, 11: 104–121, 1977.
Bankart, A.S.B.: The pathology and treatment of recurrent dislocations of the shoulder joint. Br. J. Surg., 26:23–29, 1938.
Barnes, L.: Cryotherapy: Putting injury on ice. The Physician and Sportsmedicine, 7:130, 1979.
Bateman, J.E.: The Shoulder and Neck. 1st Ed. Philadelphia, W.B. Saunders, 1972, p. 404.

————: The Shoulder and Neck. 2nd Ed. Philadelphia, W. B. Saunders, 1978, p. 506.

Bilik, S. E.: Contrast baths. In The Trainer's Bible. 8th Ed. New York, T.J. Reed & Co., 1948, p. 129.

Birnbaum, D.A.: Avulsion fracture in sports. Med. Trial Tech. Q., 26:121, 1979.

Blazina, M.E., et al.: Jumper's knee. In Orthopedic Clinics of North America. Vol. 4. No. 3. Philadelphia, W.B. Saunders, July, 1973, pp. 665–678.

Blazina, M. E., and Satzman, J. S.: Recurrent anterior subluxation of the shoulder in athletics—A distinct entity. In Proceedings of the American Academy of Orthopaedic Surgeons. J. Bone Joint Surg., 51A:1037–1038, 1969.

Burkett, L.: Causative factors in hamstring strains. Med. Sci. Sports, 2:39–42, Spring, 1970.

Clancy, W. G., Jr.: Shoulder problems in overhead-overuse sports. Am. J. Sports Med., 7:138–144, 1979.

Council on Scientific Affairs: Standard nomenclature of athletic injuries (prepared by the advisory panel on standard nomenclature of athletic injuries). Chicago, American Medical Association, 1976.

Cox, J.: Chondromalacia viewed as a "catchall." Medical Tribune, 5:14, March, 1980.

Davis, G.J., and Larson, R.L.: Examining the knee. The Physician and Sportsmedicine, 6:48–67, 1978.

DeHaven, K., Dolan, W.H., and Mayer, P.J.: Chondromalacia patella in athletes. Am. J. Sports Med., 7:11, 1979.

DeHaven, K., et al.: Throwing injuries to the adolescent elbow. Contemp. Surg., 9:67–80, 1976.

Ellison, A.E.: Skiing injuries. Ciba Clin. Symp., 29:18–36, 1977.

Francis, R.: Little League: A decade later. The Physician and Sportsmedicine, 6:88–97, 1978.

Frankel, V.H., and Nordin, M.: Basic Biomechanics of the Skeletal System. Philadelphia, Lea & Febiger, 1980.

Galway, R.D., Baupre, A., and MacIntosh, D.L.: Pivot shifts: A clinical sign of symptomatic anterior cruciate instability. J. Bone Joint Surg., 54B:763–764, 1972.

Ganong, W.F.: The Nervous System. Los Altos, Lange Medical Publications, 1977.

Grossman, R.B., and Nicholas, J.A.: Common disorders of the knee. In Orthopedic Clinics of North America. Vol. 8. No. 3. Philadelphia, W.B. Saunders, July, 1977, pp. 619–640.

Gugenheim, J.J., Jr., et al.: The Little League survey: The Houston study. Am. J. Sports Med., 4:189–200, 1976.

Hawkins, R.J., and Kennedy, J.C.: Impingement syndrome in athletes. Am. J. Sports Med., 8:151–158, 1980.

Hoppenfeld, S.: Physical Examination of the Spine and Extremities. New York, Appleton-Century Crofts, 1976.

Homer, R.: Soccer injuries: The thigh contusions. The First Aider, 48:6–7, 1978.

Hughston, J. C.: Acute knee injuries in athletes. Clin. Orthop., 23:114–133, 1962.

————: Surgical repair of acute ligamentous tears of the knee. Presented at American Academy of Orthopaedic Surgeons' postgraduate course. "The injured knee in sports with special reference to the surgical knee." Eugene, 1973.

————, and Norwood, L.A.: The posterolateral drawer test and external rotational recurvatum test for posterolateral rotary instability of the knee. Clin. Orthop., 147:82–87, March and April, 1980.

James, S.L., and Brubaker, C.E.: Biomechanics of running. Orthop. Clin. North Am., 4:605–615, 1973.

Johnson, D.: Overuse and impingement syndrome found to be common in competitive swimmers. Orthopedics Today, 2:2, 1982.

Kennedy, J.C.: The Injured Adolescent Knee. Baltimore, Williams & Wilkins, 1979.

————: Complete dislocation of the knee joint. J. Bone Joint Surg., 45A:899–904, 1963.

————, and Fowler, P.J.: Medial and anterior instability of the knee: An anatomic and clinical study using stress machines. J. Bone Joint Surg., 53A:1257–1270, 1971.

Kennedy, J.C., and Granger, R.W.: The posterior cruciate ligaments. J. Trauma, 7:367–377, 1967.

Kennedy, J.C., Hawkins, R.J., and Krissoff, W.B.: Orthopaedic manifestations of swimming. Am. J. Sports Med., 6:309–322, 1978.

Kennedy, J.C., Weinberg, H.W., and Wilson, A.S.: The anatomy and function of the anterior cruciate ligaments. J. Bone Joint Surg., 51A:223–237, 1974.

Laurin, C.A., et al.: The abnormal lateral patellofemoral angle. J. Bone Joint Surg., 60A:55–60, 1978.

Le Clerc, J.: Chronic subluxation of the shoulder. *In* Proceedings of the Dewar Orthopaedic Club. J. Bone Joint Surg., 51:778, 1969.

McCann, J.: Excise distal clavicle for separation. Medical Tribune, 16:October, 1980.

McDaniel, W.J., Jr., and Dameron T.B., Jr.: Untreated ruptures of the anterior cruciate ligament. J. Bone Joint Surg., 62A:696–705, 1980.

McNab, I., and Rathbun, J. B.: The microvascular pattern of the rotator cuff. J. Bone Joint Surg., 52B:540–553, 1970.

Madigan, R., Wissinger, H.A., and Donaldson, W.F.: Preliminary experience with a method of quadricepsplasty in recurrent subluxation of the patella. J. Bone Joint Surg., 57A:600–607, 1975.

Marshall, J.L., and Rubin, R.M.: Knee ligament injuries: Diagnostic and therapeutic approach. *In* Orthopedic Clinics of North America. Vol. 8. No. 1. Philadelphia, W.B. Saunders, July, 1977, pp. 641–688.

Merrifield, H.J., and Cowan, R.: Groin strain injuries in ice hockey. J. Sports Med., 1:41–42, 1973.

Moore, R.J., Nicolette, R.L., and Behnke, R.S.: The therapeutic use of cold (cryotherapy) in the cure of athletic injuries. J. NATA, 2:6–13, 1967.

Morton, K.S.: The unstable shoulder: Recurring subluxation. *In* Proceedings of the Canadian Orthopaedic Association. J. Bone Joint Surg., 59B:508, 1977.

Mosely, H.F.: Traumatic disorders of the ankle and foot. Ciba Clin. Symp., 17: 3–30, 1975.

Neer, C.S., II: Anterior acromioplasty for chronic impingement syndrome in the shoulder. J. Bone Joint Surg., 54A:41–50, 1972.

Neer, C.S., II, and Welsh, R.P.: The shoulder in sports. *In* Orthopedic Clinics of North America. Vol. 8. No. 3. Philadelphia, W.B. Saunders, July, 1977, pp. 583–591.

Netter plates 13 and 16. Ciba. Clin. Symp., 29:1977.

Nicholas, J.A.: Correction of lateral instability: "Nicholas method." Presented at American Academy of Orthopaedic Surgeons' postgraduate course, "The injured knee in sports with special reference to the surgical knee." Eugene, 1973.

————: The five-in-one reconstruction for anteromedial instability of the knee: indications. J. Bone Joint Surg., 55:899–922, 1973.

————: Injuries to knee ligaments: Relation to looseness and tightness in football players. J.A.M.A., 212:2236–2239, 1970.

Norwood, L.A., and Hughston, J.C.: Combined anterolateral-anteromedial rotary instability of the knee. Clin. Orthop., 147:62–67, March and April, 1980.

Norwood, L.A., DelPizzo, W., Jobe, F.W., and Kerlan, R.K.: Anterior shoulder pain in baseball pitchers. Am. J. Sports Med., 6:103–106, 1978.

Novich, M.M.: Ankle sprain; not always a minor injury. Consultant, 12:73–75, 1972.

————: The injured ankle: how serious is it? Medical Student, 3:1d–3d,12–13, 1976.

Noyes, F.R., et al.: Arthroscopy in acute traumatic hemarthrosis of the knee. J. Bone Joint Surg., 62A:687–695, 1980.

O'Donoghue, D.H.: Treatment of acute ligamentous injuries of the knee. Orthop. Clin. North Am., 4:617–645, 1973.

————: A method for replacement of the anterior cruciate ligament of the knee. J. Bone Joint Surg., 45A:905–924, July, 1973.

————: Reconstruction for medial instability of the knee. J. Bone Joint Surg., 55A:941–955, 1973.

————: Surgical treatment of injuries to the knee. Clin. Orthop., 18:11–36, 1960.

————: An analysis of end results of surgical treatment of major injuries to the ligaments of the knee. J. Bone Joint Surg., 37A:1–13, 1955.

————: Surgical treatment of fresh injuries to major ligaments of the knee. J. Bone Joint Surg., 32A:721–738, 1950.

————, et al.: Repair and reconstruction of the anterior cruciate ligaments in dogs. J. Bone Joint Surg., 53A:710–718, 1971.

O'Neil, R.: Prevention of hamstring and groin strain. Presented at Schering Symposium on Musculotendinous Injuries. Schering Corporation, 1975.

Palmar, I.: Injuries to the crucial ligaments of the knee joint as a surgical problem. Reconstr. Surg. Traumatol., 4:181–196, 1957.

————: On injuries to ligaments of the knee joint. Acta Clin. Belg. (suppl.), 8: 3–282, 1938.

Penny, J.N., and Smith, C.: The prevention and treatment of Swimmer's Shoulder. Can. J. Appl. Sport Sci., 5:195–202, 1980.

Protzman, R.R.: Anterior instability of the shoulder. J. Bone Joint Surg., 62A: 909–918, 1980.

Richardson, A.B., Jobe, F.W., and Collins, R.C.: The shoulder in competitive swimming. Am. J. Sports Med., 8:159,–163, 1980.

Rockwood, C.A., Jr.: Symposium. Shoulder Problems in the Athlete. Cassette Transcripts For Tomorrow, AOSS M 82-4.

Rockwood, C.A., Jr., and Green, D.P. (eds.): Fractures. Vol. 1. Philadelphia, J.B. Lippincott, 1975.

Rokous, J.R., Feagin, J.A., and Abbott, H.G.: Modified axillary roentgenogram: A useful adjunct in the diagnosis of recurrent instability of the shoulder. Clin. Orthop., 82:84–86, 1972.

Rothman, R.H., Marvel, J.P., Jr., and Heppenstall, R.B.: Anatomic considerations in the glenohumeral joint. Orthop. Clin. North Am., 6:341–352, 1975.

Rowe, C.R.: Acute and recurrent anterior dislocation of the shoulder. Orthopedic Clinics of North America. Vol. 2. No. 2. Philadelphia, W.B. Saunders, 1980, pp. 253–270.

————, and Marble, H.C.: Shoulder girdle injuries. *In* Fractures and Other Injuries. Edited by E.F. Cave. Chicago, Year Book Medical Publishers, 1958.

Rowe, C.R., and Zarins, B.: Recurrent transient subluxation of the shoulder. J. Bone Joint Surg., 63A:863–872, July, 1981.

Rowe, C.R., Patel, D., and Southmayd, W.W.: The Bankhart procedure: A long term end-result study. J. Bone Joint Surg., 60A:1–16, 1978.

Slocum, D.B.: Late reconstruction of the medial compartment of the knee. Clin. Orthop., 100:23–25, 1974.

————: Pes anserina transplant: Impressions of the experience of a decade. J. Sports Med., 2:123–136, 1974.

————: Rotary instability of the knee: Its pathogenesis and a clinical test to demonstrate its presence. J. Bone Joint Surg., 50A:211–225, 1968.

————, and Larson, R.L.: Pes anserinus transplantation: A surgical procedure for control of rotary instability. J. Bone Joint Surg., 50A:226–242, 1968.

————, and James, S.L.: Late reconstruction procedures used to stabilize the knee. Orthop. Clin. North Am., 4:674–689, 1973.

Smodlaka, V.: Rehabilitating the injured athlete. The Physician and Sportsmedicine, 5:43–49, 1977.

Stover, C.N.: Air stirrup management of ankle injuries in the athlete. Am. J. Sports Med., 8:360–365, 1980.

Symeonides, P.P.: The significance of the subscapularis in the pathogenesis of recurrent anterior dislocation of the shoulder. J. Bone Joint Surg., 54B:476–483, 1972.

Taylor, B.: Charley horse caused by bruising muscles on front of thigh. The First Aider, *49*:11, 1980.

————: Contrast baths. The First Aider, *50*:10–11, 1981.

Torg, J.: Little League: The theft of carefree youth. The Physician and Sportsmedicine, *1*:72–78, 1973.

Tullos, H.S., and King, J.W.: Lesions of the pitching arm. J.A.M.A., *220*:264–271, 1972.

Tullos, H.S., and King, J.W.: Throwing mechanism in sports. *In* Orthopedic Clinics of North America. Vol. 4. No. 3. Philadelphia, W.B. Saunders, 1973, pp. 709–720.

Tullos, H.BS., et al.: Unusual lesions of the pitching arm. Clin. Orthop., *88*: 169–182, 1972.

10

Examinations and Decisions on the Field

One of the most difficult and trying situations during the course of an athletic contest occurs when play is stopped because a player is ill or injured. The athlete may be limping because of an injury to his back, hip, knee, ankle, or foot. If his shoulder or any other part of his upper extremity has been injured, he may be moving it about cautiously to test the amount of mobility and extent of injury, or he may be holding it with the other hand because he is in great pain. If he has hurt his back, he may be either bent over or lying on it, afraid to move because of the pain. At times the pain may be severe enough to double him up. An athlete may have the breath knocked out of him, in which case he is usually found doubled up and gasping for air, or he may be sitting on his haunches recovering from a solar plexus punch. The injured athlete may be lying motionless on the ground in a variety of positions or writhing about in agony.

Whoever is in charge, be it coach, trainer, or physician, should make an on-the-spot examination of the athlete and a decision as to what first aid, if any, has to be administered. Is the athlete fit to remain in the game, or does he have to be removed? If he has to be removed, how will he be taken off the field? How will definitive medical care be provided if the athlete is in need of such care? A doctor who is experienced in athletic injuries can readily make examinations and decisions on the field. However, a doctor not experienced in the medical aspects of sports may find some of these problems difficult to resolve; this would be even more true of coaches and trainers in the absence of a physician. This chapter, although addressed primarily to a physician, establishes some guidelines to assist responsible personnel in the initial handling of those injuries to athletes that frequently cause a contest to be temporarily halted. This includes observations that must be made in order to recognize the nature of the injury and its severity. The responsible individual must further determine whether an athlete is fit to remain in the game or has to be removed for a medical examination and treatment. First-aid measures to cope with these athletic emergencies until qualified medical help arrives are described.

During all contact sports (e.g., boxing, wrestling, football, hockey, basketball, soccer, and lacrosse) the coach and trainer must know where to contact the team physician immediately should the need arise. This part of the pregame preparation is just as important as having a completely equipped trainer's kit. In addition, stretchers, arm and leg splints, bolt cutters shears to cut off face masks, mouthscrew for epileptic seizures, and a portable inhalator and resuscitator unit must be on hand, although out of the view of the athletes. For scheduled contests, an ambulance with a well-trained squad must be present, but out of sight of athletes and spectators. This is a must for football and boxing matches. The coach and trainer must hold certificates in Red Cross first aid and be adept at splinting fractures, bandaging injuries, closed-chest cardiopulmonary resuscitation, and other life-saving techniques that fortunately are seldom necessary to employ. They should be familiar with proper methods of lifting and transporting the injured athlete.

The team physician should be fully acquainted with the fundamentals of the sport as well as with the style of play used by his team. He should be familiar with the physical and emotional states of the players, since there are many differences among individuals exclusive of sports skills. Among these are the state of conditioning, past medical history, motivation, threshold of pain, and idiosyncrasies. This information helps in evaluating injuries and arriving at a diagnosis. During a contest, the doctor (or in his absence, the trainer) must pay close attention to the performance of the athletes rather than to the progress of the ball or game; this enables him to note quickly when an athlete is injured. Seeing the mechanism of the injury and the forces involved gives him a good understanding of the pathophysiology and the severity of the injury. He can also detect when an athlete is not performing satisfactorily. He notes when a fallen athlete does not rise quickly after a play has stopped. In boxing, the implications are obvious, since each blow carries with it a risk to the opponent.

We believe that a trainer should rush immediately toward an injured athlete without waiting for an official summons. The doctor will respond immediately if needed. This is especially important in football and boxing, where the risks and hazards are great. Game officials are not trained to render medical judgments, and they are happy to see a doctor administering first aid to a stricken athlete. Getting to an injured athlete as quickly as possible may make the difference between a minor and a serious injury, especially when unqualified teammates and officials render their questionable brand of first aid. This attitude on the part of a team physician not only lessens the effect of injuries, but helps build morale among team members.

In boxing, referees and ringside physicians should have a harmonious working relationship with each other. Voice and hand signals from the doctor to the referees will assist them in protecting the boxers. Referees should consult frequently with the ringside physician to seek aid in making decisions as to whether or not an injury is a cause for stopping a bout or letting it continue. Referees should stop bouts when the ringside physician signals them to do so. A ringside physician should have the authority to stop a bout to protect the health of a boxer.

As soon as the doctor reaches the athlete, his examination and first-aid measures begin. The doctor carries with him a capsule or perle of aromatic ammonia and a sterile gauze pad. He gently removes the mouthpiece, removable dentures, and headguard, if these are present. He places the athlete in a more comfortable position, if necessary, which provides the athlete with an opportunity to relate the history of the injury and complaints. The physician is now better able to examine the athlete, first evaluating his general appearance, adequacy of his airway, and facial expression, looking for any signs of pain, exhaustion, unconsciousness, bleeding, deformities, defects, swelling, and other objective deviations from the norm. The intensity or absence of complaints is also noted by the doctor. For a superficially dazed athlete, a whiff of ammonia usually is enough to arouse him sufficiently to push the doctor's hand away rather than to have to breathe any more of the irritating ammonia vapors. The gauze pad along with finger pressure stops bleeding from nicks and cuts.

The athlete's localized complaints guide the examiner to the site of the injury. The doctor asks the athlete questions usually associated with injuries of specific body sites. The physician correlates the athlete's responses with his personal knowledge of the happenings. Following this, the doctor palpates the site of the injury and other bony and soft tissue landmarks. Tenderness, deformities, defects, swelling, crepitus, and muscle spasm are noted. Muscle function of the injured part is tested against resistance and without resistance. Active and passive joint motion are tested.

The physician tests for joint stability before muscle spasm splints the joint, which may mask joint instability. In football and hockey, the uniform hinders the physician from accurately evaluating shoulder, back, hip, knee, ankle, and foot injuries. Many times we have wished that football pants could be unzipped about the knee so it could be exposed and more thoroughly examined. It would be asking too much for such a uniform design for the shoulder. Uniform removal is normally not permitted on the field. When in doubt, it is best to take the player out of the game, undress him, and complete the examination. A small field tent set up near the bench is ideal; this permits the athlete to be examined immediately with the parts of the uniform removed. The doctor is now able to evaluate the nature and the extent of the injury and to determine whether or not the athlete is to resume play or to start on definitive medical care.

HEAD

In all sports and particularly in football, hockey, and boxing, a blow to the head may cause an athlete to be momentarily dazed or suffer a period of unconsciousness, whether he is down or standing. A number of significant observations must be made to properly evaluate the athlete's condition. First note the general and especially the facial appearance of the athlete. Is he standing erect without any assistance? Is he shaking his head vigorously to rid his head of the "cobwebs" resulting from the blow? If his eyes are closed tightly, does he open them on command? These athletes do well with a sniff of aromatic ammonia and some deep breathing; they need not be removed from the game. However, if the athlete is standing unsteadily with wobbly knees and rubbery legs, his arms limp and his head and neck lolling around without muscle tone, and if he has to be held up by others, presenting a picture of complete defenselessness, he should be removed and not returned to the contest. If he is only temporarily dazed, he may return to the game, provided he has complete recall and there are no signs or symptoms of concussion present as described in the following paragraph.

What are the conditions of the eyes? Do they appear glassy—with a fixed, glazed stare—or do they seem out of focus? What is the condition of the pupils—are they round, regular and equal, fixed, dilated, or unequal? Pupils that are fixed, dilated, or unequal are cause for immediate removal from the game. An athlete on the ground following a head injury whose eyelids remain closed should be sent immediately to the hospital on a stretcher.

The appearance of tonic contractions (characterized by sustained muscular tension) or clonic contractions (characterized by the alternating contraction and relaxation of muscles, which results in uncoordinated movements) of the muscles of the face, neck, trunk, and extremities ending in convulsive movements of these parts is cause for immediate removal from the game on a stretcher after the player's muscles have relaxed, his color has improved, and partial consciousness has returned. In such injuries, turn the head to one side and support the chin; this prevents the tongue from falling back, which can be held in place with gauze to prevent its being swallowed. This position also allows saliva to drain from the mouth. A padded gag may be placed between the teeth to prevent the tongue from being bitten. Any bleeding from the ear associated with a head injury is sufficient to warrant removal to a hospital. Following a head injury, bleeding from the nose or mouth mixed with spinal fluid (i.e., watery, blood-tinged fluid that does not clot) and accompanied by coma or unconsciousness is probably the result of a basilar skull fracture—also cause for immediate removal by stretcher to a hospital. Fortunately, convulsive disorders and bleeding from the ear, nose, and mouth following head injuries are rare in athletics.

While the athlete is being carefully observed, he is asked a number of simple questions about orientation to time, place, and substance. He is also questioned about headaches, memory lapse, dizziness, tinnitus or visual disturbances—signs of possible brain concussion. Inappropriate responses to the questions or neurologic complaints warrant removal from the game for additional examinations and start of definitive therapy. These athletes must not be allowed back into the game.

Contusions of the head are commonplace in sports, and athletes are frequently dazed and shaken as a result. Most athletes recover quickly from such blows, and even faster when they inhale the pungent vapors of ammonia. However, when in doubt about head injuries, the doctor or other officials will do well to err on the side of conservatism, because seemingly minor head injuries may result in serious consequences. Whenever there is a suspicion of a possible brain concussion, it is best to remove the player for observation. Concomitant neck injuries must also be checked out. Never manually remove a helmet from an unconscious football player on the field. This is best done in a medical setting.

NECK

Spearing and goring is now illegal and should lessen the incidence of neck injuries with some of their devastating sequelae. Coaches should understand and constantly envision the amazingly compact and intricately knitted structures of the normal neck, with its content of spinal cord, nerve roots, and vascular channels and the exact meshing of its many moving parts. Blows have been reported that were greater than 5,000 times the force of gravity on the helmet of a football player when crashing into an opponent. Forces of this magnitude directed to the cervical vertebrae and the closely fitted surrounding musculoligamentous, nervous, and vascular structures via the head can only lead to more grim football statistics. The neck has little tolerance for such excessive forces and unnatural movements.

A player with a neck injury in any sport who also complains of pain radiating into the shoulder and upper extremity, or tingling, paresthesia, or numbness in the extremities, should be examined carefully, because he may have injured the spinal cord or nerve roots. Deformity, pain, spasm of the anterior and posterior neck muscles, tenderness, and restriction of motion in the neck may indicate a fracture or subluxation of the neck. If such are suspected, the player should be removed by stretcher with his head and neck kept perfectly immobile with sand-bags or other sturdy objects placed on both sides of the neck. He should be sent directly to the hospital under supervision. In a football player with a suspected serious neck injury, take x-ray films of the neck first. Then remove helmet by splitting it with a cast cutter. Easing off a helmet in a suspected serious neck injury must be done slowly and guardedly so as not to aggravate an existing injury. The physician should be aware of the carotid sinus syndrome, in which pressure ap-plied to the carotid sinus causes a slowing of the heart beat, thus re-ducing the flow of blood to the brain, which causes syncope (dizziness and fainting). The presence of this syndrome may indicate more seri-ous injury.

Athletes who suffer minor injuries of the neck without a concomitant head injury may be allowed to play provided the neck shows normal anatomic contours and a painless range of normal motion, and neuro-logic signs and symptoms are absent.

FACE

The face is especially vulnerable to contusions, abrasions, nicks, and cuts. Fractures of any of the facial bones are cause for immediate re-moval from the contest; contusions and abrasions usually are not. Bleeding from nicks and cuts that are superficial can be controlled with finger pressure and a gauze pad soaked with epinephrine HCL solution 1:1,000. After the bleeding has stopped, a butterfly or Band-Aid dressing is applied to the site of the injury, followed by an ice pack. Dressings of this nature are not permitted on a boxer during the course of a bout. If the cut is large or deep, the athlete should be re-moved for suturing.

EYE

Any direct blow to the eye by a ball, fist, or other missile that causes a sudden sharp pain followed by ocular disturbances such as sudden loss of vision, double vision, blurry and otherwise impaired vision, extensive tearing, or a scratchy feeling in the eye is a medical emergency. "Seeing stars" following injury to the orbit is usually due to irritation of the retina, and calls for immediate removal of the ath-lete from the contest. A complete and thorough eye examination is done and appropriate therapy started. If a physician is not present, immediate removal to a hospital on a stretcher is imperative. A patch or dressing is placed over both eyes and sandbags along both sides of the head and neck to discourage head and eye movements and reduce bleeding. An ice compress to the eye is not recommended. During the transfer, the athlete is cautioned not to blow his nose, since this may force air up one nostril, the pressure of which can easily crack the paper-thin lamina papyracea. This fragilely constructed bone is located on the medial side of the orbit; if it is broken, air goes into the soft tissues of the eyelids, causing them to swell and shut the eye tight. If the trainer recognizes a foreign body or noxious chemical, the athlete is removed from the field. The eye is washed out with tap water, and the athlete can return to the game if it is feasible.

Periorbital bleeding from nicks or cuts is not serious unless it hinders the athlete's vision. This bleeding can usually be controlled with finger pressure and a small gauze pad wet with epinephrine HCL solution 1:1,000. The athlete may continue to play provided the bleeding has stopped or is minor.

Checking the blood flow from a more serious cut about the eye during a contest so that the athlete can continue to participate usually requires a tremendous amount of skill. In boxing, first aid for cuts may be rendered only in the 60-second rest between rounds. The boxing profession has a unique paramedical corps of "cut men" (trainers) who are specialists in repairing cuts about the eyes in about 40 seconds. They are quite familiar with the effects of epinephrine HCL, Gelfoam, thrombin (USP), antiseptic powders, lanolin, petroleum jelly, and other pharmaceuticals. The procedure is basically to stop bleeding with a safe antiseptic coagulant on a swab and manual pressure followed by the application of antiseptic ointment to the cut. Epinephrine HCL solution 1:1,000 is the coagulant used most frequently. This is followed by the application of an ointment such as thymol iodide, and then by a layer of medicated petroleum jelly. These trainers are also adept in the management of puffed eyes, split lips, and bloody noses. Some of the famous trainers keep their preparations top secret.

An eye that is doctored so skillfully becomes a deliberate target for the opponent. These periorbital cuts are reopened time and time again, the renown of the "cut man" or the secretiveness of his preparation notwithstanding. Although the eye is well protected, some blows find their way to the orbit, especially if the medicated seal of a periorbital laceration is the target. If the boxer suffers recurrent episodes of periorbital cuts, the bout should be stopped because the eyebrow may be split down to the bone of the supraorbital ridge. This may cause the levator muscle of the upper lid to sever, resulting in ptosis. Recurrent periorbital cuts may lead to destruction of the tissues at this site, causing improper closing of the eyelids. Blows to the orbit may cause hemorrhage in the eyeball, retinal detachment, retinal tear, pupillary disturbances, subluxation of the lens, and other injuries. Corneal abrasions from rosin are also cause for stopping a bout. These are all medical emergencies that require a competent ophthalmologic examination and the start of definitive care.

NOSE

A severe blow to the nose that causes an obvious deformity consistent with a fracture-dislocation is reason for immediate removal from the game. If a physician is not present, the injured athlete should be taken to the nearest medical facility.

Bleeding (epistaxis) from the nose which is in the nature of a dribble is easily controlled by making the athlete sit erect to prevent swallowing or inhaling of the blood. Application of a swab soaked with epinephrine HCL solution 1:1,000 to the bleeding point of the nose followed by pressure on the nostrils and firm pinching usually stops bleeding. Packing the anterior nares with absorbent cotton coated with petroleum jelly maintains the pressure at the site of blood vessel rupture. However, if the hemorrhage is copious, which occurs infrequently, the athlete must be removed from the contest. The same routine is followed, and additional pressure is applied by pinching the nose with the fingers. If this still does not stop the bleeding, remove the athlete immediately to the hospital.

MOUTH

Although the use of soft acrylic mouthpieces has materially reduced the incidence of lacerations of the lips and gingival tissues and fractures of the teeth, these injuries are not uncommon in contact sports. When a lip injury or a tooth fracture is suspected, retract the lip and inspect the injured area. The athlete may continue to play if the pain is minimal, even if he has lost part of the tooth without pulpal exposure. An exposed pulp may be recognized as slightly pinkish soft tissue in the center of the remaining tooth, usually associated with some bleeding and severe pain. In such a case, the athlete should be removed from the game and the exposed pulp covered with a small gauze pad moistened with Eugenol. His lips must be kept closed to prevent contact between the pulp and cold air, which causes pain. In any case of a tooth injury, the athlete must be referred to a dentist following the contest.

In a severe injury that involves the actual loss of teeth, the lost teeth should be found and wrapped in sterile gauze wet with saline solution and brought along with the injured athlete to a dentist. The dentist may be able to treat these teeth endodontically, replacing and splinting them into their original position. When teeth have been luxated from their position in the alveolar bone, immediately refer the athlete to a dentist.

THROAT

Blunt trauma to the throat may injure the larynx or trachea when these structures are compressed against the fixed cervical vertebral

10

column. The thyroid cartilage (Adam's apple) is most frequently contused and causes the trachea to go into reflex spasm. The athlete cannot catch his breath and chokes and gasps for air. He should be immediately removed from the game. Remove the mouthpiece and removable dentures. Keep him out of the game until his color, composure, and normal respiration have returned. Clothing or equipment about his neck, chest or abdomen, should be loosened or removed if it constricts these parts. The application of an ice pack to the throat reduces the degree of swelling in the vocal cords and trachea. It is not unusual for a person who has been struck a blow in the throat to develop hoarseness or aphonia about 30 minutes after the accident because of swelling of the vocal cords. When this occurs, the athlete must be removed from the contest and ice applied to the throat. If normal breathing does not resume after preliminary efforts to make the athlete comfortable, artificial resuscitation should be started. The athlete usually suffers sore throat and dysphonia for a few days until all the swelling in the larynx and trachea has been resolved.

Subcutaneous emphysema in the soft tissues of the throat should alert one to the presence of a laceration of the trachea with escape of air into the soft tissues. Palpation of these tissues gives the examiner's fingers a feeling of touching something soft and crunchy. It may also be described as a crepitus. This is cause for immediate hospitalization.

CHEST

The chest wall with its supporting rib cage protects the lungs and their pleurae, the heart, and other mediastinal structures. On the right and left lower anterior aspects, it is placed anteriorly to the liver and spleen. Blows to the chest wall that result in rib fractures may tear the pleura and lung and permit a subcutaneous emphysema, pneumothorax, and hemothorax. Rib fractures occur not infrequently when a blow of sufficient force is directed to the posterolateral border of the chest, where there is maximal curvature of the rib cage. In some contact sports, except in boxing, rib fractures infrequently occur from a direct anterior blow. The athlete complains of intense pain, point tenderness, and restriction of breathing; deep breathing aggravates the pain. Careful springing of the injured rib cage increases the pain. The presence of a fine crunching feeling beneath the palpating fingers suggests subcutaneous emphysema. If a rib fracture or any of its complications is diagnosed or suspected, immediate removal of the player from the game by stretcher is indicated.

In boxing, a powerful blow to the chest under the heart may be shocking enough to knock the boxer flat on his face for a full count. This blow, made famous by Tony Zale, strikes the ventricle of the heart, causing a temporary interruption of the conduction mechanism, leading to an asystole of the heart. Because of this interruption of the heart beat, hypoxia occurs in the brain and the boxer develops a temporary syncope. Immediate removal from the ring on a stretcher and then to a hospital is indicated. Complete, rapid recovery is the rule.

Cardiac contusions frequently result from steering wheel compression of the chest in automobile accidents. The same result may be expected from a hard punch to the chest in boxing or from a golf ball striking a chest while in flight. There are no reported cases of cardiac contusion from blows to the chest in boxing in the literature. A cardiac contusion resulting from football has been reported: this injury was caused by a blow hard enough to cause a linear fracture of the sternum. An athlete who complains of chest pain that is oppressive, constrictive, or vague, and/or shortness of breath following one or several blows to the chest, should be sidelined and observed. If he has tachycardia or a weak, thready pulse, pallor, sweating, cyanosis, or a clammy feeling of the skin (signs also found in a coronary occlusion), he should be sent directly on a stretcher to the hospital. If a doctor is present, he may be able to hear pericardial friction rub, arrhythmia, murmurs, or he may be able to feel an increased venous pressure, engorged neck veins, or a paradoxical pulse. Mediastinal emphysema may be detected by a fine crunching sound, audible over the pericardium and synchronous with the heart beat. Athletes with chest pain or dyspnea who have not suffered any injury should also be examined in a like manner.

If an athlete has been struck a heavy blow to the chest wall that has resulted only in soft tissue contusions, he should be removed from the contest and given a chance to regain normal respiration. He may be returned to the game only if fractures of the ribs and sternum, costochondral separations and cardiac injuries have been ruled out by a doctor. Although repetitive blows to the chest of male athletes such as boxers do not cause mastitis, this would not be the case with female athletes who sustain blows to the breast. Women develop breast symptoms and signs (sore breasts) during jogging. Athletic bras have helped reduce these occurrences.

ABDOMEN

In athletics, a severe blunt abdominal trauma, such as that from another athlete's helmeted head, a boxer's punch, an elbow, a knee, a foot, a batted baseball, a hockey stick, or a fall, might result in any one of these three frequently disabling conditions:

1. Wind knocked out.
2. Solar plexus syndrome.
3. Ruptured viscus.

An athlete may have the wind knocked out of him by a blow to the abdomen if the abdominal muscles are not hardened by conditioning or are not braced for the force. As the blow sinks into his abdomen, he doubles up and the wind may be heard coming out of his mouth with a "whoosh." The athlete usually has a startled or painful look of surprise on his face as he struggles to breathe. If the blow is of sufficient force to knock him backwards to the ground, and if he is wearing a mouthpiece or a removable denture, these should be removed quickly to prevent him from choking. It is best to remove the athlete from the game until he has regained normal color, respiration, and composure. He can then return to the contest.

In the solar plexus syndrome, the athlete doubles up and experiences marked pain and respiratory difficulty. He feels his legs going numb. He is fully conscious of his distress and his inability to prevent his impending forward collapse to the ground; this may account for the agonized facial expressions of victims of the solar plexus blow. The athlete recovers spontaneously. Allow him to rest on his back or haunches until sensation returns to his legs and color to his face; then help him to his feet and encourage him to breathe rhythmically. Help him off the field and loosen clothing or equipment about his abdomen or chest that may restrict respiratory movements. A cold compress placed to the face and back of neck is soothing. A physician must evaluate the injured athlete as to whether or not he is fit to continue the contest, except in boxing, when he is normally counted out.

The most serious injury that could result from an abdominal blow is a ruptured viscus. If the injury is of sufficient violence, clinically recognizable neurogenic shock occurs. Abdominal pain, tenderness, abdominal wall rigidity and signs of shock, such as pallor, sweating, rapid weak pulse, and cold and clammy skin occur. It is mandatory that the athlete be moved immediately by stretcher to a hospital where appropriate care can be started. If the spleen has ruptured, pain may be referred to the left shoulder in addition to the left upper quadrant. Injuries to the liver followed by hemorrhage may cause referred pain to the right shoulder in addition to local pain. Women's abdomens do not harden with the consistency of males because they lack testosterone. The abdomen, following childbirth, needs muscular rehabilitation.

Whenever abdominal trauma produces relatively minor physical findings that are persistent and localized, a visceral injury must be suspected. A rupture of either a solid or hollow viscus not infrequently acts in this manner. Athletes who have recently recovered from infectious mononucleosis are susceptible to lacerations of the spleen from relatively minor trauma. In such injuries it is sound medical practice to hospitalize the athlete where he can be carefully observed until there is no possibility that the viscus injury has been missed. The playing field is no place for such an examination.

Colicky abdominal pain is usually due to spasm of the musculature of a hollow viscus. The type of painful sensation in abdominal trauma does not help in arriving at a diagnosis, except when it is localized. Referred pain has already been noted. In addition to nonspecific abdominal pain and discomfort, peritoneal irritation may cause symptoms of nausea and a desire to vomit. It is the persistence and localization of complaints that should make the examiner suspicious of a visceral injury.

EXTERNAL GENITALIA

The fabric athletic supporter with or without aluminum cup inserts and the more elaborate padded aluminum foulproof device used by boxers have materially reduced serious injuries of these parts. Nevertheless, blows frequently get through to the genitalia and cause temporary painful disablement. This area is abundantly supplied with sensory nerves, so that blows to this region cause excruciating pain which may take the athlete's breath away. The athlete usually doubles up and reflexly brings his arms and legs to his groin. He may remain bent over or doubled up on the ground or canvas. He usually writhes about in pain which gradually subsides, leaving him with a feeling of discomfort. The athlete may experience a strong sensation of nausea and may even vomit.

Besides being in pain, the athlete is quite agitated, but usually a whiff of aromatic ammonia does much to transfer his concern from the injured genitalia to avoiding the noxious odor of the ammonia. In the experience of the authors, this treatment settles the athlete more quickly than if he is allowed to quiet down by himself. After a short rest the athlete should be made to stand erect and to move about with instructions for deep breathing. Too much time on the ground invites self-pity. The athlete may continue to play provided there is no marked pain or objective signs of injuries to the genital organs, such as tenderness, swelling, or retraction of a testicle.

If he does not respond within a minute or two of rest or if examination reveals that one or both testicles have retracted, the athlete may be quickly revived by placing both hands under his back as he lies supine. Then he is lifted a short distance and let drop; this is done once or twice, and relief is almost instantaneous. This maneuver, called "Katsu," is frequently employed by referees in judo. The athlete is removed from the contest. He should be examined by a physician to check out the status of his genital organs and to determine whether or not he is fit to return to the contest.

MUSCULOSKELETAL SYSTEM

General Considerations. The most frequent athletic injuries of the musculoskeletal system that may result in an emergency situation have been fully explored in Chapter 9. The more common histories, symptoms, and signs that enable a doctor to arrive at a reasonably accurate diagnosis of musculoskeletal injuries have already been noted. A recapitulation of the salient features of the more frequent injuries is highlighted in this chapter to allow a rapid yet substantive appraisal of the nature and extent of an injury. In arriving at a diagnosis, a physician must take a careful and thorough history of the injury and the complaints that flow from it. This is usually sufficient to suggest a definitive working diagnosis even before a physical examination is begun.

Because pain and its various manifestations and nuances are usually the most frequent and constant symptoms following a musculoskeletal injury, it is important for the doctor to analyze their location, character, intensity, and distribution. Description of the pain depends upon the athlete's reaction to it; the doctor must be familiar with the athlete's threshold or tolerance to pain. The athlete may describe the injury in training room parlance, with which the doctor should be familiar. However, there are usually no diagnostic difficulties in connecting local pain with an evident local injury of the musculoskeletal system. Pain of varying intensity accompanies obvious fractures, joint dislocations, muscle pulls, tendon ruptures, and other injuries. The doctor must not be misled by local pain that may in fact be referred from another site. This occurs not infrequently in chest, abdominal, and peripheral nervous system injuries. Arriving at an accurate diagnosis under these conditions requires the ultimate in diagnostic skills.

The athlete may find it difficult to describe the pain accurately—pain may feel the same regardless of which structures have been injured. However, some athletic injuries produce characteristic sensations of pain. For instance, trauma to the musculoskeletal system may cause nerve root or peripheral nerve injuries that produce paresthesia—burning pain, a sensation of pins and needles, or numbness in the extremities. The sharp, swift stabs of chest pain following a rib fracture are characteristic, and cause the athlete to splint his chest to limit chest movement in an effort to avoid them. Severe pain, like something tearing in the chest, is commonly associated with intercostal muscle pull or costochondral separation. Again, the athlete splints his chest, afraid to breathe because each movement of the rib cage sets off the cycle of pain. One episode of such pain is not soon forgotten. The pain of a muscle cramp speaks for itself. No matter how severe, it usually ends abruptly as soon as treatment is started. A cramp is different from a muscle pull in a hamstring or calf muscle, which is a tearing sensation followed by a knotting up of the muscle. This is actually a painful muscle spasm. The reflex muscle spasm in the low back is frequently described as a grabbing or knotting sensation in the back muscles, which can be excruciating and crippling in intensity. Despite treatment, this type of pain lingers and subsides gradually. The pain associated with a tennis leg is characteristic, as if the calf were hit by a bat or bullet. Large and medium-sized joint dislocations are usually described as "painfully locked," which become more painful with attempted movement.

The examiner observes the athlete carefully as he finds him, noting the position of his trunk and extremities. If he is on the ground, the examiner should note if he is able to rise and move about under his own power or if he has to be helped to his feet. Does the injured part prevent him from arising to an erect position? This happens not infrequently in back, hip, and leg injuries. If the athlete is bearing weight, his posture and gait as he stands and walks should be noted. Limping may result from injuries of the back, hip, and legs. The anatomic contours of the injured part must be inspected for form, deformities, defects, swellings, and other deviations from normal. The injured part should be compared with the uninjured part, and visual findings should be checked by finger palpation. Additional findings not evident on initial inspection may be elicited in this manner.

Tenderness is a frequent and constant sign following musculoskeletal injuries. All the bony and soft tissue landmarks must be palpated for tenderness, which ranges from slight discomfort to exquisite pain. The degree of tenderness is used as an index of the severity of the injury. Point tenderness is usually found in fractures, dislocations, contusions of muscles and joints, muscle pulls, and ligament sprains and tears. This finding also has to be evaluated in light of the athlete's threshold of pain.

The injured structure is finally tested for function. With this and other assembled information, the physician is able to come to a conclusion regarding the nature and extent of the injury. He can now determine whether or not the athlete should be removed from the contest.

Fractures of shafts of the long and larger bones usually present no diagnostic difficulties. Most can easily be recognized by a deformity, swelling, or abnormal motion at the fracture site as well as the ever present pain and point tenderness. Active movement of the distal articulation usually is not obtainable. Fractures of the wrist and ankles are not as evident as shaft fractures. However, the diagnosis becomes evident when point tenderness and marked restriction of wrist and ankle motion respectively are elicited. The same is true with hand and foot fractures. In the hand, there is pain, tenderness, swelling, and marked inability to make a fist or grip properly. In the foot, there is pain, tenderness, swelling, and a painful limp upon weight-bearing. When fractures of the back are suspected, the athlete should be immediately transported in a supine position off the field by stretcher.

Fractures of the skull and neck have been covered previously (pp. 269–271).

The severity of a muscle injury usually depends upon the number of torn muscle fibers and blood vessels. Reflex muscle spasm may result, which limits the movement of the muscle and its adjacent joint. The site of the injury can be localized by palpation and active and passive motion. Activating an injured muscle against resistance increases the pain; it may also demonstrate a deformity, weakness, defect, and inability of the muscle to move an adjacent joint. Passive, gradual stretching of an injured muscle aids in localizing and grading the severity of the injury.

When a joint has been injured, the range of active and passive painless motion should be noted, as well as the site of pain on joint motion. Resistance to passive joint motion occurs because of pain and muscle spasm. If muscle spasm splints the joint, not only is the range of motion restricted, but tests to check out the joint stability are obviated. A ligament that is sprained or torn sufficiently to permit abnormal motion of a joint is best diagnosed immediately after the injury. Any delay may cause this choice finding to be missed once muscle spasm sets in.

Shoulder Injuries. These most frequently result from direct blows, falls on the point of the shoulder, and leverage forces directed to the joint from blows to and falls on an abducted, extended, and externally rotated arm. The last mechanisms are often responsible for the athlete complaining that his shoulder has "slipped out." When these injuries cause the athlete to complain of acute pain accompanied with marked limitation of arm movement at the shoulder joint, the following conditions must be suspected:

1. Contusion.
2. Shoulder dislocation.
3. Fracture of clavicle.
4. Acromioclavicular separation.
5. Sternoclavicular subluxation.

It is best to examine the athlete in a standing position. If the uniform poses no interference to the examination, the doctor should visually inspect the site of maximal pain and the anatomic contours of the bony and soft tissue landmarks, noting form, deformity, and swelling. In addition to palpating for areas of tenderness, the doctor uses his fingers to corroborate abnormal visual findings and to elicit others that might not be obvious on visual inspection. The doctor should palpate the shoulder. A visibly flattened deltoid muscle accompanied by a palpable absence of the humeral head under the deltoid muscle suggests a dislocated shoulder. A tender but normally contoured deltoid is consistent with a severe contusion of this muscle. A contused trapezius muscle is usually in spasm as well as tender.

Concomitant with inspection of the clavicle and its acromioclavicular and sternoclavicular joints, these structures are palpated for form, deformity, tenderness, swelling, and crepitus. A prominence of the outer end of the clavicle that is tender and shows some degree of laxity to finger pressure is clinically an acromioclavicular separation. In acromioclavicular injuries, the hand of the injured extremity can usually be adducted to the uninjured shoulder; this is not the case in shoulder dislocations. Local tenderness and swelling over the sternoclavicular joint, frequently described as a "lump," clinically indicate a subluxation of this joint. The injured shoulder is moved actively and passively in various planes; the ranges of pain-free motion and the site of pain are noted, as well as any abnormal motion. When any of these conditions are suspected in a football or hockey player whose uniform prevents a satisfactory examination, the player should be helped to the sidelines, supporting the injured shoulder and arm. The shirt should be cut off at the seams and the shoulder pads removed in order to do a thorough examination of the shoulder.

Contusions of the deltoid and trapezius muscles are usually not cause for removal from a contest provided no bony structures have been injured. If the blow is severe enough to anticipate marked swelling and ecchymosis or if marked restriction of shoulder motion is present, the athlete may be removed from the contest. Cryotherapy and a sling are applied to check swelling and discomfort.

In summation, an athlete who complains of acute shoulder pain and presents a marked limitation of movement of his arm at the shoulder, and crepitus, deformity, swelling or joint laxity following a shoulder injury should be walked off the field with his injured shoulder supported. If these parts have only been contused, the athlete may return to the contest as soon as he has regained a normal range of painless shoulder motion. Otherwise, the injured shoulder and its adjoining upper extremity are trussed up in a Velpeau dressing and an ice pack applied to the site of the injury. The athlete is sent directly to the hospital by ambulance.

Knee Injuries. Knee injuries result most frequently from direct blows, extension strains, and rotary forces to which the knee is so often subjected. The last mechanism is often responsible for serious ligamentous and meniscal knee injuries that occur when the athlete is running at high speed and the knee twists inwardly as the foot is fixed to the ground with or without an associated blow to the lateral side of the knee. The athlete may describe a sensation of something tearing, slipping, or feeling loose on the inner side of the knee, or he may state that he felt a snapping painful pop emanating from the knee. He may complain that his knee gave way and is locked and that he is unable to straighten it. When a knee injury causes an athlete acute sharp pain and painful limp, the following conditions must be suspected:

1. Contusion.
2. Medial collateral ligament sprains and rupture.
3. Medial meniscus tear.
4. Cruciate ligament injury.
5. Avulsion fracture of epiphysis of tibial tubercle.
6. Patellar injuries

It is best to examine the athlete in a sitting or supine position. A complete knee examination requires the use of a series of specific testing techniques that have been designed to check the integrity of particular structures of the knee. The presence or absence of abnormal physical findings determined by these tests is important in assisting the doctor to arrive at a diagnosis and to determine the severity of an injury. In a field examination, if the mechanism of the injury is known and the complaints that flow from it are definite, the doctor can proceed directly with those special tests that are applicable and dispense with those that are not. If the mechanism is unknown or obscure and the athlete is obviously disabled, a full examination must be made, not on the field, but in the privacy of a dressing or examining room.

If the uniform poses no interference to the examination the doctor should inspect the site of maximal pain and the anatomic contours of the bony and soft tissue landmarks, noting form, deformity, defect, and swelling. He should note whether the swelling is in the joint, bursal, or soft tissues. In addition to palpating for areas of tenderness, the doctor uses his fingers to corroborate the abnormal visual findings and to elicit others that might not be obvious on visual inspection. The doctor should palpate the patella and its extensor apparatus. A prominent tender tibial tubercle may be due to an avulsion fracture of the epiphysis of the tibial tubercle, with or without fragmentation. This is most frequently seen in young boys between the ages of 10 and 15 (Osgood-Schlatter's disease). At the same time, the doctor should check out the suprapatellar pouch, the prepatellar bursa, and the knee joint for effusions. Exquisite point tenderness along the course of the medial collateral ligament or at its femoral or tibial attachments suggests a sprain or rupture of this ligament. The lateral collateral ligament and its femoral and tibial attachments are palpated similarly for a sprain or rupture of this ligament. Point tenderness along the medial joint line suggests a medial meniscus injury. Palpation of the lateral joint line is performed to detect injuries to the lateral meniscus.

The physician flexes and extends the injured knee actively and passively, noting the ranges of pain-free motion. Grating, crepitus, and clicking sounds are noted if present during flexion and extension of the knee. He also tests for collateral ligament stability with the knee in extension and also in 15° of flexion, using abduction (valgus) and adduction (varus) stress tests. Rotary stress tests are also performed by the physician. Only a physician may perform stress testing of joints to evaluate integrity of ligaments. Anterior and posterior knee stability is checked by the Drawer test, which determines the integrity of the anterior and posterior cruciate ligaments. A Lachman test may be performed when a painful knee will not permit flexion. Anterior cruciate instability can be determined by this test. Patellar testing for an apprehension sign or a painful compression test may indicate a patellofemoral disorder.

Contusions of the knee are usually not cause for removal from a contest provided no bony, ligamentous, or meniscal injuries have resulted. If the blow is so severe that one can anticipate a marked effusion into the knee joint or prepatellar bursa, the athlete may be removed from the contest. An ice pack and elastic bandage to the knee check swelling and discomfort.

Athletes who suffer a sprain of the collateral ligament are frequently able to get about unaided and even to run with a painful limp, depending upon the severity of the sprain. However, when a ligament is ruptured or a medial meniscus torn and the knee locks, or there is a combination of injuries described as "O'Donoghue's unholy triad,"* or others, the athlete usually has to be helped to his feet and off the field. When these conditions are suspected in football and hockey players whose uniforms prevent a satisfactory examination, they should be helped to a dressing or examining room where the uniforms can be removed. A complete knee examination as described in the preceding paragraphs is then performed.

In summation, an athlete who complains of acute sharp pain in the knee and presents a painful limp along with swelling, tenderness, restricted knee motion, or joint instability following a knee injury should be helped off the field. First-aid measures should be started to check swelling and discomfort and a thorough medical examination should follow.

Ankle Injuries. These most frequently result from direct blows and the sudden, powerful, unexpected forces of excessive rotation, inversion, and eversion to which the ankle-foot complex is subjected in athletics. The nature and extent of the ankle injury that results from these forces also depend upon whether or not the foot was firmly fixed to the ground, plantar flexed, or dorsiflexed and the position of the leg in re-

---

* Includes tear of medial meniscus, tear of medial collateral ligament, and tear of the anterior cruciate.

lation to the foot at the moment of injury. When an injured ankle causes acute, sharp pain and painful limp, the following conditions must be suspected:

1. Contusion.
2. Tibiofibular, lateral, or deltoid ligament sprains and ruptures.
3. Fractures and/or dislocations.

The athlete is best examined in a sitting or a supine position, depending upon which is the more comfortable. If the shoes or socks pose no interference to the examination, they need not be removed. If they do, remove them quickly but gently. The doctor should inspect the site of maximal pain and the anatomic contours of the bony and soft tissue landmarks. Their location makes them easily accessible, and also they are virtually free of any swelling immediately post-trauma. The doctor notes form, deformity, and defect. The deformity of a dislocated ankle is usually quite obvious. If swelling is present, its site and amount should be noted, because it is another guide to which structures have been injured.

In addition to palpating for areas of tenderness, the doctor uses his fingers to corroborate abnormal visual findings and to others that are not obvious on visual inspection. The bony malleoli and distal thirds of the tibia and fibula are felt for tenderness and crepitus; these signs may indicate fractures at these sites, especially if accompanied by point tenderness. The course and attachments of the more frequently injured ligaments located on the front and sides of the ankle are felt for tenderness. An accurate diagnosis can be established if maximal tenderness is noted over an injured ligament. If the mechanism of injury is known, that ligament which is usually injured is palpated first. However, it takes only a few additional seconds to feel other ligaments that may have been injured as well. Ankle movements are tested for range of pain-free motion and abnormal movements, and the site of pain with these tests are noted. The anterior and posterior tibial, the peroneal, and the Achilles tendons are also inspected, palpated and tested actively and passively—these are not infrequently injured by the same forces that traumatize ligaments.

Athletes who suffer sprains or ruptures of their ankle ligaments should be helped off the field. Adhesive strappings or wraps about the ankle should be removed and a fresh elastic bandage applied with an ice pack to check swelling and discomfort. Sometimes an ankle injury may be momentarily disabling and the degree of ligamentous involvement difficult to evaluate. Rather than needlessly removing an athlete following an inconclusive examination, have him stand up and jog about. If the limp lessens or subsides and seems not to give him any difficulty, the athlete should remain in the game. If the limp worsens when he puts full weight-bearing pressure on the injured leg, he should be removed from the game and first-aid measures started to minimize the swelling.

Contusions of the ankle are usually not cause for removal of an athlete from a contest provided no bony, ligamentous, or tendon injuries have occurred. However, if the athlete continues to limp or the limp worsens after a few minutes of play, he should be removed from the contest. Adhesive strappings or wraps about the ankle should be removed and a fresh elastic bandage applied along with an ice pack to check swelling and discomfort.

Athletes who suffer fractures or dislocations must be helped off the field. The injuries should be splinted and the athlete prepared for removal to a hospital, where x-ray examinations and definitive care are started. If the diagnosis is not clear and definite, but a fracture or dislocation is suspected, the above routine must still be carried out. Adhesive strappings or wraps about the ankle should be removed and a fresh elastic bandage applied, along with an ice pack to check swelling and discomfort.

In summation, the athlete who complains of acute ankle pain and presents a painful limp along with tenderness, crepitus, deformity, restricted ankle motion, or joint instability following an ankle injury should be helped off the field. First-aid measures should be started to check swelling and discomfort.

The examiner or doctor should try to instill calmness in the injured athlete by presenting an assured, concerned manner, and gently but skillfully using his hands. He should be direct in his approach to the athlete. He must never panic, but should make light of an injury if the condition warrants it. A player who is fit should be helped up and returned to the game. If he is not fit, his clinical condition should not be discussed at the time, but he should be removed to the sidelines and then told what is wrong.

REFERENCES

Balakian, G., et al.: Team doctor tips: field, gym, general. Patient Care, *11*: 104–121, 1977.

11

Training Room Tips

Thus far we have discussed the mechanism, pathology, diagnosis, treatment and rehabilitation of those injuries that occur most frequently in athletics. The important and sensitive relationship between the trainer and the athlete is never lost sight of because, in most cases, he is the first paramedical personnel present at the time of the injury or the first to be consulted about illness. The trainer's close relationship to the athlete notwithstanding, he is neither expected nor advised to make a clinical diagnosis. However, he is in a position to render necessary first-aid measures and to obtain important clinical information from the athlete which he can relay to the doctor to help him arrive at a working diagnosis. After the physician's examination, the trainer can then render therapeutic care to the athlete as prescribed by the physician.

However, the training room can become a busy place, with athletes having a myriad of minor complaints and ailments. These can be trying times for a trainer, who may be pressured into making decisions regarding health that are both within and outside of his competency. In the supervision of a training room, the trainer can easily handle most routine ailments without consulting a physician. However, the amount of authority that a trainer is allowed to assume in health matters must be defined by the attending physician, who must know the formal training, experience and conscientiousness of the trainer. The physician must also know the trainer's limitations. In this chapter we discuss additional clinical conditions not covered previously and outline the precise areas of responsibility of the trainer in the management of injuries and sicknesses.

The trainer must refer athletes to the doctor for examination and care whenever he suspects a systemic ailment, some signs of which are high temperature, rapid pulse, hot and dry skin, coated tongue, sallow skin color, clamminess, vertigo, chronic fatigue, unexplained loss of weight, and long standing dermatitis. Only common minor skin problems, such as athlete's foot, groin itch (jock rash), or heat rash, may be handled by a trainer. Whenever the magnitude of an injury is beyond the capabilities of the trainer, the athlete must be referred to the doctor. The trainer is expected to render first aid to all injuries if a physician is not present. This includes cleansing and dressing of abrasions and lacerations. He may give the athlete ointments, lotions, or powders for athlete's foot. He may give aspirin and salt tablets.

Most trainers have their own pet theories on the causation and treatment of clinical conditions in athletics. Their tape jobs are usually modifications of standard techniques. They constantly observe and experiment, trying to develop new techniques to improve the care of the injured athlete. Some techniques that seem to work may not be physiologically sound, and a trainer should not render any service to the athlete that is not standard practice unless he discusses it with the team physician. The doctor may well see merit in the trainer's suggestion for modification and change. The trainer has an opportunity to become the good right arm of the doctor, provided the services rendered the athlete are in the best interest of the athlete and compatible with the doctor's general and specific instructions.

The following are a number of clinical conditions that the trainer may encounter in his training room.

Hernia. A hernia is commonly called a rupture because a portion of the bowel or its omentum pushes through a weakness or tear of the abdominal wall into a natural opening such as the inguinal canal. This happens as a result of a sudden rise in intra-abdominal pressure brought on by straining, lifting of a heavy weight, coughing, sneezing, or by any action or event that causes the abdominal contents to press violently against a defect in the abdominal walls.

Hernias are most commonly felt as a sudden bulge or lump generally appearing in the inguinal region, sometimes accompanied by severe pain. The indirect hernia descends through the inguinal canal sometimes even descending into the scrotum. Direct hernias may also occur. Once a hernia appears, it can only get bigger. One of the complications resulting from the untreated hernia is an irreducible or trapped hernial sac (incarcerated). Strangulation of the intestinal loop may occur, leading to an intestinal obstruction requiring emergency surgery as a life-saving procedure. If pain is present, emergency care is indicated.

Hernias also occur at the umbilical area (umbilical hernia) and through old abdominal surgical incisions (incisional hernias). Femoral hernias occur mainly in females and are located high in the anterior thigh just below the groin.

When an athlete complains of a sudden lump or bulge in the groin area, suspect a hernia. This may be accompanied by mild discomfort, a dragging sensation, or a pain with lifting of heavy objects, coughing, or strain during urination or defecation. The athlete must be referred to the team physician for an examination. He will recommend an appropriate course of treatment, which is usually surgical repair of the hernia. Trusses for athletes are not recommended as a method of treatment. Hernia repairs have now become a 1-day hospital stay operation under local anesthesia in some medical centers. Some surgeons even report doing the surgery in their offices. It is reported by one doctor that he even has them back to hard work 1 week after the operation. Such a quick return to athletics is not indicated for athletes.

Varicose Veins. Most athletes, their athletic advisory personnel, and the general population are able to recognize the appearance of varicose veins. It is the upright position of man during most of the waking hours that causes some difficulty with the venous return of blood to the heart. Increased pressure in the leg veins because of gravity, along with other anatomic and physiologic defects and even heredity, plays a role in the appearance of varicose veins.

Nature has devised an ingenious system of deep and superficial veins with their valves that helps move the blood back to the heart. The venous valves, the surrounding soft tissue and muscles as well as exercising these muscles, particularly those in the leg, aid in the venous pumping of the blood back to the heart.

Prolonged standing, an overweight condition, a weakened vein, and heredity can cause an incompetent venous valve, leading to an inability to pump blood out of the legs fast enough to reduce the high venous pressure resulting from the upright position. A back flow of blood from incompetent valves results, causing the appearance of bulging, tortuous and dilatation of veins, and varying venous patterns in the thigh and leg, especially when standing.

Varicose veins are usually evident upon inspection and may be with or without symptoms. However, if an athlete does not show any visible sign of a varicose-vein disorder but complains of leg pain, muscle cramps, easy fatigue of leg muscles, tension, or soreness in the calf, popliteal space, or ankle swelling, suspect a varicose condition. Obvious or suspected varicose-vein conditions should be referred to the team physician. The doctor may recommend external supports for the legs such as Supphose, surgical stockings, graded pressure elastic stockings, or elastic bandages. Conservative antigravity measures, such as periods of leg elevation, and avoidance of prolonged sitting or standing are advisable. The physician may recommend surgery but this is indicated only in severe and disabling cases.

Because varicose veins can lead to phlebitis, development of blood clots, varicose eczema, and varicose ulcers, the team physician will determine whether or not the athlete is fit for a particular sport. He will also advise about whether or not an athlete should return to an athletic activity following an injury or whether he should be disqualified completely.

Swollen Glands. Athletes sometimes suffer from swollen glands of the neck. These often accompany other symptoms, such as sore throat dysphagia, general malaise and fever, (either high or low grade) of a few days' duration. The neck lymph glands are generally tender to palpation.

Most times, the lymphadenopathy is part of the symptom complex of a viral respiratory infection or influenza, and after 7 to 10 days, the athlete may gradually resume training. There may be bacterial infection, however, so it is recommended that a throat culture be started immediately to rule out streptococcal pharyngitis. If the school nurse is available, she can help out.

If the symptoms do not undergo remission in a few days, or if the lymphadenopathy is generalized, that is, if the axillary or inguinal nodes are also enlarged unilaterally or bilaterally, the family physician should be consulted.

For mild symptomatology, routine, supportive care instructions are in order: home rest, force warm fluids (chicken soup), bland diet (hot cereals, etc.), paper cups and dishes to avoid infecting others, and temperature should be checked and recorded daily.

Depending on the severity of the clinical course and the results of the throat culture, the family doctor may prescribe antibiotics, penicillin for streptococcal pharyngitis, or, if there is an allergy to penicillin, the appropriate mycin drug will be prescribed.

Prolonged illness despite the institution of these measures, should be cause for concern, and further studies would be ordered by the family doctor to rule out infectious mononucleosis, hepatitis, tuberculosis, and blood dyscrasia.

It is imperative that the athlete be given adequate time for full recuperation before being permitted to participate again in competitive sports. The family doctor is the only one qualified to determine when to begin gradual resumption of athletic activities, no matter how enthusiastic the young hero may be.

Cold Sores. The herpes simplex virus causes cold sores on the mouth. These ulcerations are frequently referred to as "canker sores." These are infectious and the athlete should avoid contact with others, check temperature daily, and use paper cups and dishes. Applying warm compresses to these sores is helpful. Application of Campho-Phenique to the ulcerations seems helpful in giving relief from pain.

The physician will check for other symptoms and physical findings and will treat accordingly.

Nausea and Vomiting. These are two symptoms of the gastrointestinal tract that result from a variety of physical diseases as well as from psychic stress and emotional factors. In athletes, these symptoms have closer association with psychic stress and emotional overlay. The symptoms of nausea and vomiting may be mediated through the vomiting center. Retching or gagging is seen more often than vomiting. Nausea is not infrequently seen.

Runners frequently suffer these symptoms for a variety of reasons. Many of the competitive and even recreational runners have labile, skittish, and intense personalities. They are easily plagued by nervous indigestion, which can appear at any time before, during, or after a race. The football, tennis, hockey, soccer player, or whatever athlete may also display pregame tension, causing nausea and vomiting.

These symptoms in athletes usually result from overloaded stomachs and incompletely digested foods. During athletic competition, there is decreased blood flow to the intestine, increased acids and metabolites in the blood stream, overactivity of the vagus and sympathetic nervous system, and others. Some athletes develop these symptoms as a result of a long and hot bus ride to an event. It is similar to car sickness.

Immediate treatment is to encourage the athlete to lie down and breathe slowly for 5 or more minutes. Tell him to concentrate on rest and relaxation. Let him try a half glass of ice chips wetted down with a tablespoon of coke syrup. This does a great deal to supply the body with some needed sugar and it settles the stomach. A cold compress on the forehead and back of neck is also helpful.

If nausea and vomiting are persistent and associated with abdominal pain, weight loss, or fatigue, the athlete must be referred to the team physician for evaluation and medical workup. In such cases, gallbladder disease, peptic ulcer, and even a neurologic disorder may be the underlying cause.

Headaches. Headaches may be caused by a variety of conditions. A common cause of headache is tension of the muscles in the back of the neck; tension headaches may be precipitated by fatigue or psychic tension. Headaches may also be caused by brain tumor and head injuries. In a migraine headache, the pain may occur in one half of the head or may feel as if the head were being constricted by a metal band. An aura of spots before the eyes or nausea may precede migraine headaches. In all cases of severe, chronic, recurrent, or persistent headaches, a physician must be consulted. All headaches resulting after a head injury must be referred to the team physician.

A trainer may give an athlete aspirin for an occasional minor headache. If the headache is still present after four or five aspirins, a doctor must be consulted. Forceful head trauma by an athlete should not be handled lightly. It requires neurologic evaluation and follow-up by the team physician.

Contused Orbital Rim (Blackeye). The trainer initially applies a cold ice compress for 15 minutes to relieve discomfort. As soon as feasible, the eye must be examined by a physician.

Foreign Particles in the Eye. Athletes frequently get dirt, dust, cinders, and rosin in their eyes, and sometimes metal and wood particles. Removing any foreign body from the eye requires the instillation of one drop of ½% pontocaine for anesthesia. If the foreign body is on the conjunctiva, it can be removed with a piece of cotton wetted down with sterile water, normal saline or boric acid solution, or the conjunctiva can be flushed with normal saline solution. If the foreign body is under the eyelid, evert the lid and remove the particle with a wetted piece of cotton. A foreign body on the cornea should be removed only by a physician, who will use a foreign body spud.

Injuries of the External Ear. The external ear is frequently injured in boxing, wrestling, football, and other contact sports. If properly fitting, protective headguards are worn, the incidence of this injury is minimized. In boxing, the injury results from a hard blow or a series of blows especially during infighting. In wrestling, the outer ear may be injured by rough handling as a result of the ear being twisted, crushed, pushed, pulled, or subjected to friction when it is rubbed against the mat or gym floor. In football, blows delivered to an improperly fitted headguard may also cause an outer-ear injury.

When the outer ear is injured, the athlete feels a sudden, sharp, burning flash of pain and senses that the ear has been torn. The outer ear is swollen, reddened, tender and soon becomes black and blue (hematoma). Progressive swelling and distortion of the ear will occur.

The immediate treatment for these injuries is the continuous application of cold compresses for several hours. The swelling should not progress with the use of cold applications.

The swelling results from a subperichondrial collection of blood and serum, which strips the perichondrium away from the underlying fragile elastic cartilage, depriving it of its blood supply. Aspiration of the subperichondrial collection of blood and fluid should be carried out as promptly as it develops. Since infection is disastrous to the ear, strict aseptic precautions are essential.

Since there is almost always reaccumulation of fluid, a pressure dressing must be applied to attempt to obliterate the subperichondrial space. Irregular contours of the ear must be taken into consideration in applying a pressure dressing and the following technique is recommended: Bits of sterile cotton dipped in ether are molded into the folds of the pinna and external canal. A similar mold is built up behind the ear. A wad of mechanics waste is applied to the entire ear over the cotton and held in position with an elastic bandage. This should be changed and the ear inspected every 24 hours to observe the need for reaspiration. This is continued until fluid no longer accumulates. A similar mold can be made using collodion-soaked gauze strips molded into the contours of the ear. This cotton dressing is readily available, is easily molded into place and forms a firm compressed cotton cast. The cooling effect of the ether inhibits the reaccumulation of the hematoma.

Careful inspection for evidences of infection must be carried out daily and prompt use of adequate doses of antibacterial drugs can prevent serious deformities.

Earache. All cases of earache must be referred to a doctor for examination and care.

Nosebleed (Epistaxis). The player should sit up with his head held erect to prevent swallowing or inhaling of the blood. The trainer stops the bleeding by first applying pressure with the fingers with a cold compress on the bleeding side of the nose; closing the nostril tightly on that side will usually control bleeding. Absorbent cotton saturated with petroleum jelly can be rolled up and inserted as a pack and should be left in place for several hours. If the bleeding fails to stop in short order, the athlete should be referred to a hospital emergency room for further care because nasal fractures may be present.

Nosebleeds may occur spontaneously or as a result as trauma to the nose, face, head, or jaws. If there is deformity or if the type of injury suggests an underlying fracture, the player should be referred to a physician.

Toothache. Generally speaking, aspirin and a cold application give temporary relief of toothache. Drops of Ambusol or oil of cloves can be used if necessary if aspirin or a cold compress is ineffective. Further care should be rendered by a dentist.

Colds. Colds are common ailments caused by viruses that infect the upper and lower respiratory tracts. This subject is discussed here from the viewpoint of prevention and conservative care.

The trainer must be concerned with the sanitation of his training room. In some instances, a common drinking glass or ladle is used by the whole team. This is a reprehensible practice that could lead to cold virus infection of the entire squad. More serious illnesses, such as tuberculosis, dysentery, and influenza may also be spread in this manner. Colds may result in complications such as bronchitis, laryngitis, sinusitis, and pneumonia.

Ordinarily, the trainer can treat and advise for a minor cold. The athlete is given a conservative regimen of rest from all sports for a few days, forced fluids such as tea, soup, coffee, juices, and bland diet. Oral temperature should be taken two or three times a day by the trainer or the athlete. If the condition worsens, as evidenced by spiking or persistent temperature, deep, harsh cough, pain at the site of the sinuses or chest pain, the athlete must be referred to the physician for evaluation and care.

Abdominal Pain. This condition is manifested by a multitude of medical conditions, ranging from mild "intestinal flu" to acute appendicitis. The trainer must refer this athlete to the team physician, who can properly evaluate the complaint.

Constipation. Usually the bowels function well with a balanced diet that has sufficient roughage and adequate fluid intake. Exercise helps maintain good bowel habits.

For cases of constipation, a mild laxative such as Metamucil may be safely administered by the trainer. If there is still a need for continued laxative medication, it is best to refer the athlete to the team doctor. The trainer is cautioned not to give a laxative when acute abdominal pain is present.

Diarrhea. Diarrhea is a condition in which a person has frequent loose bowel movements. The trainer may render conservative care for minor diarrhea, which includes rest, low residue diet and one of the common, over-the-counter kaolin-pectin preparations. If the diarrhea becomes persistent, severe, or excessive, the player must consult the physician.

Hemorrhoids. Hemorrhoids are actually varicose veins at the site of the anus; these may cause pain and/or rectal bleeding. Temporary relief may be obtained by warm sitz baths, but further care should be rendered by the team physician, who may refer the patient to a specialist. The 1980 World Series of Baseball was kept on tenterhooks when George Brett of the Kansas City Royals, American League's MVP (most valuable player) in 1980, developed an acute case of painful external hemorrhoid. He was kept in action by local heat, rest, compresses, and late-inning substitution in a night game. But the following day, the hemorrhoid was surgically opened and excised.

Blister. A blister is a collection of fluid between superficial layers of skin; it usually occurs on the toes and fingers because of friction and pressure. Blisters do not occur where the skin is tough.

The trainer applies an antiseptic to the blister and aspirates the fluid by placing a 25-gauge sterile needle at the rim of the blister. He then applies a piece of adhesive over the aspirated area for 48 hours. Then he removes the tape and cuts away the dead skin with small scissors, and reapplies the tape over the same area.

Corns and Calluses. Corns and calluses are caused by a combination of factors. Mild conditions of short duration most invariably are caused by improperly fitted shoes or short stockings. Moderate to severe conditions indicate the presence of a functional disorder within the foot itself.

These excrescences should be temporarily covered with stretch-elastic tape applied by the trainer. This gives relief provided that the offending cause is removed. However, any corn or callus that does not respond to this simple treatment should be referred for professional care.

Ingrown Toenails. Ingrown toenails may occur from cutting the nails too short, but most frequently they result from pressure against the nail induced by poorly fitted shoes, stockings, or faulty foot structure. In all cases, the nail punctures the soft tissues, causing pain and swelling. If allowed to persist, infection and tissue overgrowth develop. This condition occurs most commonly in the large toe.

Prophylactically, the nails should be allowed to grow slightly beyond the nailfold border to avoid trouble. Do not trim behind this border. In mild cases, elimination of any of the pressure factors will allow resolution of the conditions. The trainer may insert a small piece of cotton under the corner of the nail to help relieve the pressure. If the pain, discomfort, or tissue overgrowth are not relieved by these measures or if infection ensues, professional care is recommended.

Foot Strain. Foot strain is caused by excessive stretching of the ligaments that hold the bones of the foot together. Although injury is usually the predisposing factor, feet that are not structurally strong are subject to this condition and present the same symptoms merely from overuse syndrome. Swelling with or without pain is the most common sign of this condition. When neglected, inflammation may also occur. X-ray films of the foot should be taken to rule in or rule out stress fracture or any other bony or periosteal disorder.

The trainer should apply cold water or ice immediately to reduce the pain and discomfort. The following day, after the pain subsides, heat and cold foot baths should be used. Physical therapy should then be used to restore strength to the overstrained areas. *Most important,* however, is never to allow weight-bearing on the injured foot without having the foot strapped. Recovery takes place much faster when strapping is used in addition to other treatments.

Skin Infections.*   *Athlete's Foot (Tinea Pedis).* This is a superficial infection of the skin of the toes and feet by various pathogenic fungi and yeast. The common fungi are *Trichophyton, Epidermophyton,* and yeast is *Candida albicans.* These organisms are commonly present on the floors of training, shower, and locker rooms, as well as about swimming pools. Athletes are highly susceptible to these because of sweating and macerated feet and toes. Clinically, the athlete complains of itching, burning, and sometimes even pain. Examination of the feet shows characteristic scales, fissures, crusts, and oozing blisters between the toes and on the plantar surfaces of the toes and feet.

---

* We gratefully acknowledge the help of Martin H. Wortzel, M.D., in the preparation of this section.

This condition may be prevented and its incidence held to a minimum by proper foot hygiene. This includes daily washing of the feet and toes with soap and water. It is essential to dry these parts thoroughly, especially between the toes, because the organisms thrive in a moist, dark environment. Athletes should avoid walking barefooted. Foot baths containing a mild fungicide solution should be installed between the shower and dressing rooms and changed regularly. Athletes should walk about the dressing room wearing shower shoes or socks. Above all, they should change their socks and shoes daily.

The trainer must use only a mild, bland treatment. Many commercial preparations are available, with directions for their topical use included in the package instructions. We have found Tinactin to be an effective ointment.

If the symptoms and signs do not respond within 7 to 10 days, the athlete must be referred to the team physician. The doctor will treat the infection more vigorously by taking appropriate cultures and, if indicated, by prescribing internal medication. Most cases of athlete's foot that do not respond within 7 to 10 days can no longer be considered a simple "fungus" infection. Rather, the skin lesions may represent a superimposed skin irritation or contact dermatitis usually from applying medication in its concentrated form, thus complicating the basic infection. In such a case, the team physician may want to refer the athlete to a dermatologist for consultation.

Jock Itch (Tinea Cruris). This is a superficial mycotic infection of the skin of the groin by the same pathogenic organisms that cause athlete's foot. It is due to the sweating and maceration of the skin of the groin coming in contact with an infected athletic supporter, soiled gear, and other contaminated athletic apparel. Rarely does a jock itch occur without an accompanying athlete's foot; however, athlete's foot may be present alone.

Clinically, the athlete complains of itching, burning, oozing, and tenderness of the groin. Examination reveals the presence of a widespread eruption involving the skin of the scrotum and inner thigh. The eruption may even advance to the perineum and up to the rectum.

This condition may be prevented by proper personal hygiene and adequate cleansing, such as frequent showers. Thorough drying of the groin and genitalia after showering is essential. An athlete should never use a soiled or sweaty athletic supporter, or sit around for a long period of time without changing his apparel.

The treatment is similar to that for athlete's foot. Recurrent jock itch or other skin eruptions should make the doctor suspect an underlying disease such as diabetes as a causative factor.

Heat Rash. This is a skin condition also known as "prickly heat." It is due to the inability of the skin to excrete sweat properly under extreme conditions of heat, excessive sweating, or maceration of the skin in the presence of superficial skin bacteria. Little pools of perspiration form at the openings of the sweat pores, giving an appearance of pinhead-sized blisters or, sometimes, a diffuse, red spotted rash. Such eruptions are seen most frequently on the upper chest, back, armpits, and sometimes the groin. These clinical findings are accompanied by complaints of burning, itching, and oozing.

Personal hygiene prevents heat rash in many instances. Heat rash is best treated with soothing emollient creams, lotions, and ointments applied topically as directed by the packaging. Athletes who do not improve substantially in 3 to 5 days must be referred to the team physician. The physician will take other measures, including a complete medical examination and suitable cultures to determine the underlying cause of the condition. He prescribes oral medication if indicated. Recurrent attacks of prickly heat may be due to a systemic condition that warrants further medical investigation.

Impetigo. This is a superficial infection of the skin most commonly caused by one of the staphylococci and occasionally by streptococci. It is spread in those contact sports in which direct skin contact between athletes takes place. In a sport such as wrestling, the infection may be transmitted also by contact with a contaminated mat or other gear.

Itching, burning, and oozing of the skin are common complaints. Physical examination reveals reddish rings or segments with honey-colored heaped-up, crusted areas on the surface of the lesions. Occasionally, the crust comes loose, revealing a reddish, oozing, and pus-like skin lesion. The exudate is highly contagious, both to the athlete and to his physical contacts. Impetigo lesions are most frequently seen on the exposed portions of the face, neck, and sometimes hands.

Strict personal cleanliness is the best prevention. Keeping fingernails short and manicured is essential. Wrestling equipment and gear should be thoroughly cleansed with a commercial disinfectant and aired frequently to rid it of contamination. An athlete with impetigo or any questionable eruption on the exposed surfaces of the face, neck, or hands should not be permitted to compete until the dermatitis has been checked out by the physician. The doctor will decide whether or not the athlete is fit to compete. This is done not only to protect an athlete's adversary, but also to protect the athlete from auto-inoculation (spreading of the eruption on his own person).

Impetigo must be treated by a doctor. He will prescribe internal and external antibiotics plus local compresses of an antiseptic soothing preparation, such as Burow's solution, silver nitrate, and others.

Furuncle (also known as a "boil"). This is a deep seated staphylococcal infection of the skin transmitted by contact from another person or infected source. The condition is characterized by pain, redness, and tenderness localized around a hair follicle. It is first noticed as a cherry-sized swelling that soon enlarges. It develops a central area of pus which liquefies and escapes to the surface through a central slough site of necrosis. A large furuncle with several areas of drainage is considered a carbuncle; a single drainage site is also known as a boil. Prevention is best achieved by adherence to strict personal cleanliness.

Treatment for a furuncle must be supervised by a physician, who applies warm compresses and prescribes internal and external antibiotics. Recurrent furuncles should make the physician suspect the presence of an underlying diabetes.

Swimmer's Itch. This is caused by the reaction to certain larvae that penetrate the skin. The most common one is the Schistisome larva. The early eruption is hive-like and then, as the larva burrows into the skin, severe itching sometimes develops and an acute inflammatory reaction ensues with redness and swelling—sometimes even with crusting due to the scratching.

The condition is found in shallow, swampy ponds, and along the shoreline of small lakes (campsites).

It is self-limited because man is a coincidental host and all that is needed is a mild anti-itch lotion (such as Calamine) and antihistamines. The person should avoid the contaminated area in the future. If infection is severe or persists, the care of a physician is needed.

Ganglion. A ganglion is a small, soft-tissue cystic lesion that is palpable, benign, and thin-walled. It contains a clear, thick, mucinous fluid that arises from the lining of a joint, aponeurosis, or tendon sheath. It is commonly seen on the dorsum of the wrist and, infrequently, near joints of fingers and dorsum of the foot. The ganglion may be pea-size or larger, depending on when the patient is first treated. Although the etiology is still unclear, there is sufficient clinical experience to state that among younger patients, trauma plays a significant role. In older patients, colloid degeneration that occurs in local connective tissue may lead to the ganglion's appearance.

When consulting the trainer or physician, the patient complains of a lump, which feels soft or hard depending on when the patient seeks help. Treatment usually starts with repeated felt-pad pressure dressings placed snugly over the lump and with advice to reduce activity at this site. If this treatment fails, the team physician attempts aspiration under aseptic precautions, and a pressure dressing is placed snugly over the injection site. Some physicians also use a sclerosing solution. If aspiration is unsuccessful, complete surgical excision of the mass and its connection to the tendon sheath or joint is performed by the team physician in a hospital setting.

Bruise. These result from a blow (contusion) that injures the subcutaneous tissue and causes visible black and blue marks (ecchymoses)

Crutch Gaits

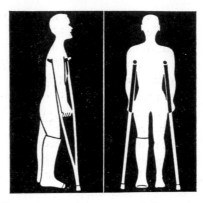

Balance is basic to all crutch gaits. To maintain balance the body must be kept in good alignment with head held high, shoulders back, and stomach and buttocks in.

Crutches must fit the patient properly. Generally they should be 2 inches longer than the distance from the armpit to the floor—fitting comfortably under the arm when tips are placed 4 to 6 inches to front and side of user. Hand grips should be adjusted so that weight can be borne by hands and *not by shoulders*. Heavy rubber tips to prevent skidding are a must.

Non-Weight-Bearing

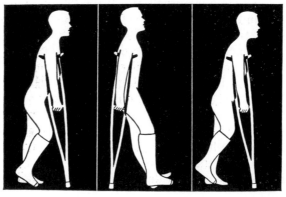

This is the preferred gait for patients unable to bear any weight on one lower extremity.

● With crutches placed 12 to 15 inches in front of good foot and 4 to 6 inches to the side, balance on good leg, supporting weight on hands.

● Pushing down on hand grips, swing both legs through crutches so that heel is carried no farther than 12 to 15 inches beyond crutches.

● As good foot touches floor, bring both crutches forward to starting position and repeat steps rhythmically.

Toe Touching

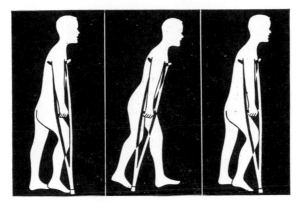

This gait is used when toe is allowed to touch the ground for balance.

● Line up injured extremity even with crutches.

● Bearing most of weight on hands, step forward so that good leg is in front of crutches.

● Bring crutches forward and repeat procedure.

Partial Weight-Bearing

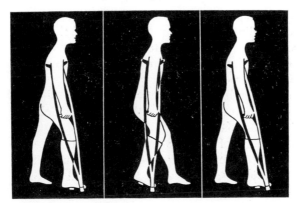

This gait is recommended for patients who can put limited weight on an injured leg (such as those in walking cast).

● Keeping weight on strong leg, place injured limb between crutches.

● With bulk of weight on crutches, take step with good leg.

● Bring crutches and damaged leg forward simultaneously, and repeat steps in rhythm.

Fig. 11-1.   Crutch gaits for a patient who has one disabled limb.
(Courtesy of Wyeth Laboratories, Philadelphia, Pennsylvania).

caused by ruptured blood vessels in the fatty layer of the subcutaneous tissue.

The trainer applies cold (ice) compresses to the injured area to relieve pain and check swelling; these are continued periodically for 48 hours. After the swelling has stopped, hot compresses, hot baths or showers are indicated to help resorption of traumatic exudates. When a limb has been bruised, the use of an elastic bandage around the injured area gives some support and comfort and helps prevent swelling.

Open Wounds. During the course of athletic competition, an athlete frequently sustains abrasions, slide burns, strawberries, and lacerations of various sizes and shapes. Relatively minor wounds may be adequately handled by the trainer. Generally speaking, the wounds should be cleansed with an antiseptic liquid soap, peroxide and then covered with a sterile Telfa dressing. Any wound more than minor in nature and extent must be examined and therapy started by the doctor. He may in turn refer the athlete back to the trainer to apply fresh dressings.

Splinters. A splinter occurs when a piece of wood becomes imbedded under the skin. Removal of a splinter depends on whether the splinter is made of hard wood or soft wood. The site of entry of the hard-wood splinter is washed with soap and water, and the area is prepared with alcohol. The tweezers should be antiseptically prepared before removing the splinter.

A soft-wood splinter breaks up at the site of skin entrance. This is best treated by immersing the site in warm salt water to soften the skin. Frequently, the splinters can then be removed with a pair of antiseptically prepared tweezers.

After the splinter has been removed, the area should be cleansed once more with an antiseptic, and a Band-Aid, which aids in the prevention of infection, should be applied.

Crutches. The use of crutches and crutch gaits is a daily fact of life in a busy training room. Trainers should be given instructions on how to provide an injured athlete with proper-sized crutches, as well as information on crutch gaits. The crutch-gait schematic by Wyeth (Fig. 11–1) is easy to follow for trainers and athletes and should be posted on the training-room bulletin board.

Appendix

PRESEASON CONDITIONING PROGRAM—
SAMPLE LETTERS TO FOOTBALL CANDIDATES

The following letters* are examples of "reminders" sent by the trainer or coach to prospective football candidates, along with the preseason conditioning program and suggestions for summer conditioning. Similar letters with appropriate modifications might be sent to participants of other sports.

First Letter (June)

Dear _____:

I have been informed by the Head Football Coach, _____ that you will be participating in our athletic program this fall as a football player.

I expect each candidate to report in tip-top condition—to play a regulation game if it were necessary. Watch your weight, work hard and faithfully, and you will have no trouble reporting in excellent condition.

I suggest that you follow the enclosed conditioning program, so you will be able to pass the test that will be given immediately following your physical examination. It is highly desirable that you be able to run the mile in less than 6.30; however, if you are now over 6.30, run every day until you have posted the desired time.

I am looking forward to meeting you personally.

Second Letter (July)

To All Varsity Football Candidates:

Now is the time to take inventory of yourself. You must check to see if you have worked hard enough for the ultimate in conditioning that you need

* Adapted in part from Dayton, O.W.: Athletic Training and Conditioning. New York, Ronald Press, 1960.

in September. Did you do enough exercise to be in good physical condition by the 15th of August? If not you'll have to go a little harder during the remaining time to catch up. Unfortunately, you cannot make up what has been lost, but it is possible to catch up by working a little harder.

The more intensive the training routine, the more efficient the body will be. I urge you to follow the conditioning program rather than exercising in "spurts." If you do not take the time now to get in condition and stay in condition, the chances of making the team will be lessened. Do not subject yourself to being disabled early in the season by reporting out of shape. The football season is a short one; take advantage of the time you have. Believe me, it's a great game when you are in shape to play it. By the same token, it's pretty tough when you are not in condition.

Condition, attitude, spirit and cooperation will win many a ball game.

Injury Form to Send Athlete to Physician or Dentist

Date _____

Time _____

Sport _____

Name _____

Injury _____

How did injury occur? _____

_____

When did injury occur? _____

Trainer's impressions: _____

_____

_____

Sent to Dr. _____

_____

Athletic Trainer

Authorization for Treatment

Date _____

This is to authorize treatment for _____ by

(Athlete's Name)

_____ for injuries received while

(Doctor or Hospital)

participating in athletics.

Approved by _____

Athletic Trainer

To Be Completed by Athletic Trainer

Name of Group Policy Holder _____

Group Policy Number _____

Name of Insurance Company _____

Mailing Address for Claims _____

Authorization to Refrain from Practice

Name _____ Date _____

This athlete has the following injury: _____

_____

He should: _____ Discontinue all athletic activity.

_____ Discontinue body contact only.

_____ Continue full athletic activity.

It is anticipated that he can resume:

_____ Full activity.

_____ Partial activity.

in _____

_____

Team Physician

Authorization to Return to Practice

Name _____ Date _____

This athlete has recovered sufficiently from the following injury

_____

that he can resume:

_____ Full activity.

_____ Partial activity (drills,

no body contact).

_____

Team Physician

Training Room Treatment Record

Date	Name	Complaint.	How Sustained	Diagnosis	Treatment	Games/ Practice Missed	Physician's Signature

Third Letter (August)

To All Varsity Football Candidates:

Now is the time to cut down on your outside activities; also, to get into a good sleeping routine. At least eight hours of sleep is necessary. Park the car and do a little more walking than usual. Golf and tennis are great sports for summer conditioning. Check your weight and do not let it increase. Watch your diet; good simple food in moderation is essential to building good bodies.

Active games of any type are excellent ways of getting in shape. Organize a touch football game in your community or play handball at the local playground. If you are close enough to a beach, running in the sand is an excellent way to strengthen your legs.

We cannot wait for you to get in shape. The games are scheduled and must be played. The season offers a wonderful opportunity. If you are not ready, someone else will be. WILL YOU BE READY? Remember, August can be an easy month. Do not let the people down who are counting on you this season.

BE READY!

Glossary

Before the relatively recent involvement of the medical profession in sports medicine, a vocabulary of great descriptive and communicative value concerning athletic injuries had developed among coaches, athletes, and trainers. This "training room language," although not scientifically oriented to anatomy and pathology, did express in a meaningful manner the effect of an injury on the performance of an athlete. Unfortunately, in many instances it emphasized the concern over whether or not an athlete could play; the medical care of an injury took a secondary role.

When the medical profession became intimately involved in athletic medicine, primarily through the AMA Committee on the Medical Aspects of Sports, physicians found the training room parlance confusing and unacceptable, primarily because it was not based on sound anatomic and pathologic concepts. Moreover, the primary concern of the physician is to allow only physically fit persons to participate in sports, and to sideline those who are not.

In order to clean up this situation, the Subcommittee for Classification of Sports Injuries of the AMA Committee on the Medical Aspects of Sports published an excellent volume: *Standard Nomenclature of Athletic Injuries.* Although this book is recommended for physicians and others concerned with sports, we believe it is asking too much at this time to expect coaches, trainers and physicians to communicate with each other solely in these terms. This book represents a giant step in the right direction, but a preliminary background in anatomy, physiology, pathology and kinesiology greater than that which now exists for coaches and trainers must be attained before all the concerned parties can verbalize at the level recommended in the book.

A far more effective means of removing this language barrier would be to have doctors become familiar with training room language. By gradually using correct anatomic and pathologic phrases to discuss athletic injuries, physicians can thus bring a greater awareness of scientific terminology to athletics. Therefore, we present here some of the more common expressions used to describe athletic injuries, in an attempt to familiarize the readers with those terms that are scientifically oriented and those that represent training room jargon and colloquialisms.

Abduction. Movement of a part away from the midline of the body. Opposed to adduction.

Abrasion. Superficial wound of the skin resulting from friction or scraping the skin against a hard surface, such as floor burn, mat burn, strawberry, etc.

Achilles tendon (Tendo Achilles). Anatomically, this is the common tendon of the gastrocnemius and soleus (calf muscles) which inserts into the posterior portion of the os calcis (heel bone).

Acute. Sharp, abrupt, sudden, such as acute pain; a course that is relatively severe and short.

Adduction. Movement of a part toward the midline of the body. Opposed to abduction.

Anterior. Situated in front of or in the forward part.

Articulation. The site at which bones meet to form a joint.

Athlete's foot (dermatophytosis, foot ringworm, tinea pedis). An infection of the feet caused by one of several fungi.

Avulsion. A tearing or pulling away of a part of a structure.

Backward extension. Backward movement of the arm at the shoulder from a zero starting position.

Baseball finger. Dropped finger due to an avulsion of the distal insertion of the extensor tendon with or without a bony fragment, resulting from a direct blow to the tip of the finger. Also known as "mallet" and "hammer finger."

Basketweave. A method of taping for protection, usually applied to ankles. (See Figs. 9-3, 9-4.)

Bursa. A small closed sac, lined by specialized connective tissue, which contains synovial fluid. Bursa are usually located over bony prominences where muscles or tendons move over the projection of bone. They facilitate gliding movements by diminishing friction.

Butterflies. An upset stomach usually due to pregame tension and anxiety.

Cartilage. A specialized form of connective tissue with varying amounts of intercellular matrix that is nonvascular and found in various parts of the body. In training room parlance, cartilage in the knee joint is commonly referred to as gristle-like padding; anatomically, these cartilages are known as the medial and lateral semilunar cartilages (menisci).

Caudad. Towards the tail, or downwards. Opposite of cephalad.

Cauliflower ears. A very descriptive term for such ears, because they look like the surface of cauliflower. This condition results from a replacement of the elastic cartilage by fibrocartilage or fibrous tissue following trauma to the lateral surface of the auricle. This condition is also known as a "tin ear," and is frequently seen in boxers, wrestlers, and occasionally in football players.

Cephalad. Towards the head, or upwards. Opposite of caudad.

Charley horse. Contusion of the quadriceps muscle characterized by pain and swelling (intramuscular bleeding).

Chronic. Marked by long duration; continued; not acute. In athletics, may also refer to a recurrent injury, or one that has not responded to treatment.

Compression point. Points on the body where pressure can be applied to control arterial bleeding.

Contusion. A bruise of superficial or deeper tissues without a break in the covering skin or membrane; caused by external violence.

Cotton mouth. A condition of discomfort and dryness in the mouth, caused by dehydration or emotional tension.

Counterirritant. An agent that is applied locally to produce an irritation or mild inflammation of the skin in order to reduce an inflammatory process in deeper and adjacent structures.

Dislocation. Complete displacement of a bone from its normal position in a joint.

Distal. Remote; farther away from a point of reference; opposed to proximal.

Dorsiflexion (Extension). This motion refers only to the wrist and ankle joints. In the wrist, it is a cephalad movement of the back of the hand at the wrist from a zero starting position. In the ankle, it is a cephalad movement of the foot at the ankle from a zero starting position (e.g., as when walking on the heel).

Ecchymosis. An extravasation of blood under the skin.

Epiphysis. That part of a bone that is concerned with growth in length (e.g., the ends of long bones).

Epistaxis. Nosebleed.

Eversion. Turning the sole of the foot outwards, away from the midline of the body.

Extension. Return motion to the zero starting position in a true hinge joint, such as an elbow, interphalangeal and less typical hinge joint such as the knee. Opposite of flexion.

Flexion. Motion away from the zero starting position in a true hinge joint, such as the elbow, interphalangeal, and less typical hinge joint such as the knee. See also **Palmar flexion** and **Plantar flexion.**

Fungicide. A chemical agent that destroys fungi.

Funny bone. A contusion of the ulnar nerve in the ulnar notch, causing a temporary burning sensation and numbness along the inner (ulnar) aspect of the forearm, which may also involve the small and ulnar half of the ring finger. Also known as "crazy bone."

Galled skin. An area of irritated and raw skin caused by sweat and friction. Galled areas are inviting to bacteria and fungi.

Germicide. A chemical agent that destroys pathogenic microorganisms.

Glass jaw. A term used in the boxing trade to describe boxers who are easily knocked out by a blow to the head, especially the chin. This characteristic response is related to the peculiarities of the boxer's neurophysiologic make-up.

Hamstring muscles, tendons. The muscles in the back of the thigh (biceps femoris, semitendinosus, and semimembranosus) that extend from the pelvis to the upper foreleg, and their tendons. Their main action is to flex the leg at the knee.

Heel lock. A processes of anchoring the heel in taping or wrapping an ankle.

Hematoma. A circumscribed collection of blood following trauma.

Hematuria. Presence of blood in the urine.

Hip pointer. A contusion of the iliac crest, which is quite painful and usually very tender to finger palpation.

Horizontal extension. Backward movement of the arm at the shoulder with the arm in an abducted position.

Hot spot. A hot or irritated feeling on the foot that occurs just before a friction blister forms.

Inflammation. A reaction of tissues to injury and infection, characterized by heat, swelling, redness, pain and sometimes loss of function.

Inversion. Turning the sole of the foot inward, toward the midline of the body.

Isometric. A form of muscular contraction in which the muscle length does not change.

Isotonic. A form of muscular contraction in which the length of the muscle changes.

Javelin thrower's elbow. A clinically painful and disabling elbow condition unique to javelin throwers. The ulnar collateral ligament is sprained or the tip of olecranon is injured; it may include a fracture.

Jock itch (tinea cruris). An irritated area between the legs, complicated by a fungus infection.

Laceration. A cut or tear of skin or other body tissues, usually accompanied by bleeding.

Lateral. On the outer side, as distinguished from the inner (medial) side.

Ligament. A band of strong fibrous connective tissue that connects joint ends of bones. Ligaments strengthen joints by providing stability while allowing freedom of movement.

Little Leaguer's elbow. Avulsion fracture of the epiphysis of the medial epicondyle of the humerus, as seen in Little League pitchers.

Louisiana wrap. A method of wrapping the ankle that uses the heel lock.

Lumbosacral. Refers to the area of the back where the lumbar and sacral areas are in contact. Commonly referred to as the small of the back.

Luxation. Dislocation.

Massage, manual. The use of hands in friction, kneading, stroking and other techniques in the manipulation of soft tissues to effect beneficial changes.

Medial. Pertaining to the middle, or internal, as distinguished from the lateral (outer) side.

Meniscus. Semilunar cartilage. See **Cartilage.**

Muscle, striated. Voluntary contractile tissue whose special function is to move and stabilize joints.

Myalgia. Muscle pain.

Myositis ossificans. The formation of new bone, following trauma, in tissues that normally do not undergo such a process. Most frequently seen in the quadriceps muscle following a severe blow to the thigh.

Nail avulsion. Dislodgement of the nail from its bed by trauma.

Neuritis. Inflammation or irritation due to infection or mechanical pressure on a nerve, causing pain, tenderness and paresthesia along the course of the nerve.

Osteomyelitis. Infection of a bone.

Palmar flexion. Refers only to the wrist. Caudad movement of the hand at the wrist from a zero starting position with the palm down.

Perichondrium. The membrane that covers the surface of a cartilage.

Pharyngitis. Sore throat.

Pinched nerve. Usually results from a compression or traction trauma to a nerve root causing a contusion of this root; usually associated with neck injuries from blocking and tackling. Transient root-like pain with dermatomal paresthesia. hypalgesia and/or weakness in the muscles innervated by this root are characteristic.

Plantar. Refers to the sole of the foot.

Plantar flexion. Refers only to the ankle. Caudad movement of the foot at the ankle from a zero starting position (e.g., as when walking on the toes).

Plantar wart. An epidermal tumor of viral origin seen on the sole of the foot.

Posterior. Behind or in back of.

Proximal. Nearest to; closer to point of reference; opposed to distal.

Reduction. To bring back to the normal position, as in reducing a dislocated shoulder or a fractured bone. Closed reduction is done without incision; open reduction is done through an incision.

Rhinitis, acute. Common cold. A catarrhal inflammation of the nasopharynx due to a virus.

Scoliosis. Lateral curvature of the spine.

Shin splint. Clinically painful and disabling condition of the lower leg that is unique to athletes and results from a strain of the tibialis anterior muscle. This injury is usually associated with running and jumping on hard surfaces or uneven terrain early in the season.

Sock pack. A treatment that uses a counterirritant salve and an athletic sock. Usually used on ankles, shins, and elbows.

Spasm. An involuntary contraction of one or more muscles.

Sprain. An injury of the supporting ligaments and other attachments of a joint following a sudden twisting, wrenching or external force applied to the joint.

Sprinter's fracture. Avulsion of the ischial tuberosity by strong contraction of the hamstring muscles.

Stone bruise. A painful bruise that results from contusion of the bone. Also known as bone bruise. In baseball catchers, it occurs in the palm of the hands. In broad jumpers, basketball players, football players and others, it occurs on the plantar aspect of the heel or ball of the foot.

Stoved finger. Painful, tender, stiff and sore proximal interphalangeal joint following a sprain of this finger joint from a blow on the tip of the finger by a ball.

Strain. An injury of muscles or tendons as a result of overstretching, over-exertion or powerful contraction against resistance. In training room parlance, these are better known as a pull or tear.

Strapping. The use of adhesive tape to support or protect a joint. Also called taping.

Strawberry. An abrasion that results from sliding on the ground, usually seen in baseball.

Subluxation. Partial or incomplete dislocation.

Superficial. Refers to the surface, as in superficial injuries—those that do not go below the skin.

Tape burn. Superficial skin irritation from adhesive tape.

Tendinitis. Irritation, inflammation, and swelling of a tendon, caused by excessive use.

Tendinomyositis. A combination of tendinitis and adjacent myositis in muscle groups that take origin from a bone by a common tendon (i.e., superficial group flexor muscles of forearm).

Tendon. A band of fibrous connective tissue of great tensile strength and flexibility that forms the end of muscle and inserts into a bone controlling the direction of muscle pull.

Tennis elbow. A localized condition of tendinomyositis of the supinator and extensor group of muscles that arises from the lateral epicondyle of the humerus. This condition is not only seen in tennis players, but in golfers, fishermen, and squash players, among others.

Tennis leg. Rupture of the plantaris tendon that occurs while playing tennis and other sports.

Tenosynovitis. Inflammation of the tendon sheath.

Tetanus. A serious infection caused by a tetanus spore, which inhabits the soil. All players should be immunized against tetanus. Also known as lockjaw.

Thrombophlebitis. Inflammation of the wall of a vein, associated with the formation of a thrombus (blood clot).

"Went out." An expression frequently used to refer to a dislocation of a joint. The athlete actually feels the bones of the joint go out of place.

Wrapping. The use of cloth or elastic bandages to support or protect a joint.

Zero starting position. A defined anatomic position from which all joint motions are measured. This is also referred to as a neutral position.*

---

* Joint motion—Manual of Orthopaedic Surgery, American Orthopaedic Association, 1966.

Index

Page numbers in *italics* indicate figures; numbers followed by "t" indicate tables.